Tai Chi Ball Qigong

FOR HEALTH AND MARTIAL ARTS

DR. YANG, JWING-MING AND DAVID GRANTHAM

Tai Chi Ball Qigong

FOR HEALTH AND MARTIAL ARTS

YMAA Publication Center
Wolfeboro, N.H., USA

YMAA Publication Center
PO Box 480
Wolfeboro, NH 03894
1-800-669-8892 • www.ymaa.com • info@ymaa.com

Paperback edition	**Ebook edition**
ISBN-13: 978-1-59439-199-6	ISBN-13: 978-1-59439-241-2
ISBN-10: 1-59439-199-8	ISBN-10: 1-59439-241-2

POD 0312

Anatomy drawing Figures 2-4, 2-5, 4-23, 5-36, and 5-43 are are used with permission from the LifeART Collection of Images © 1989-1997 by Techpool Studios, Cleaveland, OH.

Publisher's Cataloging in Publication

Yang, Jwing-Ming, 1946-

    Tai chi ball qigong : for health and martial arts / Yang, Jwing-Ming, David Grantham. -- Wolfeboro, N.H. : YMAA Publication Center, c2010.

    p. ; cm.

    ISBN: 13-digit: 978-1-59439-199-6 ; 10-digit: 1-59439-199-8
    Includes glossary of Chinese terms.
    Includes bibliographical references and index.
    Text in English; prefatory material in Chinese and English.

    1. Qi gong. 2. Tai chi. 3. Qi (Chinese philosphy) 4. Medicine, Chinese. 5. Mind and body. I. Grantham, David W., 1965- II. Title.

RA781.8 .Y364 2010   2010941229
613.7/148--dc22   1011

To Grandmaster Kao, Tao (高濤). Dr. Yang's first Taijiquan teacher.

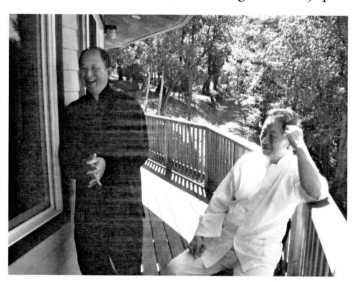

Editorial Notes

Using the book and DVD together. Throughout this book, you will see this icon on certain pages. The DVD icon tells you that companion material is found on the DVD. The larger words indicate the type of content (eg. Lecture, Follow Along, etc.), the smaller words indicate the precise menu selection you should choose on the DVD. There are two companion DVDs for this book. *Tai Chi Ball Qigong 1* DVD contains courses 1 and 2. *Tai Chi Ball Qigong 2* DVD contains courses 3 and 4.

Both DVDs are available from YMAA or many other retailers worldwide.

Romanization of Chinese Words. This book primarily uses the Pinyin romanization system of Chinese to English. Pinyin is standard in the People's Republic of China, and in several world organizations, including the United Nations. Pinyin, which was introduced in China in the 1950's, replaces the Wade-Giles and Yale systems. In some cases, the more popular spelling of a word may be used for clarity.

Some common conversions:

Pinyin	Also Spelled As	Pronunciation
Qi	Chi	chē
Qigong	Chi Kung	chē gōng
Qin Na	Chin Na	chǐn nǎ
Jin	Jing	jǐn
Gongfu	Kung Fu	gōng foo
Taijiquan	Tai Chi Chuan	tī jē chüén

For more information, please refer to *The People's Republic of China: Administrative Atlas, The Reform of the Chinese Written Language,* or a contemporary manual of style.

The author and publisher have taken the liberty of not italicizing words of foreign origin in this text. This decision was made to make the text easier to read. Please see the comprehensive glossary for definitions of Chinese words.

Contents

Editorial Notes   **vi**

Contents   **vii**

Foreword   **ix**

Preface   **xv**

How To Use This Book (如何使用這本書)   **xxi**

Acknowledgments   **xxiii**

Chapter 1: General Qigong Theory   **1**

1.1 Introduction (介紹)   1

1.2 What is Qi and What is Qigong? (何謂氣？何謂氣功？)   1

1.3 Categories of Qigong (氣功之分類)   6

1.4 Theory of Yin and Yang, Kan and Li (陰陽坎離之理論)   13

1.5 Qigong and Health (氣功與健康)   18

1.6 Qigong and Longevity (氣功與長壽)   20

Chapter 2: Qigong Training Theory and Procedures   **25**

2.1 Introduction (介紹)   25

2.2 Five Regulatings (五調)   26

Chapter 3: General Introduction to Taiji Ball Qigong   **57**

3.1 Introduction (介紹)   57

3.2 History of Taiji Ball Qigong (太極球氣功之歷史)   58

3.3 Taiji Ball Qigong and Health (太極球氣功與健康)   60

3.4 Taiji Ball Qigong and Martial Arts (太極球氣功與武術)   62

Chapter 4: Theory of Taiji Ball Qigong   **65**

4.1 Introduction (介紹)   65

4.2 What is Taiji in Taiji Ball Qigong? (太極球氣功之太極)   65

4.3 Theory of Physical Conditioning (強身之原理)   75

4.4 Theory of Inner Qi's Cultivation (內氣培養之理論)   76

4.5 Martial Grand Qi Circulation (武學大周天)   86

4.6 Other Benefits (其他益處)   93

4.7 Conclusions (結論)   94

Chapter 5: Taiji Ball Qigong Training   97

5.1 Introduction (介紹)   97

5.2 Taiji Ball Qigong Training Contents and Procedures (太極球氣功練
習之內含與程序)   97

5.3 Warm-Up (軟身)   107

5.4 Internal Training (內功)–Breathing Exercises   119

5.5 External Training (外功)–Fundamental Stances   125

5.6 External Training (外功)–Exercises   128

Chapter 6: Applications of Taiji Ball Qigong   227

6.1 Introduction (介紹)   227

6.2 Self-Practice (自我練習)   228

6.3 Train with Partners (*Yu Ban Tong Lian,* 與伴同練)   243

6.4 Advanced Taiji Ball Training (高級太極球之練習)   266

Conclusion   269

Appendix A: Translations and Glossary of Chinese Terms   271

Appendix B: Tai Chi Ball Qigong DVD 1 & 2   285

Index   289

About the Author   297

Foreword 陰陽太極球氣功序

by Kao, Tao 高濤

太極球顧名思義是屬於太極拳多項輔助教材中之一環。昔時，太極
球的練習是非常的普遍。可惜現在近乎失傳。俊敏與他多年的學
生，David Grantham，寫的這本書當可以將這球藝傳至下一代。本人
習楊氏太極拳逾四十年之久。緣當本人十二歲在上海拜河南樂奐之老
師習拳時，母親一再叮嚀，祇要認真練拳，決不可練武打搏擊技巧。
因本人外公（高重威）因諳武功在蘇州開設鏢局。某次得罪綠林人
士，竟遭人暗算而喪命。年僅三十六歲而已。

When you ponder the name and meaning of Taiji Ball, it can be understood that
it is one of many assistant training training tools of Taijiquan. Taiji Ball was once
popular, but now it is almost lost. This book by Jwing-Ming and his longterm student
David Grantham should preserve the art for the next generations. I have practiced
Yang style Taijiquan more than 40 years. When I was 12 years old, I began learning
from Master Yue, Huan-Zhi (樂奐之) from Henan (河南). My mother reminded me
repeatedly that when I practiced the art, I should only focus on the forms and should
not train the skills of the fighting techniques. The reason for this was because my
grandfather, Kao, Zhong-Wei (高重威), was killed in a fight at the age of 36. Because
of his high Gongfu skills, he had an escort company. One time, he offended a martial
artist and was plotted against, and lost his life.

吾弟子俊敏，1963 年在新竹唸高中時，即隨余習拳。同時亦隨南派白
鶴拳老師曾金灶為師。嗣後又拜山東，青島李茂清老師習北派長拳。
由於酷愛我國拳術，更以數十年時光，追研各種刀、槍、棍棒以及擒
拿術等技能。今在美國東西兩岸開設武館多處，名楊氏武藝協會。在
全球也多達五十多處，開館授徒。

My student, Jwing-Ming, learned Taijiquan from me while he was studying in
high school at Xinzhu (新竹) city in 1963. At the same time, he was also practicing
southern southern-style White Crane from Master Cheng, Gin-Gsao (曾金灶). Later,
he studied northern style Long Fist (長拳) from Master, Li, Mao-Ching (李茂清) of
Qingdao, Shandong Province (山東，青島). I saw that he was so in love with learning Chinese martial arts. Since then, he spent a few decades studying various weapons
such as saber, spear, staff, and various qin na techniques. Presently, he has opened many
schools around the world named "Yang's Martial Arts Association (YMAA)." I am happy to see that he has created more than 50 of his schools spreading around the world to
preserve the traditional arts.

本人親臨其設在加州北部地區之 Miranda 山莊的楊氏武藝協會加州
特訓中心。見有七位洋弟子，每天練拳完畢，已是滿頭大汗，仍不得
休息。立即各持一木球，放置手掌，然後上下、左右、前後邁步運
轉。據俊敏謂太極係一圓形體，將球在兩掌心間翻滾運轉。此時全神
灌注，拋除雜念，形成裡應外合，內靜意專。猶如太極隨個人之意念
在上肢翻騰變化。此時無聲勝有聲，氣場充滿身，必可達到相當的境
界。

I personally came to the YMAA CA Retreat Center, located in Miranda, northern
California. I saw six of Jwing-Ming's disciples, who after finishing fist training were
covered in sweat. Instead of stopping to rest, they immediately picked up a wooden
ball between their palms to train Tai Chi Ball. They manipulated the ball with up-
down, left-right, and forward-back stepping. Taiji has a shape of roundness, and when
the ball is between the palms, one is able to rotate and circle it. At this time, the entire
mind and spirit are concentrated and all random thoughts leave the mind. The external
and internal bodies harmonize and the mind is calm. The Taiji follows the concentration and manifests through the upper limbs with tumultuous changes. At this time,
soundless is more precious than soundness. The Qi field has reached its abundant level
around the entire body.

吾本人習拳，祇求健身防身。雖無功夫可言，但數十年未曾一病。應
拜習拳之賜益也。今年已實足七十九歲，仍在淡水社區指導鄰居拳術
及養生法。

I practice martial arts only to strengthen my body and also for self-defense. Though
my Gong Fu is so little it is not worth mentioning, I have never gotten sick in the last
few decades. All of these benefits are gained from practicing Taiji and Qigong. Now,
I have passed 79 years of age, and I am still teaching my neighbors Taiji and also the
techniques of nourishing Qigong for longevity.

俊敏父子之兩大武術館在美國東西兩地，除一名華人外，餘皆為
洋人。由於教規嚴格，洋弟子們執師禮甚恭。一次偷懶，受罰。三次
犯錯，立刻開除。反觀我國青年學子喜習西洋歌舞，樂器或通宵達旦
上網及電玩。難怪國有之拳術、書法等國粹漸趨式微。俊敏在八年前
傾其全部資蓄在美加州北部，購得此二百四十畝土地，建造首座傳統
武館，其發揚我國國粹之心血與毅力，值得讚揚。

Jwing-Ming and his son Nicholas have established prominent martial headquarters
schools on both coasts of the United States. Except for one Chinese student, all of
the disciples at the Retreat Center are Westerners from the U.S., as well from as Chile
and Switzerland. Because of his strict teaching manners, all of Jwing-Ming's students
are very polite and respect their teacher humbly. If one is lazy, the first time he will be
punished. If one makes the same mistakes three times, he will be expelled from school.

When I look at youngsters in China today, they like to imitate Western culture with pop music, fashion, the Internet, and playing computer games for hours into the night without sleeping. No wonder our country's quintessence, such as traditional martial arts, calligraphy, and painting, has declined. Jwing-Ming has spent all of his life savings to purchase 240 acres of mountain land in northern California and build this first traditional training center. His hard work and perseverance in preserving and propagating our country's quintessence is worth great praise.

Humble Teacher
Kao, Tao
May 7, 2010

愚師
高濤　謹撰
二零一零，五月七日

Foreword
by Pat Rice

As we who inhabit the world of qigong and taijiquan strive to improve our understanding and to find methods for training that are both achievable and effective, we welcome another volume by Dr. Yang, Jwing-Ming. We find inestimably excellent guidance in Dr. Yang's works. All of his productions, whether in the format of books, videos, or workshops and seminars, are the ultimate in information and practicality and are examples of excellence. He has a very able collaborator in David Grantham, co-author of this book. In each succeeding book by Dr. Yang, we get an update on his understanding and interpretation of the theories that provide the substructure for experience. This current work on taiji ball qigong exemplifies his growing mastery in these areas. As he achieves more clarity for himself and finds deeper correlations within systems, we are the beneficiaries of his advancements. He continually researches the volumes of historical documents and steadily conducts intense personal experimentation in the actual physical training. With the same attentiveness, he is a keen observer of others: long-term and one-time students, learners with varied abilities, colleagues and associates at all levels of experience, and his own teachers and mentors. He applies scientific principles to the human energy field, combines this information with wisdom gathered from ancient sources and his own investigations and introspections, and then explains it all in language that facilitates our own endeavors.

His style of explication makes the information accessible; the personal touch of directly addressing the reader—"*you*"—reassures us that we can comprehend the complexities, that we can perform these exercises, and we can achieve the desired benefits. He has respect for us, his readers, but makes no assumptions about our level of expertise, and he speaks to us neither over our heads nor beneath our dignity. He and David Grantham explain as clearly as possible in the medium of paper and print what we are supposed to do and feel, and why.

They introduce the material with a solid foundation of theory and principles. In particular, they summarize and condense previous discussions in foregoing works, organizing the information clearly and concisely, and finally set it all into place as the basis for the training methods in *Taiji Ball Qigong*.

Play with a ball has been a component of most human cultures. Such activities serve many purposes, among them recreation, entertainment, physical cultivation, organized sport, and martial training. In *Taiji Ball Qigong*, we are introduced to purposes beyond the ordinary: not only the development of good health, but also the potential for longevity, spiritual growth, and even enlightenment. Granted, similar outcomes may possibly be derived from common uses, but in training with the taiji ball, these are specifically stated as purposes. In a unique combination of ball handling and qigong theory, patterns of physical movement are interwoven with esoteric aspects of internal energy. With these as foundation and as actualization, a portal is opened into a vast domain of possible rewards.

As director of a Taste of China, an organization that since 1983 has promoted

Chinese martial arts and health arts and has sponsored international seminars, as well as national and international tournaments, I have been pleased to include Dr. Yang as one of the most popular presenters. His depth of knowledge and his superb teaching style make him among the most valuable members of this community since its inception and of others nationally and internationally. Dr. Yang has consistently been very well received as he presented information on a variety of topics associated with Chinese health practices in general, and on taijiquan and qigong specifically. He introduced us to taiji ball qigong in 2002 over a weekend workshop, and we had a glimpse of the benefits and pleasures to be gained from this exercise. He not only taught the theoretical foundation and the core training exercises and led us through many of the drills; he also described the qualities to be developed and the correlations to internal qi development.

Dr. Yang is able to convey ideas not only in a classroom and from an active video, but also with his co-author, in this book. Here they teach effectively through the medium of written words and graphics. Always a master teacher, he is true to the ideals of the past and its histories and legends, hoping to maintain the standards exemplified by famous martial artists and desiring great achievements for every student; at the same time he accepts the realities of us as individuals, with our limitations and personal variables. In all instances, he has a manifest desire to be helpful, to provide true and usable information. He assists us in our struggle to learn, supports us in our desire to do well, encourages us as we make small gains, and befriends us in our hopes for reaching lofty goals. All these generosities we encounter when we are fortunate enough to have interactions with him, but we also find his great spirit shining from these pages.

The ancient saying that "words are helpful at first, only doing leads to understanding" perfectly describes the ideal approach to these exercises. I hope this book and these authors inspire you to learn the theory and to practice the movements and that you will ultimately realize the benefits that can accrue from taiji ball qigong.

Pat Rice
Director, A Taste of China
Winchester, Virginia
January 2010

Preface
by Dr. Yang, Jwing-Ming (楊俊敏博士)

Qigong study and practice have become very popular since being introduced into Western society in the 1970s. However, many challenges still remain:

1. Many people are still skeptical about the science of qigong and only a few books explain qigong scientifically, bringing scientific theory and ancient experience together.

2. Few scholars and scientific researchers are pursuing and verifying this qigong science. Qigong is new to Western society, and few convincing scientific results are reported in scholarly studies and papers.

3. Many people are still in traditional and religious bondage, preventing them from opening their minds to another spiritual culture. Qigong is a science of inner feeling and spiritual cultivation. If you cannot jump out of your traditional matrix, you cannot accept this science, which has been studied by Chinese and Indian societies for more than four thousand years.

4. Few qualified qigong practitioners can read, understand, and accurately translate the abundant ancient qigong documents into Western languages. I estimate that less than one percent of the ancient documents have been translated into Western languages. Most have been hidden in Buddhist and Daoist monasteries, and have only been revealed in recent decades.

5. Many qigong practitioners have used qigong as a tool to abuse and mislead their followers. This has led people into superstitious belief and blind worship, making scientific scholars doubt the truth of qigong practice.

Chinese qigong derives from more than four thousand years of experience in healing and prevention of disease, and in spiritual cultivation. Four major schools have emerged: medical, scholar, religious, and martial. Qigong is one major essence of Chinese culture that cannot be separated from its people.

Western science has developed from its focus on the material world. That which can only be felt is considered unscientific. Inner feeling and development are ignored. To Chinese, feeling is a language that allows mind and body to communicate, extending beyond the body to communicate with nature (heaven and earth) or Dao (道). This feeling has been studied and has become the core of Chinese culture. It is especially cultivated in Buddhist and Daoist society, where the final goal is to attain spiritual enlightenment, or Buddhahood. Through more than two thousand years of study and practice, this cultivation has reached such a high level that it cannot yet be interpreted by material science. I believe it will take some time to break through this barrier and for Western scientists to accept this concept.

From my more than 42 years of qigong practice and from studying many ancient documents, I am at last confident that I have derived and understood the map of this qigong science. I believe that as long as a "Dao searcher" (Xun Dao Zhe, 尋道者) is willing to study this map, even without guidance from a qualified master, he should still be able to stay on the correct path of study.

*   *   *

Dr. Yang has interpreted this map in several books:
1. *Qigong for Health and Martial Arts*, YMAA Publication Center, 1985, 1998
2. *Eight Simple Qigong Exercises for Health*, YMAA Publication Center, 1988, 1997
3. *The Root of Chinese Qigong–The Secrets of Qigong Training*, YMAA Publication Center, 1989, 1997
4. *Qigong–The Secret of Youth*, YMAA Publication Center, 1989, 2000
5. *The Essence of Taiji Qigong–Health and Martial Arts*, YMAA Publication Center, 1990, 1998
6. *Arthritis Relief—Chinese Qigong for Healing and Prevention*, YMAA Publication Center, 1991, 2005
7. *Qigong Massage–General Massage*, YMAA Publication Center, 1992, 2005
8. *The Essence of Shaolin White Crane*, YMAA Publication Center, 1996
9. *Back Pain Relief*, YMAA Publication Center 1997, 2004
10. *Qigong Meditation–Embryonic Breathing*, YMAA Publication Center, 2004
11. *Qigong Meditation–Small Circulation*, YMAA Publication Center, 2006

When I was in high school in the early 1960s, taiji ball qigong practice was often seen in the early mornings in many parks in Taiwan, especially in Taipei. However, when the Taiwan society adopted a more Western style, this kind of practice gradually disappeared. Today, it is very rare to find anyone practicing openly. Due to this reason, it is even more difficult to find a qualified teacher who really knows the theory, principle, and the correct way of taiji ball qigong practice.

When I was studying physics in Taiwan University between 1968–1971, I often went to Taipei Park to learn and practice with those martial artists who were willing to share their knowledge with the public openly. I found an old man, Mr. Zhao (趙) who was teaching and practicing taiji ball qigong in the park. After obtaining his approval, I joined the practice for nearly eight months. When I was accepted to teach physics in Tamkang College (淡江學院), which was located at Tamsui town (淡水鎮), I had to stop my practice. Since then, I had not had any chance to practice again until I came to United States in 1974.

From Mr. Zhao, I learned about 24 basic training patterns. After nearly twenty years of teaching and practicing taiji ball qigong in the United States and other countries, I developed these 24 patterns further into 48 patterns. I believe I have made this training program more complete. From these 48 basic patterns, countless combinations of practice have become possible.

I mentioned taiji ball qigong training in my books, *Advanced Yang Style Tai Chi Chuan, Vol. 1 and 2*, in 1986, which has brought wide attention to this practice. The results were the 2004 *Taiji Ball Qigong* videotape and DVD production by YMAA Publication Center. Since 2003, more and more of taiji ball qigong practices have been revealed to the public by different styles, thus offering many possibilities for discovery and discussion. I hope the readers of this book will keep their minds open and continue to absorb more knowledge from other sources.

Taiji ball qigong practice can benefit your martial capability, and also condition your physical and mental bodies to a higher tuned state. From understanding the theory, I personally believe that taiji ball qigong most likely effectively prevents or heals both breast and prostate cancer.

In this book, Mr. Grantham and I have summarized these 48 basic patterns and some applications. We hope this book is able to offer you some foundation and guidelines of taiji ball qigong theory and practice.

Dr. Yang, Jwing-Ming

Preface
by David W. Grantham

On occasion, I have had people ask me about taiji ball qigong. As I explained what it is to them, I began to realize that taiji ball qigong actually surrounds us everywhere in today's society. Although the theory may not be as deep, you see taiji ball theories applied in basketball, soccer, hackey sacks, medicine balls, and even in the rubber exercise balls used today in aerobics classes. Each and every one utilizes the concentration of the mind and the physical training of the body to reach higher levels of skill.

In this book Master Yang, Jwing-Ming and I hope to expose you to the theories and exercises of taiji ball qigong. The book begins with a brief explanation of qi and qigong in Chapter 1. Chapter 2 follows up on this theory with the five regulations common to qigong practice. We then explore the history of taiji ball qigong as well as its relationship to health and martial arts in Chapter 3. This is followed with the theories of qigong applied to taiji ball training both internally and externally in Chapters 4 and 5. Finally, in Chapter 6, we show you applications of these exercises in solo and partner practices. With this knowledge, you will be able to increase the flow of qi and strengthen your body.

Taiji ball qigong is a vital tool for health and martial arts training. It is our hope that this book will assist in reintroducing it into our society.

David W. Grantham

How To Use This Book (如何使用這本書)

This book is to be used in conjunction with the *Taiji Ball Qigong* DVD series by Dr. Yang, Jwing-Ming. While the DVD can provide you with the continuous actions, this book is able to offer you a clear explanation of the theory and movements. With both DVD and book, you will be able to reach a high level of practice without an instructor. However, if you have the chance, you should attend seminars. Often, seminars can lead you to the deep and profound feeling needed, which cannot be attained with the DVD and book alone.

During the course of practice, you should always ask yourself questions, such as "What is the purpose of the exercise?" "Why am I practicing it this way?" "What are my goals for this training?" and "What is the theory behind it?" Only with this kind of attitude can you remain humble and continue learning and pondering.

Upon reaching a high level in both action and understanding, you should keep the mind open and continue to absorb taiji ball theories and practices from other sources. In this case, you will obtain different views of the taiji ball practice; see it from various angles.

Finally, *taiji ball qigong* is an art, which can bring you great health benefits and improved martial arts capabilities. Since it is an art, it leaves room for creativity. The deeper, creative arts originate from profound feeling and understanding. Therefore, once having reached a grave level of feeling and understanding, you should be capable of creating different patterns or even comprehending new theory. This allows for further development of the already existing arts to a more precocious level. Only then can the arts survive, through preservation and development.

Acknowledgments

Thanks to Nick Boston, Nicholas C. Yang, and Eric Hinds for helping with this book.

CHAPTER 1

General Qigong Theory
(般氣功之理論)

1.1 Introduction (介紹)

To understand taiji ball qigong, first you must know what qi and qigong are. You should also understand different categories of qigong and its basic theory of yin-yang and kan-li. Only then will you be able to comprehend how and why qigong is able to bring you health, longevity, and even spiritual enlightenment. This chapter will help you build this theoretical foundation. Only if you understand this chapter, can your practice of taiji ball qigong reach its deep meaning and purpose.

1.2 What is Qi and What is Qigong? (何謂氣？何謂氣功？)

In this section, we discuss the general concept of qi, both the traditional understanding and modern scientific explanations, and the concept of qigong.

1.2.1 A General Definition of Qi

Qi is the energy or natural force that fills the universe. The Chinese believe in three powers (*san cai*, 三才) of the universe: heaven (*tian*, 天), earth (*di*, 地), and man (*ren*, 人). Heaven (the sky or universe) has heaven qi (*tian qi*, 天氣), the most important of the three, consisting of forces exerted by heavenly bodies, such as sunshine, moonlight, gravity, and energy from the stars. Weather, climate, and natural disasters are governed by heaven qi (*tian qi*, 天氣). Every energy field strives to stay in balance. When the heaven qi loses its balance, it tries to rebalance itself through wind, rain, tornadoes, and hurricanes, enabling a new energy balance to be achieved.

Earth qi (*di qi*, 地氣) is controlled by heaven qi. Too much rain forces a river to flood or change its path. Without rain, vegetation will die. The Chinese believe earth qi is made up of lines and patterns of energy, as well as the earth's magnetic field and the heat concealed underground. These energies must also be in balance; otherwise disasters such as earthquakes occur. When earth qi is balanced and harmonized, plants grow and animals thrive.

Finally, each individual person, animal, and plant has its own qi field, which continually seeks balance. Losing qi balance, an individual sickens, dies, and decomposes. All natural things, including humankind and our human qi (*ren qi*, 人氣), are determined by the natural cycles of heaven qi and earth qi. Throughout the history of qigong, people have been most interested in human qi and its relationship with heaven qi and earth qi.

In China, qi is also defined as any energy that demonstrates power and strength, be it electricity, magnetism, heat, or light. Electric power is called electric qi (*dian qi*, 電氣), and heat is called heat qi (*re qi*, 熱氣). When a person is alive, his body's energy is called human qi (*ren qi*, 人氣).

Qi also expresses the energy state of something, especially of living things. The weather is called heaven qi (*tian qi*, 天氣) because it indicates the energy state of the heavens. When something is alive it has vital qi (*huo qi*, 活氣), and when dead it has dead qi (*si qi*, 死氣) or ghost qi (*gui qi*, 鬼氣). When a person is righteous and has the spiritual strength to do well, he is said to have normal qi or righteous qi (*zheng qi*, 正氣). The spiritual state or morale of an army is called its energy state (*qi shi*, 氣勢).

Qi can represent energy itself, or else the state of the energy. It is important to understand this when you practice qigong, so your mind is not channeled into a narrow understanding of qi, limiting your future understanding and development.

1.2.2 A Narrow Definition of Qi

Now let us look at how qi is defined in qigong society today. Among the three powers, the Chinese have been most concerned with qi affecting health and longevity. After four thousand years of emphasizing human qi, when people mention qi they usually mean qi circulating in our bodies.

In ancient Chinese medical and qigong documents, the word qi was written "炁". This character consists of two words. The "旡" on top means "nothing," and ",,,," at the bottom means "fire." So qi was originally written as "no fire." In ancient times, physicians and qigong practitioners attempted to balance the yin and yang qi circulating in the body so there was "no fire" in the internal organs. Each internal organ needs a specific amount of qi to function properly. If it receives an improper amount, usually an excess which makes it too yang or "on fire," it starts to malfunction. In time, this causes physical damage. The goal of qigong at that time was to attain a state of "no fire," which eventually became the word qi.

In more recent publications, the qi of "no fire" has been replaced by the word "氣," which is also constructed of two words, "气" which means "air" and "米" which means "rice." Later practitioners realized that post-birth qi is produced by breathing in air and consuming food. Air is called "kong qi" (空氣), literally "space energy."

For a long time, people debated what type of energy circulates in our bodies. Many believed it to be heat; others believed it to be electricity, while others assumed it was a mixture of heat, electricity, and light. This debate continued into the 1980s when the concept of qi gradually became clear. Today, science postulates that, with the possible exception of gravity, there is actually only one type of energy in the universe, namely electromagnetic energy. Light and heat are also manifestations of electromagnetic energy. The qi in our bodies is actually bioelectricity, and our bodies are a living electromagnetic field.[1] Thus, the qi is affected by our thoughts, feelings, activities, the food we eat, the quality of the air we breathe, our lifestyles, the natural energy that surrounds us, and also the unnatural energy which modern science inflicts upon us.

The following scientific formula represents the major biochemical reaction in our body:

$$\text{glucose} + 6O_2 \longrightarrow 6CO_2 + 6H_2O$$
$$\Delta G^{\circ\prime} = -686 \text{ Kcal}$$

(energy content)
$\longrightarrow$ Heat
$\longrightarrow$ Light
$\longrightarrow$ Bioelectricity (qi)

As you can see, rice is glucose, air is oxygen, and qi is bioelectricity.

1.2.3 A General Definition of Qigong

In China, the word "gong" (功) is often used as a shorter form of "gongfu" (*kung fu*, 功夫), meaning energy and time. Any study or training which requires energy, time, and patience to achieve is called gongfu. Qigong is a science which studies the energy in nature. The main difference between this energy science and Western energy science is that qigong focuses on the inner energy of human beings, while Western energy science pays more attention to the energy outside the human body. When you study qigong, it is worthwhile to consider the modern scientific point of view, and not restrict yourself to traditional beliefs.

The Chinese have studied qi for thousands of years, recording information on the patterns and cycles of nature in books such as *The Book of Changes,* 1112 B.C. (*Yi Jing,* 易經), which describes the natural forces of heaven (*tian,* 天), earth (*di,* 地), and man (*ren,* 人). These three powers (*san cai,* 三才) manifest as heaven qi, earth qi, and human qi, with their definite rules and cycles. The rules are unchanging, while the cycles return to repeat themselves. The *Yi Jing* applies these principles to calculate changes in natural qi, through a process called the eight trigrams (*bagua,* 八卦). From the eight trigrams are derived the 64 hexagrams. The *Yi Jing* was probably the first book describing qi and its variations in nature and man. The relationship of the three natural powers and their qi variations were later discussed extensively in the book, *Theory of Qi's Variation* (*Qi Hua Lun,* 氣化論).

Understanding heaven qi is very difficult, and was especially so in ancient times. But since natural cycles recur, accumulated experience makes it possible to trace the natural patterns. Understanding the rules and cycles of heavenly timing (*tian shi,* 天時) helps describe changes in the seasons, climate, weather, and other natural occurrences. Many of these routine patterns and cycles are caused by the rebalancing of qi. Various natural cycles recur every day, month or year, while others return only every twelve or sixty years.

Earth qi forms part of heaven qi. From understanding the rules and structure of the earth, you understand the process whereby mountains and rivers are formed, plants grow and rivers move, and also where it is best to build a house and which direction it should face to be a healthy place to live. In China, geomancy teachers (*di li shi,* 地理師) or wind water teachers (*feng shui shi,* 風水師) make their living this way. The term wind water (*feng shui,* 風水) is used because the location and character of wind and water are the most important factors in evaluating a location. These experts use the accumulated body of geomantic knowledge and the *Yi Jing* to help make important decisions such as where and how to build a house, where to bury the dead, and how to arrange homes and offices to be better and more prosperous places in which to live and work.

Human qi has been studied most thoroughly, encompassing many different aspects. The Chinese believe human qi is affected and controlled by heaven qi and earth qi, and that they in fact determine your destiny. By understanding the relationship between nature and people, and also human relations (*ren shi*, 人事), you may predict wars, the destiny of a country, a person's desires and temperament, and even their future. The people who practice this profession are called calculate life teachers (*suan ming shi*, 算命師).

However, the greatest achievement in the study of human qi is in regard to health and longevity. Since qi is the source of life, if you understand how qi functions and know how to regulate it correctly, you may live a long and healthy life. As a part of nature, you are channeled into its cycles, and it is in your best interest to follow the way of nature. This is the meaning of Dao (道), which can be translated as the Natural Way.

Many different aspects of human qi have been researched, including acupuncture, massage, herbal treatment, meditation, and qigong exercises. Their use in adjusting human qi flow has become the root of Chinese medical science. Meditation and moving qigong exercises are used to improve health and cure certain illnesses. Daoists and Buddhists also use meditation and qigong exercises in their pursuit of enlightenment.

In conclusion, the study of any of the aspects of qi, including heaven qi, earth qi, and human qi, should be called qigong. However, since the term is usually used today only in reference to the cultivation of human qi through meditation and exercises, we will conform to this narrower definition.

1.2.4 A Narrow Definition of Qigong

The narrow definition of qi is the energy circulating in the human body. Qigong studies and trains the qi circulating in the body. Qigong includes how our bodies relate to heaven qi and earth qi, and the overlapping fields of acupuncture, herbal treatment, martial arts qigong, qigong massage and exercises, and religious enlightenment qigong.

In ancient times, qigong was called "tu-na" (吐納), meaning "to utter and admit," namely, focused breathing. Qigong depends on correct breathing. The well-known Daoist, Zhuang Zi (莊子) said, "Blowing to breathe, utter the old and admit the new. The bear's natural movement, and the bird's extending (of the neck), are all for longevity. This is favored by those living as long as Peng Zu (彭祖) who practiced dao-yin (導引, guide and lead), and nourish the shape (cultivate the body)."[1] Peng Zu was a legendary qigong practitioner during the reign of Emperor Yao (堯) (2357-2205 B.C.), said to have lived for 800 years. Qigong was also called dao-yin, meaning to use the mind and physical movement to guide and lead qi circulation. The movements imitate the natural movements of animals such as bears and birds. A famous medical qigong set passed down from that time is called the Five Animal Sports (*Wu Qin Xi*, 五禽戲), which imitates the movements of the tiger, deer, bear, ape, and bird.

Qigong defines twelve major channels (*shi er jing,* 十二經) in the body, branching into many secondary channels (*luo,* 絡), similar to the blood circulatory system. The primary channels are like arteries and veins, while the secondary ones are like capillaries. The twelve primary qi channels are also like rivers, while the secondary channels are like streams flowing in and out of the rivers. Qi is distributed throughout the body through this network, which connects the extremities to the internal organs and the skin to the bone marrow. The internal organs of Chinese medicine do not necessarily correspond to the physical organs as understood in the West, but rather to a set of clinical functions related to the organ system.

The body also has eight vessels (*ba mai,* 八脈), called strange meridians (*qi jing,* 奇經), that function like reservoirs and regulate the qi circulation. The famous Chinese Daoist medical doctor Li, Shi-zhen (李時珍) described them in his book, *The Study of Strange Meridians and Eight Vessels* (奇經八脈考): "The regular meridians (12 primary qi channels) are like rivers, while the strange meridians (eight vessels) are like lakes. When the qi in the regular meridians is abundant and flourishing, they overflow into the strange meridians."[2]

When qi in the eight reservoirs is full and strong, it will be so in the rivers. Stagnation in any channel leads to irregularity in the qi flow to the extremities and organs, and illness may develop. Every channel has its own particular qi flow, the strength of which can be affected by your mind, the weather, time of day, food you have eaten, and even your mood. For example, qi in the lungs tends to be more positive and yang in drier weather. When you are angry, the qi flow in your liver channel will be irregular. Qi strength in different channels varies throughout the day in a regular cycle, and at any particular time one channel is strongest. For example, between 11 A.M. and 1 P.M. the qi flows most strongly in the heart channel. The qi level of the same organ differs from one person to another. For more detail on the relationship of the qi flow and time of day, refer to the book, *Qigong for Health and Martial Arts*[3], published by YMAA Publication Center.

When the flow of qi in the twelve channels is irregular, the eight reservoirs act to stabilize it. When one experiences a sudden shock, qi in the bladder becomes deficient. The reservoir immediately regulates it to recover from the shock, unless the reservoir qi is also deficient, or if the shock is too great; in this case, the bladder contracts, causing urination.

A sick person's qi tends to be either too positive (*yang,* 陽) or too negative (*yin,* 陰). A Chinese physician would prescribe herbs to adjust the qi, or insert acupuncture needles at various points to adjust the flow and restore balance. The alternative is to practice qigong, using physical and mental exercises to adjust the qi.

In scholar society, qigong is defined differently, focusing on regulating disturbances of the emotional mind into a state of calm. This relaxes the body and enables qi to rebalance and circulate smoothly, so mental and physical health may be attained.

In Daoist and Buddhist society, qigong is the method to lead qi from the lower dan tian (下丹田), or elixir field, to the brain for spiritual enlightenment or Buddhahood. This place in the abdomen stores qi in a bioelectric battery. Religious qigong is considered the highest and most rigorous level of Chinese qigong training.

In martial arts society, qigong is the theory and method of manifesting qi to energize the physical body to its maximum efficiency and power. Martial arts qigong originated from religious qigong, especially *Muscle/Tendon Changing* and *Marrow/Brain Washing* Qigong (*Yi Jin Jing* and *Xi Sui Jing*, 易筋經、洗髓經), and the goal of the most profound level of martial arts qigong training is the same as that of religious qigong, namely spiritual enlightenment.

1.3 Categories of Qigong (氣功之分類)

In this section, we would like to discuss the scope of human qigong, and the traditional concept of nei dan (內丹, internal elixir) and wai dan (外丹, external elixir), to clarify the differences between the styles of qigong practice around the world.

1.3.1 Scope of Qigong Practice–Physical and Mental (氣功練習之規範)

If we trace qigong history back to before the Chinese Qin and Han dynasties (秦、漢) (255 B.C.–A.D. 223), we find the origin of many qigong practices in dancing. Dancing exercises the body and maintains it in a healthy condition. Matching movement with music harmonizes the mind, either to energize or calm it down. This qigong dancing was later passed to Japan during the Han dynasty and became the very elegant, slow, and refined dancing still practiced in the Japanese Royal Court today.

African and Native American dancing, in which the body is bounced up and down, also loosens the joints and improves qi circulation. Any activity that regulates qi circulation in the body, even jogging or weight lifting, may be regarded as qigong. Additional aspects of qigong include the food we eat, the air we breathe, and even our emotions and thoughts.

In Figure 1-1, the vertical axis to the left represents qi used by the physical body (yang), and the right vertex, that of the mind (yin). The more to the left an activity is represented, indicates it requires more physical exertion and less mental effort. This

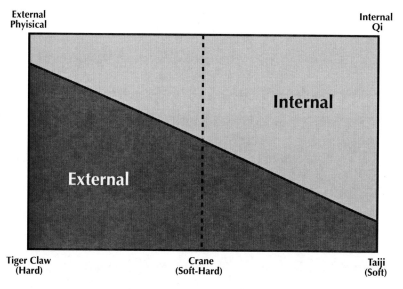

Figure 1-1. The range of defined qigong

could be aerobics, unfocused dancing, walking, or jogging, where the mind is used less than the body. These activities do not require special training and are classified as secular qigong. At the mid-point of the graph, mental and physical activities are combined in equal measure. This would be the slow-moving qigong commonly practiced, in which the mind is used to lead qi in coordination with movement. With slow, relaxed movements, the qi led by the mind may reach deeper into the ligaments, marrow, and internal organs. Deep internal feeling can lead qi there significantly. Taijiquan, White Crane, Snake, and Dragon are typical systems of qigong, cultivated intensively in Chinese medical and martial arts societies.

At a deeper level of practice, the mind becomes critically important. It is actively involved while you are in deep relaxation. This level is cultivated primarily by scholars and religious qigong practitioners. There may be some physical movement in the lower abdomen, but the main focus is to cultivate a peaceful and neutral mind, and pursue the final goal of spiritual enlightenment. This practice includes sitting chan (*ren*, 坐禪，忍), Embryonic Breathing Meditation (*Tai Xi Jing Zuo*, 胎息静坐), Small Circulation Meditation (*Xiao Zhou Tian Jing Zuo*, 小周天静坐), Grand Circulation (*Da Zhou Tian*, 大周天), and Brain Washing Enlightenment Meditation (*Xi Sui Gong*, 洗髓功).

Different qigong practices aim for different goals. For a long, happy life, you need health of mind and body. The best qigong for health is at the middle of our model, to regulate both body and mind. You may practice the yin side through still meditation, and the yang side through physical activity. This balances yin and yang and abundant qi may be accumulated and circulated.

From this we may conclude:

1. Any activity able to improve qi circulation is qigong.
2. Qigong, which emphasizes the physical side, will improve physical strength and qi circulation, conditioning the muscles, tendons, and ligaments.
3. Qigong activating both physical and mental aspects can reach deeper levels, enhancing physical strength and qi circulation. By coordinating the relaxed physical body with the concentrated mind, qi may circulate deep inside the joints, internal organs, and even the bone marrow.
4. Qigong, which focuses on achieving a profound meditative state, may neglect physical movement, causing physical strength to degenerate.

1.3.2 External and Internal Elixirs (Wai Dan and Nei Dan) (外丹與內丹)

Qigong practices can be divided according to their training theory and methods into two general categories, wai dan (外丹), external elixir, and nei dan (內丹), internal elixir. Understanding the differences between them gives you an overview of qigong practice.

1.3.2.1 Wai Dan (External Elixir) (外丹)

Wai means external, and dan means elixir. External here refers to the extremities and the superficial parts of the torso as opposed to the torso at the center of the body, which includes the vital organs. Elixir is the life-prolonging substance for which Chinese Daoists searched for millennia. They first thought it was something physical, which could be prepared from herbs or from chemicals purified in a furnace. After thousands of years of experimentation, they found the elixir within, namely qi circulating in the body. To prolong your life, you must develop the elixir in your body, cultivating, protecting, and nourishing it.

In wai dan qigong practice, you exercise to build qi in your arms and legs. When enough qi accumulates there, it flows through the twelve primary qi channels clearing obstructions and into the center of the body to nourish the organs. A person who works out, or has a physical job, is generally healthier than one who sits around all day.

Massage, acupuncture, and herbal treatment are all wai dan practices. Massaging the body produces qi, stimulating the cells to a more energized state. Qi is raised and circulation enhanced. After a massage, you are relaxed, and the higher levels of qi in the muscles and skin flow into the torso and internal organs. This is the theoretical foundation of tui na (推拿), push and grab, qigong massage. Acupuncture may also enhance qi, regulating the internal organs.

Any stimulation or exercise that generates a high level of qi in the limbs or at the surface of the body, which then flows into the center of the body, can be classified as wai dan (Figure 1-2).

1.3.2.2 Nei Dan (Internal Elixir) (內丹)

Nei means internal. Nei dan means to build up the elixir internally, inside the body instead of in the limbs, in the vessels rather than the channels. Whereas in wai dan, qi is built up in the limbs or skin and then moved into the body through primary qi

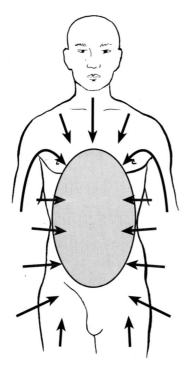

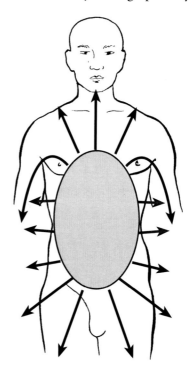

Figure 1-2. External elixir (wai dan) Figure 1-3. Internal elixir (nei dan)

channels, nei dan exercises build up qi inside the body and lead it out to the limbs (Figure 1-3). This is accomplished by special breathing techniques during meditation. First, one builds abundant qi in the lower dan tian, the bioelectric battery; then one leads it to the eight vessels for storage. As a result, qi in the twelve primary channels can be regulated smoothly and efficiently.

Nei dan is more profound than wai dan, and more difficult to understand and practice. Traditionally, nei dan qigong practices were passed down more secretively than wai dan, especially at the highest levels such as marrow/brain washing, which were passed down to only a few trusted disciples.

1.3.3 *Schools of Qigong Practice* (氣功練習之門派)
Qigong has four major categories according to the purpose of training:
- Curing illness
- Maintaining health
- Enlightenment or Buddhahood
- Martial arts

Most styles serve more than one of these purposes. For example, Daoist qigong aims for longevity and enlightenment, but you need to maintain good health and cure sickness. Knowing the history and principles of each category helps one understand their essence more clearly.

1.3.3.1 *Medical Qigong–for Healing*
In ancient China, most emperors respected scholars and their philosophy. Doctors were not highly regarded because they made their diagnosis by touching the patient's body, which was considered characteristic of the lower social classes. Although doctors were commonly looked down upon, they quietly passed down the results of their research to following generations. Of all the groups studying qigong in China, doctors have been researching it the longest. Since the discovery of qi circulation in the human body about four thousand years ago, Chinese doctors have devoted major efforts to its study, developing acupuncture, acupressure, and herbal treatment.

Many Chinese doctors also created sets of qigong for maintaining health or curing specific illnesses. Doing only sitting meditation with breathing, as practiced in scholar qigong or Buddhist Chan meditation, is not enough to cure illness. They believed in movement to increase qi circulation. Although a calm and peaceful mind is important for health, exercising the body is more important. They learned through practice that people who exercised properly got sick less often, and their bodies degenerated less quickly than people who just sat around. Specific movements increase qi circulation in specific organs, and are used to treat specific illnesses and restore normal function.

Some movements are similar to the way certain animals move. For an animal to survive in the wild, it must instinctively protect its body, especially accumulating its qi and preserving it. We humans have lost many of these instincts over time, in separating ourselves from nature.

A typical, well-known set of such exercises is Five Animal Sports (*Wu Qin Xi*, 五禽戲) created nearly two thousand years ago by Hua Tuo (華佗) (ca. A.D. 145–208). (Others say it was by Jun Qing (君倩). Another famous set is Eight Pieces of Brocade

(*Ba Duan Jin*, 八段錦). It was developed by Marshal Yue, Fei (岳飛) during the Southern Song dynasty (南宋) (A.D. 1127–1280), who was a soldier and scholar rather than a doctor.

Before physical damage manifests in an organ, there is first an abnormality in qi circulation. Excess yin or yang is the root of illness and organ damage. In a specific channel, abnormal qi circulation leads to organ malfunction. If the condition is not corrected, the organ degenerates. The best way to heal is to adjust and balance the qi before there is any physical problem. This is the major goal of acupuncture and acupressure treatment. Herbs and special diets also help regulate the qi.

As long as the illness is limited to qi stagnation and there is no physical organ damage, qigong exercises can be used to readjust qi circulation and treat the problem. Ulcers, asthma, and even certain kinds of cancer, are often treated effectively with simple exercises. But if the sickness is already so serious that the organs have started to fail, the situation is critical and specific treatment is necessary. This can be acupuncture, herbs, or even an operation.

Over thousands of years of observing nature, qigong practitioners went even deeper. Qi circulation changes with the seasons, so they helped the body during these periodic adjustments. In each season, different organs have characteristic problems. For example, at the beginning of fall, the lungs adapt to breathing colder air, making us susceptible to colds. Other organs are also affected by seasonal changes, and by one another. Focusing on these seasonal qi disorders, they developed movements to speed up the body's adjustment. These sets were originally created to maintain health, and later were also used for curing sickness.

1.3.3.2 Scholar Qigong–for Maintaining Health

Before the Han dynasty (漢朝) (206 B.C.–A.D. 221), two major scholar societies arose. One was founded by Confucius (Kong Zi, 孔子) (551–479 B.C.), during the Spring and Autumn Period (Chun Qiu, 春秋) (722–484 B.C.) His philosophy was popularized and expanded by Mencius (Meng Zi, 孟子) (372–289 B.C.) during the Warring States Period (Zhan Guo, 戰國), (403–222 B.C.). Scholars who practice his philosophy are called Confucians (*Ru Jia*, 儒家). Their basic philosophy consists of loyalty (*zhong*, 忠), filial piety (*xiao*, 孝), humanity (*ren*, 仁), kindness (*ai*, 愛), trust (*xin*, 信), justice (*yi*, 義), harmony (*he*, 和), and peace (*ping*, 平). Humanity and human feelings are the main subjects, and Confucian philosophy is the root of much of Chinese culture.

The second major scholar society was Daoism (*Dao Jia*, 道家), established by Lao Zi (老子) in the sixth century B.C. His book, the *Classic on the Virtue of the Dao* (*Dao De Jing*, 道德經), describes human morality. During the Warring States Period, his follower Zhuang Zhou (莊周) wrote a book called *Zhuang Zi* (莊子), which led to the forming of another strong branch of Daoism. Before the Han dynasty, Daoism was considered a branch of scholarship. However, in the East Han dynasty (東漢) (A.D. 25–168), traditional Daoism was combined with Buddhism imported from India by Zhang, Dao-ling (張道陵), and began to be treated as a religion. Daoism before the Han dynasty should be considered scholarly Daoism rather than religious.

With regard to qigong, both schools emphasized maintaining health and preventing disease. Many illnesses are caused by mental and emotional excesses. When your mind is disturbed, the organs do not function normally. For example, depression may cause stomach ulcers and indigestion. Anger may cause the liver to malfunction. Sadness may lead to stagnation and tightness in the lungs, and fear can disturb the normal functioning of the kidneys and bladder. To avoid illness, you need to balance and relax your thoughts and emotions. This is called regulating the mind (*tiao xin*, 調心).

Both schools emphasize gaining a peaceful mind through meditation. In still meditation, the primary training is getting rid of thoughts to clear the mind. As the flow of thoughts and emotions slows down, you feel mentally and emotionally neutral, leading to self-control. In this state of "no thought," you even relax deep down into your internal organs, and your qi circulation is smooth and strong.

This still meditation is very common in Chinese scholar society, which focuses on regulating the mind, body, and breath, so qi flows smoothly and sickness may be averted. Their training is called xiu qi (修氣), which means cultivating qi. This is very different from the religious Daoist qigong of the East Han dynasty, called lian qi (練氣), meaning to train qi to make it stronger.

Qigong documents from Confucians and Daoists are mainly limited to maintaining health. Their aim is to follow natural destiny. This is quite different from that of religious Daoists after the East Han dynasty, who believed one's destiny could be changed. They believed it is possible to train your qi to make it stronger and to extend your life. Chinese scholar society maintained that "in human life, seventy is rare."[4] Few common people in ancient times reached seventy years of age as a result of harsh conditions. They also said, "Peace with heaven and delight in your destiny" (*an tian le ming*, 安天樂命), and "cultivate the body and await destiny" (*xiu shen si ming*, 修身俟命). Compare this with the philosophy of the later Daoists, who said, "One hundred and twenty means dying young."[5] They proved by example that life can be extended and that your destiny can be resisted and overcome.

1.3.3.3 Religious Qigong–for Enlightenment or Buddhahood

Religious qigong, though not as popular as other categories in China, has achieved the greatest accomplishments. It was kept secret in the monasteries and only revealed to seculars, or lay people, in the last century.

Religious qigong is mainly comprised of Daoism and Buddhism. The main purpose of their training is striving for enlightenment or Buddhahood. They seek to rise above normal human suffering and escape from the cycle of reincarnation. They believe all human suffering is caused by the seven passions and six desires (*qi qing liu yu*, 七情六慾). The seven passions are happiness (*xi*, 喜), anger (*nu*, 怒), sorrow (*ai*, 哀), joy (*le*, 樂), love (*ai*, 愛), hate (*hen*, 恨), and desire (*yu*, 慾). The six desires are the six sensory pleasures of the eyes, ears, nose, tongue, body, and mind. If you are bound to them, you will reincarnate after death. To avoid this, they train to be spiritually independent of the body and physical attachments. Thereby, they enter the heavenly kingdom and gain eternal peace. This rigorous training is called "unification of heaven and man" (*tian ren he yi*, 天人合一). It is extremely difficult to achieve in the everyday world, so practitioners generally shun society and move into the solitude of the mountains—where they can concentrate all their energies on spiritual cultivation.

Religious qigong practitioners train to strengthen internal qi, to nourish their spirit (*shen*, 神) until it can survive the death of the body. Marrow/Brain Washing Qigong training enables them to lead qi to the brain, where the spirit resides, and to raise the brain cells to a state of higher energy. This training used to be restricted only to a few advanced priests in China and Tibet. Over the last two thousand years, Tibetan and Chinese Buddhists, and the religious Daoists, have followed the same principles, becoming the three major religious schools of qigong training.

This religious striving, toward enlightenment or Buddhahood, is recognized as the highest and most difficult level of qigong. Many practitioners reject the rigors of this religious striving, and practice Marrow/Brain Washing Qigong solely for longevity. It was these people who eventually revealed the secrets of Marrow/Brain Washing to the outside world, as described in *Qigong–The Secret of Youth,* published by YMAA Publication Center.[6]

1.3.3.4 *Martial Qigong–for Fighting*

Chinese martial qigong developed from Da Mo's *Muscle/Tendon Changing* and *Marrow/Brain Washing Qigong Classic* (*Yi Jin Jing* and *Xi Sui Jing,* 易筋經 and 洗髓經), written in the Shaolin Temple (*Shaolin Si,* 少林寺) during the Liang dynasty (梁朝) (A.D. 502-557)). Shaolin monks training this qigong improved their health and greatly increased their martial power and effectiveness. Since then, many martial styles have developed further qigong sets, and many internal martial styles have been created based on qigong theory. Martial artists have played a major role in Chinese qigong society.

When qigong theory was first applied to martial arts, it was used to increase the power and efficiency of the muscles. The mind (yi) generated from clear thinking leads qi to the muscles to energize them to function more efficiently. The average person generally uses his muscles at about 40% efficiency. Training a strong yi to qi to the muscles effectively, one may energize the muscles to a higher level, increasing fighting effectiveness.

Acupuncture theory enabled fighting techniques to reach even more advanced levels. Martial artists learned to attack vital cavities, disturbing the enemy's qi flow to cause injury and death. Central to this technique is understanding the route and timing of qi circulation in the body, allowing one to have a better knowledge of effectively striking cavities accurately and to the correct depth. These techniques are called dian xue (點穴, pointing cavities) or dian mai (點脈, pointing vessels).

While most martial qigong practices also improve the practitioner's health, there are some which, although they build up some special skill useful for fighting, also damage the practitioner's health. An example of this is Iron Sand Palm (*Tie Sha Zhang,* 鐵砂掌). Although it builds amazing destructive power, it can also harm your hands, causing qi circulation in the hands and internal organs to be affected.

Many martial styles have developed from Da Mo's sixth century qigong theory and methods. They can roughly be divided into external and internal styles. The external styles emphasize building qi in the limbs for physical martial techniques, following the practices of wai dan qigong. The concentrated mind is used during the exercises to energize the qi. This significantly increases muscular strength and the effectiveness of the martial techniques. Qigong trains the body to resist punches and kicks by leading qi to energize the skin and the muscles, enabling them to resist a blow without injury. This training is called Iron Shirt (*Tie Bu Shan*, 鐵布衫) or Golden Bell Cover (*Jin Zhong Zhao*, 金鐘罩). Martial styles that use wai dan training are called external styles (*wai jia*, 外家). Hard qigong training is called hard gong (*ying gong*, 硬功). Shaolin gongfu is a typical example of a style using wai dan martial qigong.

Although wai dan qigong increases the martial artist's power, training the muscles can cause overdevelopment, leading to energy dispersion (*san gong*, 散功). To prevent this, when an external martial artist reaches a high level of external training, he will start training internal qigong, which specializes in curing the energy dispersion problem. "The external styles are from external to internal and from hard to soft."[7]

In contrast, internal martial qigong is based on the theory of nei dan. Qi is generated in the torso instead of the limbs, and later led to the limbs to increase power. To lead qi to the limbs, the techniques must be soft and muscle-use kept to a minimum. Nei dan martial training is much more difficult than wai dan. For more detail, refer to the books, *Tai Chi Theory and Martial Power*[8] and *Taijiquan Theory of Dr. Yang, Jwing-Ming*[9] published by YMAA Publication Center.

Several internal martial styles were created in the Wudang (武當山) and Emei (峨嵋山) mountains. Popular ones are Taijiquan (太極拳), Baguazhang (八卦掌), Liuhebafa (六合八法) and Xingyiquan (形意拳). Even internal martial styles, called soft styles, must sometimes use muscular strength while fighting. Utilizing strong power in a fight requires qi to manifest externally, using harder, more external techniques. "Internal styles are from internal to external and from soft to hard."[10]

Although qigong is widely studied in Chinese martial society, the main focus is on increasing fighting ability rather than on health. Good health is considered a by-product of training. Only recently has health started receiving greater attention in martial qigong, especially in the internal martial arts.

1.4 Theory of Yin and Yang, Kan and Li (陰陽坎離之理論)

The most important concepts in qigong practice are the theories of yin and yang, and of kan and li. These two different concepts have become confused in qigong society, even in China. If you understand them clearly, you have grasped an important key to qigong practice.

1.4.1 What are Kan and Li?

The terms kan (坎) and li (離) occur frequently in qigong documents. In the eight trigrams, kan represents water (*shui*, 水) while li represents fire (*huo*, 火). Kan and li training have long been of major importance to qigong practitioners.

Although kan-li and yin-yang are related, kan and li are not yin and yang. Kan is water, which cools your body down and makes it more yin, while li is fire, which warms your body and makes it more yang. Kan and li are the methods or causes, while yin and yang are the results. When kan and li are adjusted correctly, yin and yang are balanced and interact harmoniously.

Qigong practitioners believe your body is always too yang, unless you are sick or have not eaten for a long time. Excess yang leads the body to degenerate and burn out, causing aging. Using water to cool down your body, you can slow the aging process and lengthen your life. Qigong practitioners improve the quality of water in their bodies, and reduce the quantity of fire. You should always keep this subject at the top of your list for study and research. If you earnestly ponder and experiment, you will grasp the trick of adjusting them.

Water and fire represent many things in the body. First, qi is classified according to fire or water. When your qi is not pure, causing your body to heat up and your mind to become unstable (yang), it is classified as fire qi (*huo qi*, 火氣). The qi, which is pure and can cool your physical and spiritual bodies, making them more yin, is water qi (*shui qi*, 水氣). Your qi should never be purely water. It should cool down the fire, but never quench it. That would signify death.

Fire qi agitates and stimulates the emotions, generating from them the emotional mind called xin (心), which is considered the fire mind or yang mind. On the other hand, the mind that water qi generates is calm, steady and wise. It is called yi (意), and considered to be the water mind or wisdom mind. If your spirit is nourished primarily by fire qi, although your spirit may be high, it will be scattered and confused. If the spirit is nourished and raised up mainly by water qi, it will be a firm, steady yin mind. When your yi governs your xin effectively, your will, as strong emotional intention, can be firm.

Your qi is the main cause of the yin and yang of your body, mind and spirit. To regulate yin and yang, you need to regulate water and fire qi at their source.

To analyze kan and li and adjust them efficiently, apply modern science to marry the past and the present, and give birth to the future. The reliance of modern medicine on drugs is the worst way to cure illness or gain health. The best way is to solve the problem at its root. Ancient China did not have our modern medical chemistry, and had to develop other ways to adjust the body's water and fire. We could learn much from them. For example, many arthritis patients today rely on medicine to reduce pain. While this reliance may offer temporary relief from pain, it does not cure the problem. When the medicine is gone, the pain resumes. Chinese medical qigong cures arthritis by rebuilding the strength of the joints. Patients increase qi circulation with slow, easy exercises, and massage to strengthen the joints. These practices readjust the yin and yang balance, allowing the body to repair the damage and increase the strength of the joints. This approach addresses the root of the problem. If you are interested in this subject, please refer to the book, *Arthritis Relief–Qigong for Healing & Prevention*, published by YMAA Publication Center.[11]

Nevertheless, many modern medical practices conform to kan and li theory. Fever is treated by applying medicine and ice cubes to reduce one's temperature. Ice cubes are also used to reduce swelling caused by injuries. Whether you follow ancient or modern medicine, the basic theory of healing remains the same, namely the adjustment of kan and li. Medical chemistry has brought us much that is marvelous, but also many problems.

The key is found in understanding the circulation of qi, or bioelectricity, in the body. Regulating it strengthens the body and maintains health, allowing doctors to correct irregular qi even before the appearance of physical symptoms, and increasing the quality and duration of life.

1.4.2 The Keys to Kan and Li Adjustment

Here we discuss how kan and li relate to your breathing, mind, and spirit, and the keys to regulating them in qigong practice. Combining them, we construct a secret key which opens the qigong treasure.

1.4.2.1 Kan and Li of Breathing

In qigong, breathing is considered a strategy to lead the qi. By directing your breath, you can lead qi to the skin or marrow. Breathing slowly can calm the qi flow, while rapid breathing can invigorate it. When you are excited, your body is yang, and you exhale longer than you inhale. This leads qi to the skin, where excess qi dissipates through sweat. When you are sad your body is yin, and you inhale longer than you exhale. This preserves qi by leading it inward, and you feel cold. Through breathing you adjust the body's yin and yang, so breathing has kan and li classifications.

Inhaling is a water (*kan*) activity, because you lead qi inward to store it in the bone marrow. This reduces guardian qi (*wei qi*, 衛氣) and the qi in the muscles and tendons, calming the body's yang. Exhaling is a fire (*li*) activity, because it brings qi out to energize the muscles, tendons, and skin, enhancing guardian qi by making the body more yang. When the body is more yang than its surroundings, its qi is dissipated.

Yin and yang should be balanced so your body functions harmoniously. The trick is using breathing strategies. Usually inhalation and exhalation should be equal. When you are excited, your body is too yang, so you may inhale longer and deeper to calm your mind and lead qi in to make it more yin.

Exhalation leads qi to the skin and to the five extremities; the crown (*baihui*, Gv-20, 百會), the two cavities at the center of the palms (*laogong* P-8, 勞宮), and the two cavities near the centers of the soles (*yongquan* K-1, 湧泉), to exchange with your surroundings. Inhalation leads qi deep inside to reach the internal organs and marrow. Table 1-1 summarizes how different breathing strategies affect yin and yang in their various manifestations.

1.4.2.2 Kan and Li of the Mind

According to Chinese tradition, one has two minds, xin (心) and yi (意). Xin means heart, the mind generated by emotional disturbance, or, the emotional mind. The Chinese word yi is comprised of three characters. The top one means establishing (*li*, 立), the middle one means speaking (*yue*, 曰), and the bottom one means heart (*xin*, 心). That means the emotional mind is under control as you establish communication with your heart. Yi can be translated as the wisdom mind. Xin makes you excited and disturbs your emotions, making your body yang, so it is considered li. Yi makes you calm, peaceful, and able to think clearly (yin), so it is considered kan.

In qigong training, the mind is the general who directs the battle, decides on fighting strategy (breathing), and directs the movement of the soldiers (qi). As a general, you control your xin (emotional mind) and use your yi (wisdom mind) to judge the situation and decide on the proper strategy.

In qigong, your yi dominates the situation and generates a thought. This thought executes the strategy (breathing) and is the force moving the qi. When your mind is excited and energized, the strategy is more offensive (emphasize exhalation) the qi circulation is more vigorous and expansive. This aggressive mind is considered a fire mind, making your body more yang. When the strategy is more defensive, emphasize inhalation. Qi circulation will be calmer and more condensed. A calm or relaxed mind is a water mind, since it makes your body more yin.

The mind's kan and li are more important than breathing, because the mind determines the strategy. Regulating mind and breathing are the two basic techniques for controlling your body's yin and yang. Regulation of the body and mind cannot be separated. When the mind is regulated, the breathing can be too, and when breathing is regulated, the mind enters a deeper level of calm.

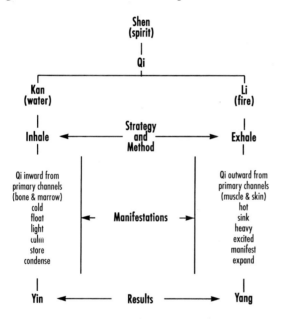

Table 1-1. The Effects of Breathing Strategies on the Body's Yin and Yang in Their Various Manifestations

1.4.2.3 Kan and Li of the Shen

We now consider the most decisive element in winning a battle, the shen (神) (spirit). Shen is the morale of the general's officers and soldiers. There are many cases throughout history of armies winning battles against great odds because the morale of their soldiers was high.

It is the same in qigong training, where the shen determines how successful your qigong practice will be. Your yi, the general who makes the strategy, must be concerned with raising the fighting morale (shen) of the soldiers (qi). When morale is high the soldiers are led efficiently and strategy is executed effectively.

Using yi to raise shen is the primary key to successful qigong training. Shen is the headquarters which governs qi, together with the yi. Yi and shen are closely related and cannot be separated.

When yi is energized, shen is also raised. You want to raise your shen but not let it become excited. When shen is raised, the strategy is carried out effectively. If the shen is excited, the body becomes too yang, which is not desirable in qigong practice. When you practice qigong, you want to keep your shen high at all times, to govern the strategy and the qi. This enables you to regulate kan and li.

Shen is the control tower which adjusts kan and li, but does not have kan and li itself. Some practitioners consider raised shen to be li (fire) and calm shen to be kan (water).

Now, let us draw a few important conclusions from this discussion:
- Kan (water) and li (fire) are not yin and yang. Kan and li are methods that regulate yin or yang.
- Qi itself is only a form of energy and does not have kan and li. When qi is excessive or deficient, it can make the body too yang or too yin.
- When you adjust kan and li in the body, the mind is the first concern. The mind can be kan or li. It determines the strategy (breathing) for withdrawing qi (kan) or expanding it (li).
- Breathing has kan and li. Inhaling is kan as it makes the body more yin, while exhaling, which makes the body more yang, is li.
- Shen does not have kan and li. Shen is the key to making the adjustment of kan and li effective.

1.4.3 The Keys to Adjusting Kan and Li
The keys to kan and li adjustment are mentioned repeatedly in the ancient documents. The first key is that shen and breathing mutually rely on each other. The second key is that shen and qi mutually combine.

1.4.3.1 Shen and Breathing Mutually Dependent (Shen Xi Xiang Yi, 神息相依)
Breathing is the strategy which directs qi in various ways, controlling and adjusting kan and li, which in turn control the body's yin and yang. Shen is the controlling influence which makes strategy work most efficiently. Shen governs strategy directly, and controls kan and li and the body's yin and yang indirectly. The success of your kan and li adjustment depends upon your shen.

When shen matches respiration, it leads qi directly to condense and expand in the most efficient way. Shen must match the breathing for it to be raised up or calmed down, and the breathing must rely on shen to make the strategy work. Shen and breathing are dependent on each other and cannot be separated. This training is called shen xi xiang yi (神息相依), which means shen and breathing depend on each other. When shen and breathing match each other, it is called shen xi (神息) or spirit breathing because it seems your shen is actually doing the breathing.

Shen xi xiang yi is a technique in which, when shen and breathing are united, shen controls the qi directly.

1.4.3.2 Shen and Qi Mutually Combine (Shen Qi Xiang He, 神氣相合)
When shen and breathing match each other as one, the qi is led directly, so shen and qi become one. This is called shen qi xiang he, which means shen and qi mutually harmonized. Shen governs qi directly and efficiently. Harmony of shen and qi is the result of shen and breathing being mutually dependent.

Da Mo believed that to have a long and peaceful life, shen and qi must coordinate and harmonize with each other. He said, "If one does not keep mother (qi) and son (shen) together, though qi breathes internally, shen is labored and craves the external, so shen is always debauched and dirty and thus not clear. If shen is not clear, original harmonious qi will disperse gradually, and they cannot be kept together."[12] The spirit is very important, and regulating shen is one of the highest levels of qigong practice. To reach a high degree of harmony, you must first regulate your emotional mind. Unfortunately, this is difficult to achieve in secular society.

1.5 Qigong and Health (氣功與健康)

When we discuss the relationship between qigong practice and health, we should first define health. There are two aspects of health, the yang side of physical health, which can be seen, and the yin side of mental health, which can only be felt. More than half of today's sickness is caused by mental problems such as depression, stress, and mental fatigue. There are several reasons:

1. Due to our changing social structure, the pressure of living in today's society is greater than ever. Our modern lifestyle only started in the twentieth century. Before then, industry did not heavily dominate the social structure, and many people lived as farmers. The struggle of living in a society demanding more money and material enjoyment dominates our thinking and generates great pressure. In a few short decades, we have become slaves to money. We have lost the original lifestyle that connected us with nature and spiritual feeling. We are facing a revolution that is changing the old life style to the new one, generating many mental problems.

2. Medical science has advanced to a high level and controls most common illnesses, but is still limited to the yang side of understanding. It lacks interest in and knowledge of the bioenergetic aspect of body, mind, and spirit. Because of this, we miss half of human science and are unable to solve several problems and illnesses. We cannot effectively cure problems such as cancer and AIDS. Also, lacking understanding of our mental and spiritual center, we cannot solve mental illness. Many scientists believe that we understand less than 12% of the function of the brain.

3. Due to the decline of religious belief, seculars have lost their guide in understanding the meaning of life. The general public is more knowledgeable and religious dogma is questioned more seriously than ever. Religious authorities cannot offer an educational program that is persuasive to the new open-minded generation. Most churches still preach with methods used for thousands of years. This is very unfortunate since many people have become lost in today's new society. Many Westerners cannot find new meaning in their lives from traditional religion, so they turn to Eastern religions and philosophy, hoping to find answers and peace.

4. Internal cultivation, such as meditation, has been largely ignored. Many people build up a facade in order to hide their true selves from others around them. We lie, and hide our fears and guilty feelings deep in our subconscious mind. Going to confession (Western way), or removing our mask through meditation (Eastern way), were traditional ways of releasing pent-up emotions and balancing our feelings. Today, many people have lost these two most powerful methods of relieving mental imbalance induced by suppressed emotions and feelings of guilt.

Our mental condition is closely related to our health. Many diseases are caused by mental imbalance, which results in the disharmonious qi circulation in the body. To have good health, you need a strong body but also a healthy mind. Qigong for healing and fitness is based on this concept.

To maintain physical strength, qigong exercises that condition the muscles, tendons, ligaments, and bones were developed. Before Da Mo (達磨) (A.D. 483–536), many exercises were developed by doctors to regulate sickness and facilitate healing. Da Mo brought a different concept as recorded in the *Muscle/Tendon Changing Classic* (*Yi Jin Jing*, 易筋經). Since then, based on this training, countless wai dan qigong styles were created.

Meditation was also developed by different schools to regulate the mind into peace and harmony. Meditation not only brings a peaceful mind, but also builds up abundant qi to circulate in the body.

Modern medical science has improved health and significantly extended lives. But today's scientific achievement is still in its infancy. Many problems have arisen due to new social structures and environmental changes. The pressure generated in today's society has caused many mental problems, and many new diseases have emerged. For example, the increase of breast cancer is caused by going against the course of nature. Even fifty years ago, many women could expect to bear at least ten children. There was a constant qi exchange between mothers and babies. Today we control birth and most women will not bear more than three babies in their lifetime. Qi is trapped in the breast area and generates cancer cells. We should understand one important thing. The body we have now has developed through millions of years of evolution. It is impossible for us to fit into the new lifestyle created only in the last few decades.

Similarly, lower back pain is caused by lack of exercise. Physical labor was the traditional way of maintaining strength and health, but now machines have replaced most of it, and naturally, the torso degenerates rapidly. Again, common knee problems are generated by lack of walking, which was required in daily activity until fifty years ago. Automobile transport has caused degeneration of our knees.

Human sperm production has decreased significantly over the last two decades, caused by our new lifestyle.[13] Traditionally, people went to bed shortly after sunset and woke up at dawn. Our bodies adapted to nature over millions of years. In our new lifestyle, we often do not go to bed before midnight. According to qigong theory, the qi in our bodies manifests as physical action during daytime. Qi nourishes our brain and sexual organs through the spinal cord at night. If we go to sleep by 9 P.M., it takes two to three hours of natural breathing during sleep to lead qi from the surface to nourish deep inside. By midnight it is ready to nourish the brain and sexual organs. Brain energy is recharged, and sperm and sexual hormones are produced. The modern lifestyle has introduced a new time schedule that precludes the natural production of hormones. If we continue in this manner, problems may become even more significantly serious.

Countless other problems have been generated by new products, which cause material and energetic pollution. Through lack of understanding of human energy and its vulnerability to this pollution, we live in a world at great risk of physical and mental imbalance. To solve these problems, we must first achieve awareness before we can awaken others. Profound and significant studies need to be conducted and acted upon.

1.6 Qigong and Longevity (氣功與長壽)

To many seculars, longevity means long life, without regard to health or the meaning of life. Most of the people today want to live long physically even though they are in pain mentally and physically. Longevity is important to them, not happiness. Others search for the meaning of life to make longevity more meaningful. They look for a way to extend physical life and at the same time keep mental peace in harmony with the physical body. For them, qigong for longevity was developed.

To religious Daoists, longevity is considered very important and crucial to reaching enlightenment. They believe it takes many lifetimes to reach enlightenment to be reunited with the Dao. They believe, as do the Buddhists, that the physical body is only born for the spirit to temporarily reside in, for further spiritual cultivation. The physical body has no further purpose or meaning. To Buddhists, the physical body is unimportant, and they often ignore its condition, emphasizing only the cultivation of the mind and the spirit. But Daoists believe that if you live longer in each lifetime, you will have more time for spiritual cultivation, and need not reincarnate as often before reaching enlightenment. So they take good care of the physical body. To some religious people, the meaning of longevity is to provide a longer time for spiritual cultivation.

Then, what are the keys or requirements to reach longevity? How do we reach this goal? These questions have been searched for many generations. Now let us summarize some key points of longevity from past human experiences.

1.6.1 Key points of longevity:
- There must be balance and harmony of the qi body (yin) with the physical body (yang). When there is balance and harmony of yin and yang, excess energy is minimized. Health is maintained and longevity reached through a healthy lifestyle, and by keeping yin and yang in balance through qigong training.
- Follow the way of the Dao, adjusting your body to fit in with natural cycles such as the time of day and the change of the seasons. Avoid artificial material or energetic pollution.
- Understand the physical body and qi body scientifically. Through this, you can find a way to slow down the aging process and the key to attaining spiritual enlightenment.

These concepts were also discussed in medical qigong society. One of the oldest medical classics, *Yellow Emperor's Inner Classic: Simple Questions* (黃帝內經・素問) said,

The ancient people who knew the Dao, modeled themselves after yin and yang, matched the ways of nature, controlled their eating and drinking, lived with regularity, did not labor without knowing their limit, and so were able keep the shape (body) and the shen (spirit) together. Therefore, they end their heaven years (the age granted by heaven) completely and pass hundred years, then gone.[14]

For a healthy body, concern yourself with the harmony of yin and yang and follow the natural way. Only then can you reach longevity.

Let us summarize how we reach these goals with qigong.

1.6.1.1 Physical body

1. Keep the bone marrow clean: The majority of blood cells are produced by the bone marrow. Once we reach thirty, the bone marrow starts to degenerate rapidly, causing the quantity and quality of blood production to decrease. Blood cells carry nutrients, oxygen, and the qi required to replace old cells with new ones. Without enough healthy blood cells, cell replacement stagnates and degeneration of the body sets in.
   Degeneration of bone marrow results from deficiency of qi. Without abundant qi, blood production from bone marrow is slow and deficient. Bone Marrow/Washing Qigong teaches how to lead qi to the bone marrow, as described in the book, *Qigong–The Secret of Youth* available from YMAA Publication Center.

2. Maintain health of the body, especially the torso: For health and longevity, we need physical and mental health. Without a strong healthy body, even though you have abundant energy, you still cannot manifest this energy into physical form.
   A healthy physical body depends heavily on the condition of your torso, especially the spine. Through the spinal cord, our brain controls the entire body. Any spinal problem disturbs the smooth control by your brain. Along the spine there are two qi vessels, one being the spinal cord (thrusting vessel, 衝脈) and the other outside the spine just under the skin (governing vessel, 督脈). They distribute qi to the central nervous system and out to the limbs. If your spine is healthy, qi circulation will not be stagnant. Most blood cells are produced in the spinal marrow and the pelvis. When qi circulates abundantly, degeneration of bone marrow is slowed and production of healthy blood cells is maintained.

3. Provide the best quality food and air for cell replacement: Approximately one trillion cells in our bodies die each day. To replace them, we must provide good quality food and air, or else the new cells will be unhealthy causing us to age faster. Deep breathing is one of the main keys to keeping cells healthy.

4. Boost hormone production in the body: Hormones (original essence) act as catalysts to expedite a smooth metabolism. When hormone production slows down, cell replacement does too, and our bodies degenerate faster.

1.6.1.2 Qi and the Mind

1. Accumulate qi at the real lower dan tian, which produces elixir qi and also stores it. From this energy center, qi is distributed throughout the body. The lower dan tian has a similar structure to the brain, with the capacity for memory.[15,16] The lower dan tian and the upper dan tian (brain/mind) are connected through the spinal cord and the central nervous system, where electric conductivity is highest and resistance is lowest. Though there are two brains, their function can be considered as one. The lower brain can store bioelectricity. When the mind generates a thought (EMF, electromotive

force), qi is led to the body for action. When the qi stored at the real lower dan tian is abundant, the life force is strong; otherwise we are weak and die young.

2. Accumulate qi in the eight vessels. The qi accumulated in the lower dan tian is distributed to the eight vessels, or qi reservoirs, which, in turn, regulate the qi's circulation in the twelve primary qi channels, or qi rivers. Small circulation meditation is one of the most important methods used to increase qi and smoothly circulate it.

3. Circulate qi smoothly in the twelve primary qi channels. Only when qi is distributed everywhere smoothly can the cells in the body obtain proper qi nourishment and our life force be strong. To reach this goal, balance exercise (yang) with relaxation (yin).

4. Maintain an emotionally neutral state. In Chinese scholar qigong, regulating the emotional mind is most important. Aging is caused by imbalance of qi distributed in the body, caused, in part, by emotional disturbance. Set yourself free from emotional bondage to live peacefully and harmoniously.

5. Raise up the spirit of vitality. When your spirit is high, your life force is strong. To raise the spirit of vitality, having stored abundant qi at the real lower dan tian, lead it up to the brain to nourish the spirit. This raises the spirit and leads to enlightenment.

6. Understand the meaning of life. Analyze your life and try to understand its meaning. Without understanding, you are rudderless and confused, leading to depression and low spirits. When you have a goal in life, your thinking and activities are meaningful.

1.6.1.3 Mental Body

1. Humbly learn from ancient experiences, which offer guidelines for the future. They have shown what is possible and where the problems may be. If our scientific dignity ignores this accumulated experience, we may repeat their mistakes. One who is wise remembers both past successes and failures.

2. Make life meaningful. Many people have no meaning in their lives, making them depressed and unhealthy. To direct them, we must establish non-religious spiritual centers where they can meditate and recognize the spiritual role of their existence. Through meditation, the mind can be clear and peaceful, providing an environment for self-recognition. This is the first step to self-understanding and the path of spiritual enlightenment.

3. Raise up the spirit of vitality. When we recognize ourselves, we will see how to fit into this society and raise the spirit of vitality. Using scientific methods to activate more brain cells and open the third eye, we may be able to shorten the path to enlightenment. Our spirit of vitality will be high, the most important invisible factor in longevity.

1.6.2 Longevity and Spiritual Cultivation

According to Buddhism, you may need hundreds or even thousands of lifetimes to cultivate the spirit and see the true nature of reality in order to reach enlightenment. In each life, you might improve only a little. Before you are twenty years old, you start to feel your spiritual identity, the first step to spiritual recognition. Throughout life, you collect information and experiences, filter them, and finally understand their meaning. The spirit learns new ideas. If you die in your twenties, you have only a few years for cultivation. The best time for spiritual cultivation is from the age of thirty, when you have a few advantages for spiritual cultivation:

1. Understanding the world better. By age thirty, you have been educated and have experienced the world. You may adjust to their circumstances and become serious about spiritual life.

2. Better financial situation. With financial security, the mind is calmer and not trapped in the circle of daily survival, so it can focus more on the spiritual than the material side.

3. Better mental preparation. By thirty, you are more mature both mentally and spiritually, making yourself more ready for spiritual cultivation.

4. A more logical mind. By age thirty, your knowledge and judgment have developed logical thinking, which is crucial for correct spiritual development. Spiritual cultivation, guided by imagination, can lead you away from the true nature of reality, and into deeper bondage of emotional confusion. The longer you live, the more time for cultivation and development of your spiritual understanding to a higher level. If you die young, you have only a short time for cultivation, and progress will be limited in this lifetime.

Notes

1. 《莊子刻意》：〝吹呴呼吸，吐故納新，熊經鳥伸，為壽而已矣。此導引之士，養形之人，彭祖壽考者之所好也。〞

2. 李時珍《奇經八脈考》：〝蓋正經猶夫溝渠，奇經猶夫湖澤，正經之脈隆盛，則溢于奇經。〞

3. *Qigong for Health and Martial Arts*, Dr. Yang, Jwing-Ming, YMAA Publication Center, Boston, 1985.

4. 人生七十古來稀。

5. 一百二十謂之夭。

6. *Qigong—The Secret of Youth*, Dr. Yang, Jwing-Ming, YMAA Publication Center, Boston, 1989.

7. 外家由外而內，從硬到軟。

8. *Tai Chi Theory and Martial Power*, Dr. Yang, Jwing-Ming, YMAA Publication Center, Boston, 1986.

9. *Taijiquan Theory of Dr. Yang, Jwing-Ming*, Dr. Yang, Jwing-Ming, YMAA Publication Center, Boston, 2003.

10. 內家由內而外，從軟到硬。

11. *Arthritis Relief 3rd edition,* Dr. Yang, Jwing-Ming, YMAA Publication Center, Boston, 2005.

12. 《達摩大師住世留形內真妙用訣》：〝若不知子母相守，氣雖呼吸於于內，神常勞役于外，遂使神常穢濁而神不清，神既不清，即元和之氣漸散，而不能相守也。〞

13. "Silent Sperm," Lawrence Wright, *The New Yorker*, January 15, 1996, p. 42.

14. 《黃帝內經素問·上古天真論》：〝上古之人，知其道者，法于陰陽，和于術數，食飲有節，起居有常，不妄作勞，故能形與神俱，而盡終其天年度百歲乃去。〞

15. "Complex and Hidden Brain in the Gut Makes Cramps, Butterflies and Valium," Sandra Blakeslee, Science, *New York Times,* January 23, 1996.

16. *The Second Brain: The Scientific Basis of Gut Instinct and a Groundbreaking New Understanding of Nervous Disorders of the Stomach and Intestine*, Michael D. Gershon, New York, Harper Collins Publications, 1998.

CHAPTER 2

Qigong Training Theory and Procedures
(氣功練習之理論與過程)

2.1 Introduction (介紹)

Whether you practice internal elixir (*nei dan*, 內丹) or external elixir (*wai dan*, 外丹) qigong, there are five regulating processes to reach the final goal of practice. These are regulating the body (*tiao shen*, 調身), regulating the breathing (*tiao xi*, 調息), regulating the emotional mind (*tiao xin*, 調心), regulating qi (*tiao qi*, 調氣), and regulating the spirit (*tiao shen*, 調神). These five are commonly called five regulatings (wu tiao, 五調).

The Chinese word tiao (調), which is translated as "regulating," consists of two words, namely, yan (言), which means speaking or negotiating, and zhou (周), which means to be complete, perfect, or round. Tiao means to adjust or to fine tune until it is complete and harmonious with others. It is like tuning the notes of a piano to be in harmony with one another. Tiao means to coordinate, cooperate, and harmonize by ongoing adjustment. All five aspects, body, breathing, mind, qi, and spirit, need to be regulated until harmony is achieved.

The key to regulating is through feeling, which is the language of the mind and body. The deeper and more sensitively you feel, the more profoundly you can regulate, and vice versa. It requires significant effort to reach the finest stage of feeling and regulating. This training of inner feeling is called gongfu of self-internal observation (*nei shi gongfu*, 內視功夫), internal feeling or awareness. The more refined your gongfu, the deeper you harmonize with others.

At the beginning, your mind is focused on regulating and on making it happen, so it is not natural or smooth. Later it becomes regulating without regulating. "The real regulating is without regulating."[1] It is like learning to drive, with your mind on the road and the controls of the car. This is the stage of regulating. Once you are experienced, your mind does not have to regulate. You drive without driving, and everything happens naturally and smoothly. With the five qigong regulatings, you practice until regulating is unnecessary. Then your feeling is profound, and regulating is achieved naturally and automatically.

Next, we will discuss these five regulatings and the importance of mutually coordinating them, as they pertain to all qigong practice.

2.2 Five Regulatings (五調)

2.2.1 Regulating the Body (Tiao Shen, 調身)

A tense posture affects qi circulation and disturbs the mind. "When shape (posture) is incorrect, qi will not be smooth. When qi is not smooth, the yi (wisdom mind) is not at peace. When yi is not at peace, then qi is disordered."[2]

The purposes of regulating the body are to:

1. Find the most natural and comfortable posture for practice. This allows the qi and breathing to flow smoothly, so the mind relaxes and focuses on raising the spirit.

2. Provide the best conditions for self-internal feeling. When your body is well regulated, your feeling can reach a profound level. When mind and body communicate, your judgment will be accurate, and your mind circulates qi effectively.

3. Coordinate body and mind, using yi (意), wisdom mind, and correct feeling.

2.2.1.1 Relaxation in Regulating the Body

Relaxation is a major key to success in qigong practice. It opens your qi channels, and allows qi to circulate smoothly and easily.

Each stage has two aspects, mental and physical. Mental relaxation precedes physical relaxation. There are two minds, the emotional (xin, 心) and the wisdom mind (yi, 意). The xin affects your feelings and the condition of your body. The yi leads you to a calm and peaceful state, which allows you to exercise sound judgment. Your wisdom mind must first relax, so it can control the emotional mind and let it relax too. When the peaceful wisdom mind and emotional mind coordinate with your breathing, the physical body also relaxes.

2.2.1.2 Yin and Yang in Regulating the Body

To regulate the body into a desired state, apply the concept of yin and yang in your practice, adjusting them using kan (坎, water) and li (離, fire). When your mind is calm and your breathing is long and smooth, your body more deeply relaxes and qi can circulate smoothly. The deep, calm mind and long breath are kan (water), making your physical body more yin and your qi body more yang. The physical body is cooler, while the qi body is more assertive.

By contrast, when you are excited, with short and heavy breathing, your physical body will also be tense, hot, and energized. Qi stagnates so it can manifest into physical form. The excited mind and heavy breathing is li (fire), making your physical body yang, and the qi body more yin. The physical body is excited and the qi circulation is slow and stagnant. Depending on your purpose, you regulate your body accordingly. To make your body more yang and build up external strength, use li. To internalize and make your qi body more yang, use kan to make it happen.

2.2.1.3 Regulating the Body and the Spirit

When you practice, relax your body as much as possible so your mind can be calm, the qi can circulate smoothly, and your feeling can be centered and balanced. Harmonize your mind and body, and build up a firm root. Then the spirit can be raised. Relaxing the body is the first step in raising the spirit.

2.2.2 Regulating the Breathing (Tiao Xi, 調息)

Once regulating your body reaches the stage of regulating without regulating, focus on the breathing. The body can be regarded as a battlefield, with qi as soldiers, the mind as the general, and the spirit as fighting morale. Breathing is regarded as the strategy. When breathing methods are correct, qi is led effectively. Since ancient times, qigong breathing methods have been studied and practiced, and kept top-secret, only being passed down orally in each style. Embryonic Breathing (Tai Xi, 胎息) is the crucial key to storing qi at the real lower dan tian (zhen xia dan tian, 真下丹田) and for cultivating spiritual enlightenment. Embryonic Breathing is very important in internal elixir qigong (nei dan qigong, 內丹氣功). It is discussed more extensively in the book, Qigong Meditation—Embryonic Breathing, published by YMAA Publication Center.[3]

2.2.2.1 Purposes of Regulating the Breathing

1. To convert nutrition, or food essence, into qi efficiently: The source of post-birth qi is mainly from food. According to the biochemical formula, the more oxygen we inhale, the more efficient the biochemical reaction and the more energy generated. The body converts this energy into heat, light, and bioelectricity (qi).

$$\text{glucose} + 6O_2 \longrightarrow 6CO_2 + 6H_2O$$
$$\Delta G^{\circ'} = -686 \text{ kcal}$$

2. To improve metabolism, which is the efficiency of cell replacement: Approximately one trillion cells die every day in a healthy person.[4] As mentioned before, to slow the aging process, they must be replaced each day, for which oxygen is one of the elements required. Without it, the new cells will be deformed and unhealthy. Dead cells (carbon) must also be disposed of. The respiratory system supplies the oxygen and removes the dead cells. Inhaling and exhaling deeply allows cell replacement to proceed smoothly.

3. To serve the strategic purpose of regulating yin and yang: Breathing is a kan and li method with which you may adjust the body's yin and yang. Inhalation makes the body more yin, while exhalation makes it more yang.

4. To coordinate and harmonize the body, mind, qi, and spirit: Breathing, as one of the five important regulatings, plays the important role of coordinating and harmonizing the others. Concentrating in a deep, profound inhalation can calm you and condense your spirit. Focusing on exhalation can raise the body's energy, excite the mind, and raise the spirit. Correct breathing assists in leading qi more efficiently.

2.2.2.2 Breathing and Qigong

There are eight qi vessels (*mai*, 脈), which function like reservoirs, and twelve primary qi channels (*jing*, 經), which function like rivers in your body. In addition, there are millions of tiny channels called luo (絡) branching out from the twelve channels to the surface of the skin, to generate a shield of guardian qi (*wei qi*, 衛氣). This qi is responsible for hair growth and for defending against negative outside influences. These tiny channels also enter the bone marrow (*sui qi*, 髓氣) to keep it healthy and producing blood cells. They also establish pathways for qi exchange and communication between internal organs.

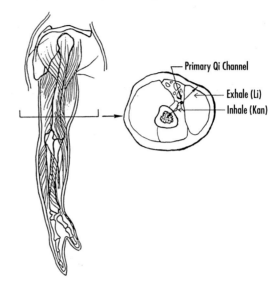

Figure 2-1. The expansion and condensing of qi during breathing

Qi circulates naturally and automatically without qigong training. Qigong practice coordinates the mind and breathing to generate electromotive force, to control the qi circulation more efficiently. As you exhale, you expand the qi and lead it from the primary channels to the skin, and the body becomes more yang. When you inhale, you draw in qi and lead it from the primary channels to the bone marrow, and the body becomes more yin (Figure 2-1). When inhalation and exhalation are balanced, yin and yang are balanced.

As you get older, your breath becomes shorter, and less qi is led to the skin and bone marrow. Qi stagnates there, and the skin starts to wrinkle, while the hair turns gray or

Table 2-1. General Rules of Breathing to Regulate Kan-Li and Yin-Yang

Kan-Li	Methods	Consequence
Kan	Inhalation	Yin*
Li	Exhalation	Yang*
Kan	Inhale then hold the breath	Yin
Li	Exhale then hold the breath	Yang
Kan	Soft, slow, calm and long breath	Yin
Li	Heavy, fast and short breath	Yang
Kan	Normal Abdominal Breathing (Buddhist Breathing)	Yin
Li	Reverse Abdominal Breathing (Daoist Breathing)	Yang

*Yin and yang are relative, not absolute. After defining a reference standard or level, compare them with each other.

Yin*: Cold, calm, body relaxed, and qi body energized

Yang*: Hot, excited, physical body tense, and energized

falls out. Fewer blood cells are produced, and they are not as healthy as before. Because they carry less nutrition and oxygen through the body, you get sick more often and age faster. The first key to maintaining youth is regulating your breathing to control kan and li, and thus the yin and yang of your body.

2.2.2.3 Breathing Methods

Normal Breathing (*Pin Chang Hu Xi,* 平常呼吸). Normal breathing is also called chest breathing (*xiong bu hu xi,* 胸部呼吸), in which the breath is controlled by emotion. Regulate it by relaxing the lungs. Concentrate until the practice is neutral, calm, and peaceful. The breathing can be long and deep while the body relaxes, and the heartbeat slows down. You may practice in any comfortable position, ten minutes each morning and evening until one day, you notice that your mind does not have to pay attention to the chest. Then concentrate on feeling the result of the training. When you exhale, you feel the pores of the skin open, and when you inhale, the pores close. It seems that all the pores are breathing with you. This is a low level of skin or body breathing. The feeling is very comfortable. When you can do this comfortably and automatically, you have regulated your chest breathing.

You should practice until you reach a level of regulating without regulating (*wu tiao er tiao,* 無調而調), which is known as "the real regulating." Then you will be practicing all the time because you have built up a natural habit for your breathing. The most powerful qigong practice is one that you have integrated into your lifestyle, including your breathing behavior.

Normal Abdominal Breathing (*Zheng Fu Hu Xi,* 正腹呼吸). Normal abdominal breathing is called Buddhist breathing (*fo jia hu xi,* 佛家呼吸). Control your abdominal muscles and coordinate them with the breathing. When you inhale, the abdomen expands, and when you exhale, it withdraws. Practice until the process becomes smooth, with the body relaxed. Concentrate on your abdomen initially to control the abdominal muscles. Afterward, the process becomes natural and smooth, and you are ready to build up qi at the false lower dan tian (*jia xia dan tian,* 假下丹田 and *qihai,* Co-6, 氣海).

The next step is to coordinate your breathing with the movements of your huiyin (Co-1, 會陰, perineum). When you inhale, gently push the huiyin down, and when you exhale, hold it up (Figure 2-2). Hold up the huiyin gently, without tensing; it

Table 2-2. Normal Abdominal Breathing

Body Neutral (Inhalation and exhalation are of equal length.)

    Yin —Inhalation (Abdomen expands, huiyin pushed out gently)

    Yang—Exhalation (Abdomen withdraws, huiyin held up gently)

Body Yin

    —Inhalation longer (Abdomen expands, huiyin pushed out gently)

    —Exhalation (Abdomen withdraws, huiyin relaxed)

Body Yang

    —Inhalation (Abdomen expands, huiyin pushed out gently)

    —Exhalation longer (Abdomen withdraws, huiyin held up strongly)

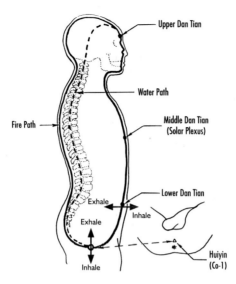

Figure 2-2. Normal Abdominal Breathing

should remain relaxed. Tensing impedes qi circulation and causes tension in the ab-domen, which can generate other problems. Initially, use your mind to control the muscles of the abdomen and perineum. Later, your mind does not need to be there to make it happen, and you regulate without regulating. You feel a wonderful, comfort-able feeling at the huiyin, and the qi is led more strongly to the skin than when you did "chest breathing." It will feel as though your whole body is breathing with you.

Reverse Abdominal Breathing (*Fan Fu Hu Xi, Ni Fu Hu Xi,* 反腹呼吸 · 逆腹呼吸). Reverse abdominal breathing is called Daoist breathing (*Dao jia hu xi,* 道家呼吸). Start this training after you have mastered Buddhist breathing. It is called reverse abdominal breathing because the movement of the abdomen is the reverse of Buddhist breathing. The abdomen withdraws when you inhale and expands when you exhale (Figure 2-3). Buddhist breathing is more relaxed, in contrast with Daoist breathing, which is more aggressive. Daoist breathing makes the body more yang, while Buddhist breathing makes it more yin.

Many people wrongly believe that reverse breathing is against the Dao, or nature's path. This is not true. It is simply used for different purposes. If you observe your breathing patterns, you notice you use reverse breathing in two types of situations.

First, when emotionally disturbed, you often use reverse breathing. When you laugh, you make the sound "ha" (哈), using reverse breathing. Your abdomen expands, exhalation is longer than inhalation, guardian qi (*wei qi,* 衛氣) expands, and you get hot. This is the natural way of releasing excess energy from excitement or happiness. When you cry, you make the sound "hen" (哼) while inhaling, your abdomen with-draws, and inhalation is longer than exhalation. Guardian qi shrinks and you feel cold. This is the natural way of preventing energy loss from inside your body. When you are sad, your spirit and your body's energy are low.

The second occasion in which you use reverse breathing is to energize the body, such as when pushing or lifting something heavy. You inhale deeply to take in more oxygen,

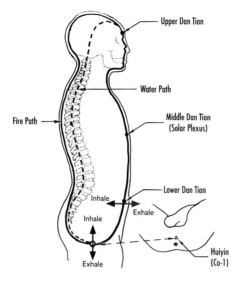

Figure 2-3. Reverse Abdominal Breathing

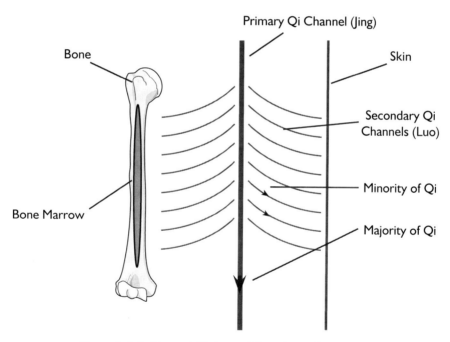

Figure 2-4. In Normal Abdominal Breathing, the majority
of the qi circulates in the primary qi channels

and then exhale while pushing the object, which is reverse breathing. When you are disturbed emotionally or have aggressive or strong intentions, you use reverse breathing naturally.

With practice, you can lead the qi to the skin more efficiently than with Buddhist breathing. You can also lead it to the bone marrow to enhance the marrow qi (*sui qi*,

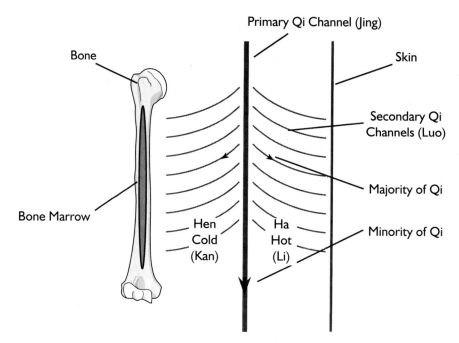

Figure 2-5. In Reverse Abdominal Breathing, the majority of the qi is lead to the skin surface and bone marrow

髓氣). Compare normal abdominal breathing with reverse abdominal breathing to see how qi is led in these two different breathing strategies.

In normal abdominal breathing, qi circulates mainly in the primary qi channels (*jing*, 經), connecting the internal organs to the extremities. Some also spread out through the secondary qi channels (*luo*, 絡), to reach the skin and bone marrow (Figure 2-4). Because most qi remains in the primary qi channels, the body is not energized and stays relaxed, enabling a state of deep relaxation. Normal abdominal breathing (*kan*, 坎) makes the body yin, while reverse abdominal breathing (*li*, 離) makes it yang.

In reverse abdominal breathing, most qi is led sideways through the luo to the skin and bone marrow, while much less circulates in the primary qi channels (Figure 2-5). Skin breathing (*ti xi, fu xi*, 體息・膚息) and marrow breathing (*sui xi*, 髓息) can be achieved more aggressively through reverse abdominal breathing.

In reverse abdominal breathing, when you inhale, you withdraw your abdomen and hold up your huiyin, while moving the diaphragm downward. Tension generated at the stomach area may cause pain, like when you laugh loudly or cry. So before practicing it, first practice normal abdominal breathing for a while, to relax and control the abdominal muscles. Use small movements at the beginning before increasing the scale of abdominal movement.

Embryonic Breathing (*Tai Xi*, 胎息). Embryonic Breathing has always been an important component in internal elixir qigong practice. It is the breathing method that allows you to store qi in the real lower dan tian (*zhen xia dan tian*, 真下丹田)

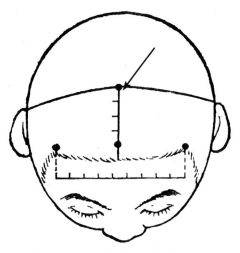

Figure 2-6. The baihui (Gv-20) cavity

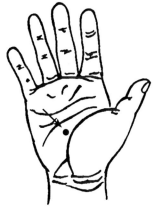

Figure 2-7. The laogong (P-8) cavity

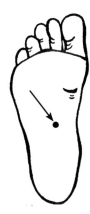

Figure 2-8. The yongquan (K-1) cavity

Table 2-3. Reverse Abdominal Breathing

(Emotionally unsettled, the mind has intention of yin or yang)

Body Neutral*

    Yin —Inhalation (abdomen withdraws, huiyin held up gently)

    Yang —Exhalation (abdomen expands, huiyin pushed out gently)

       *Inhalation and exhalation are of equal length.

Body Yin

       —Inhalation longer* (abdomen withdraws, huiyin held up firmly)

       —Exhalation (abdomen expands, huiyin relaxed)

      *Hen sound can enhance the body's yin.

Body Yang

      - Inhalation (abdomen withdraws, huiyin held up gently)

      - Exhalation longer* (abdomen expands, huiyin pushed out firmly)

      *Ha sound can enhance the body's yang.

and charge your bio-battery to a high level. Your vital energy is raised, the immune system strengthened, and the body reconditioned. More importantly, once abundant qi is stored, you can lead it upward through the spinal cord (*chong mai*, 衝脈) to nourish the brain and raise the spirit. This is the crucial key of spiritual enlightenment. Embryonic breathing is also crucial in skin breathing and marrow breathing, which is closely related to our immune system and longevity. Again, if you are interested in this subject, please refer to the book, *Qigong Meditation–Embryonic Breathing,* available from YMAA Publication Center.

Skin–Marrow Breathing (*Fu Sui Xi,* 膚髓息). Skin breathing (*fu xi,* 膚息) is sometimes called body breathing (*ti xi,* 體息). Actually, body breathing involves breathing with the whole body, not just the skin. When you exhale, you lead qi to the muscles and skin, and when you inhale, you lead qi to the marrow and internal organs. You feel your whole body transparent to qi, as though it had disappeared. Skin-marrow breathing is closely related to Embryonic Breathing. When qi is led to the real lower dan tian, you are also leading it to the bone marrow, and when it is led to the girdle vessel (*dai mai,* 帶脈), you are also leading it to the skin.

Five Gates Breathing (*Wu Xin Hu Xi,* 五心呼吸). The five gates are the head (upper dan tian and baihui, Gv-20, 百會), the two laogong (P-8, 勞宮) cavities on the palms, and the two yongquan (K-1, 湧泉) cavities on the soles of the feet (Figures 2-6, 2-7, and 2-8). Beginners should use the baihui gate located at the top of the head. Using this gate will make it easier to communicate with natural qi. Later, use the third eye (*tian yan,* 天眼).

Having built up qi at the real lower dan tian, you harmonize your breathing and lead the qi to the yongquan cavities. For yongquan breathing (*yongquan hu xi,* 湧泉呼吸), you may adopt any posture, even lying down and using normal abdominal breathing. Inhale, leading qi from yongquan to the real lower dan tian, and exhale, leading it back to yongquan (Figure 2-9). When you inhale, the abdomen and huiyin (Co-1, 會陰) expand, and when you exhale, they withdraw. Even though the mind is involved, it does not aggressively lead the qi, and relaxation is paramount.

To lead qi to the yongquan aggressively, reverse abdominal breathing is more effective, and the best posture is standing. Inhale, leading qi from the yongquan cavities to the real lower dan tian, and when you exhale, your mind leads the qi back to the yongquan, while you slightly squat down and imagine pushing your feet down into the ground (Figure 2-10). When you inhale, withdraw the abdomen and hold up the huiyin, and when you exhale, they expand.

Yongquan Cavity Breathing is also called sole breathing (*zhong xi,* 踵息) described by the well-known Daoist scholar, Zhuang Zi (莊子), during the Chinese Warring States Period (戰國) (403–222 B.C.). He said, "The breathing of the ancient truthful persons (*zhen ren,* 真人) (Daoists) was deep and profound. They used the soles to breathe, while seculars used the throat."[5] These documents verify that yongquan breathing was practiced more than two thousand years ago. For medical qigong, yongquan breathing is one of the most effective methods to regulate abnormal qi in three of the yin organs, namely, liver, kidneys, and spleen.

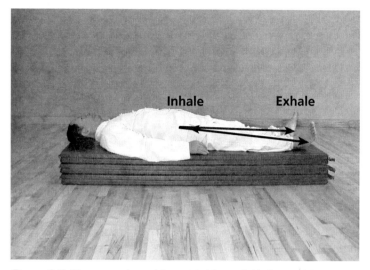

Figure 2-9. Yongquan breathing with Normal Abdominal Breathing

With yongquan breathing well established and having reached the real regulating of no regulating, combine it with the laogong breathing at the center of your palms. These two gates regulate the heart and lungs. Use normal abdominal breathing or reverse abdominal breathing. Inhale, leading qi from the four gates to the real lower dan tian, and exhale, leading it back again (Figure 2-11).

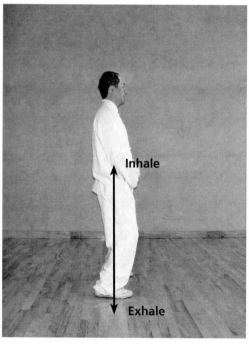

Figure 2-10. Yongquan breathing with Reverse
Abdominal Breathing

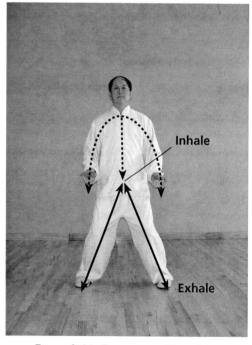

Figure 2-11. Four gates qi breathing

Four Gates Breathing is a common method of grand qi circulation (*da zhou tian*, 大周天). Once you reach a profound level, add the fifth gate, which elevates the practice into spiritual breathing (*shen xi*, 神息).

Spiritual Breathing (*Shen Xi*, 神息). Spiritual breathing is also called Fifth Gate Breathing (*Di Wu Xin Hu Xi*, 第五心呼吸), baihui breathing (*baihui hu xi*, 百會呼吸), or upper dan tian breathing (*shang dan tian hu xi*, 上丹田呼吸). It means to breathe through the third eye and is crucial in opening the third eye for enlightenment.

Reaching the level of spiritual breathing pre-supposes regulating your body, breathing, mind, and qi, and now the spirit. Your qigong practice and the search for spiritual enlightenment have reached the final stage and are approaching maturity. According to *The Complete Book of Principal Contents of Life and Human Nature* (性命圭旨全書), "What is spiritual breathing? It means the maturity of cultivation."[6] That means cultivating the interaction of kan and li has reached the stage of regulating without regulating, and all the cultivations have become natural. We will discuss this subject further in the forthcoming books on the subjects of qigong meditation and spiritual enlightenment.

There are some other breathing methods trained in Daoist qigong, such as Turtle Breathing (*Gui Xi*, 龜息) and Hibernation Breathing (*Dong Mian Xi*, 冬眠息). Because they are not related to taiji ball training and we do not have a profound understanding of the practices, they are not discussed here.

2.2.2.4 Final goals of regulating the breathing

The Complete Book of Principal Contents of Life and Human Nature (性命圭旨全書) says, "Regulate the breathing, you must regulate until the real regulating ceases. Train the spirit, you must train until the spirit of being without spirit."[7] Practice Embryonic Breathing until you achieve regulating without regulating. It is the same in cultivating your spirit. First, aim for spiritual neutrality and enlightenment. Afterward, no further enlightenment is necessary.

The Correct Theory of Becoming a Heavenly Fairy, A Frank Discussion of Taming the Breathing (天仙正理·伏氣直論) states, "When ancient people talked about the way of regulating the breathing, it is to follow the rules of nature's to and fro (circulation) without stubbornly keeping the shape of to and fro. This means to match the breathing as if there were no breathing."[8] The goal of regulating the breath is to follow nature without stagnation and practicing until regulating becomes unnecessary.

2.2.3 Regulating the Mind (Tiao Xin, 調心)

Regulate the emotional mind (*xin*, 心) until it is under control. This is the most difficult subject to train in qigong. It sets your mind to deal with itself, and since everyone has his own way of thinking, it is also the most difficult subject to explain.

The methods of regulating the mind have been widely studied, discussed, and practiced in all Chinese qigong societies, which include scholar, medical, religious, and martial arts groups. First, we will define the mind and then the purposes of regulating it. We then will discuss the Buddhist and Daoist point of view, and finally we will analyze methods of practice.

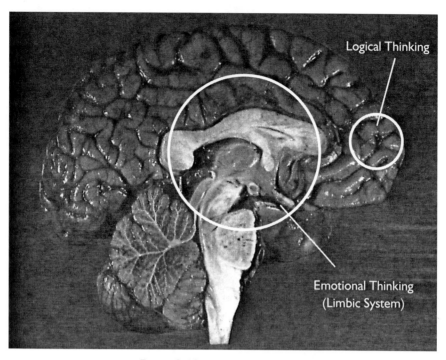

Figure 2-12. Brain and emotions

2.2.3.1 Two Minds, Xin and Yi (心・意)

Chinese society describes two minds. Xin, the emotional mind (心, heart), is yang, making you confused, scattered, depressed, or excited. Yi, the other mind (意, intention), relates to rational and logical thought. It is yin, making you calm, concentrated, and able to feel and ponder deeply. The word yi (意) consists of three words. li (立) on top means to establish, yue (曰) in the middle means to speak, and xin (心) at the bottom means the heart. So yi means to establish communication while the emotional mind is under control.

Xin and yi are directed by different parts of the brain.[9,10] Magnetic resonance imaging (MRI) has determined that the prefrontal cortex of the brain controls logic and judgment, while the limbic system near the center of the brain governs emotional thinking (Figure 2-12). According to the Director of the Center for Brain Research and Informational Sciences at Radford University in Virginia, the prefrontal cortex controls executive functions and is the seat of civilization.

By the age of twenty, the limbic system is fully functional, while the prefrontal cortex is still being formed. In adults, emotional responses are modulated by the prefrontal cortex, the part of the brain just behind the forehead that acts as a mental traffic cop, keeping tabs on many other parts of the brain, including the limbic system. The yi generated by the prefrontal cortex determines wise, clear thought and judgment, and calm, logical behavior, while the xin from the limbic system leads to confusion and emotional behavior. The key to making the prefrontal cortex mature earlier and faster than normal, is to use it as early as possible. Learning mathematics, physics, philosophy, or listening to classical music, leads qi to the front of the brain for faster development. Meditation to open the third eye, which focuses the mind at the front of the brain, also stimulates development of the prefrontal cortex.

We use yi to control, coordinate, and harmonize the xin. In scientific terms, we develop the prefrontal cortex to a powerful level, to control and direct the thinking generated by the limbic system of the brain.

2.2.3.2 Purposes of Regulating the Mind (調心之目的)

The purposes of regulating the mind vary from one school to another. Qigong practitioners in scholar and medical societies aim for a calm, peaceful, and harmonious mind so emotions do not disturb qi circulation. Thoughts affect qi circulation in the organs. Happiness and excitement affect the heart, while anger affects the liver. The kidneys are affected by fear and the lungs by sadness. (Table 2-4) Regulating your emotional mind to harmony and peace benefits your health.

According to the ancient medical book, *Thousand Golden Prescriptions for Emergencies* (備急千金要方),

> *Contemplate too much, then the spirit is tired. Obsess too much, then aspirations are dispersed. Too much desire, then the will is confused. Involved too much in affairs, then the body is fatigued. Talk too much, then qi is deficient. Laugh too much, the internal organs can be injured. Worry too much, then the heart is fearful. Too much joy, then expectations stop. Too much happiness, then (one) makes mistakes and is disordered. Angry too often, then circulation in hundreds of vessels is unsteady. Too many favors, then bewitched and ignore regular affairs. Too much wickedness, then gaunt without happiness. Without getting rid of these twelve 'too much,' then the control of flourish and protection (spirit and health) are lost, and blood and qi circulation disordered. This is the root of losing the life.[11]*

Wrong sentiments are the root of sickness. In medical and scholar qigong, regulating the mind to be calm, neutral, and not disturbed by emotions is the main task of practice.

Daoist and Buddhist religious groups, having regulated the emotional mind to a peaceful state, also aim for Buddhahood and enlightenment. Having controlled the emotional mind and developed their wisdom mind to a profound stage, they search for the meaning of life and nature.

Martial arts qigong practitioners raise the spirit of vitality and build a highly concentrated mind to lead qi efficiently and to develop the sense of enemy, which is critical in battle. While your mind is calm and clear, your spirit is raised to a state of high alertness.

Whatever the goals of each school, the principles of training are the same.

To Harmonize Body and Mind. To achieve a calm meditative mind, first attend to the condition of your body. When it is tensed and energized, breathing is rapid and your mind excited. Body and mind must coordinate and harmonize with each other. This is called the balance of the body and the xin (*shen xin ping heng*, 身心平衡). *The Complete Book of Principal Contents of Life and Human Nature* (性命圭旨全書) said, "When the body is not moving, the xin is peaceful. When xin is not moving, the

	WOOD 木	FIRE 火	EARTH 土	METAL 金	WATER 水
Direction	East	South	Center	West	North
Season	Spring	Summer	Long Summer	Autumn	Winter
Climactic Condition	Wind	Summer Heat	Dampness	Dryness	Cold
Process	Birth	Growth	Transformation	Harvest	Storage
Color	Green	Red	Yellow	White	Black
Taste	Sour	Bitter	Sweet	Pungent	Salty
Smell	Goatish	Burning	Fragrant	Rank	Rotten
Yin Organ	Liver	Heart	Spleen	Lungs	Kidneys
Yang Organ	Gall Bladder	Small Intestine	Stomach	Large Intestine	Bladder
Opening	Eyes	Tongue	Mouth	Nose	Ears
Tissue	Sinews	Blood Vessels	Flesh	Skin/Hair	Bones
Emotion	Anger	Happiness	Pensiveness	Sadness	Fear
Human Sound	Shout	Laughter	Song	Weeping	Groan

Table 2-4. Emotion and Internal Organs

spirit abides by itself."[12] The first step in regulating the mind is to calm the body, so the mind can be calm. When the emotions are calm, the wisdom mind can function efficiently, and the spirit of vitality can be raised.

To Harmonize the Breathing and the Mind. Regulating the emotional mind (*xin*) is done by the wisdom mind (*yi*). Xin is compared to a monkey or ape, while yi is compared to a horse (*xin yuan yi ma*, 心猿意馬). A monkey is weak, unsteady, and disturbing, generating confusion and excitement. A horse, though powerful, can be calm, steady, and controlled.

Thousands of years of experience in meditation have shown that in order to 'tame the monkey mind' and lead it into a cage, you need a banana. This banana is the breathing. As you focus on your breathing, your emotional mind becomes restrained and calm. When your breathing becomes long, slender, soft, and calm, your mind becomes calm, and vice versa. Mind and breathing mutually affect each other, working harmoniously to reach a high level of meditation. This is called "xin and breathing mutually rely on each other" (*xin xi xiang yi*, 心息相依).

The Complete Book of Principal Contents of Life and Human Nature (性命圭旨全書) said, "To conform with the Daoist's deep profound breathing, xin and breathing rely on each other mutually. When breathing is regulated, xin can be calm."[13] To have a calm emotional mind, first regulate your breathing through Daoist Breathing methods.

Questions From A Buddhist Guest About Listening to the Heart (聽心齋客問) explains,

> *The xin has been relying on affairs and objects for a long time; separated from its residence, it cannot be independent. Therefore, use gongfu of regulating the breath to restrain xin. Xin and breathing can then mutually rely on each other. Regulating does not mean to use yi, but only a thought of one inhalation and one exhalation. Once Xin separates from its residence, it is without others and without self, and breathing cannot be regulated. Keep the breathing soft and continuous as though existing, yet not existing (regulating without regulating). After a long time, it will be become proficient naturally.[14]*

This paragraph explains that our emotional mind concerns itself with human affairs and objects around us and is influenced by them. Then it is confused and cannot be independent. The way to restrain it is to regulate the breathing, until the emotional mind and the breathing are mutually dependent on each other. You should not have an intention (yi), but simply pay attention to the breathing. After you have practiced for a period of time, you will be able to breathe softly, naturally, smoothly, and continuously. The xin will stay at its residence without disturbance.

Use the Mind to Build Up, Store, and Lead Qi Circulation. In religious and martial qigong, one of the main goals is using the mind to build up qi, store it, and lead its circulation. To build up and store qi in the real lower dan tian (*zhen xia dan tian*, 真下丹田), practice Embryonic Breathing (*Tai Xi*, 胎息), and keep your mind in this qi residence. If your mind is away from this center, qi is led away from it and consumed. "Keep the yi at the dan tian" (*yi shou dan tian*, 意守丹田).

After building up abundant qi, use your mind to lead it. "Use the yi to lead the qi" (*yi yi yin qi*, 以意引氣). In nei dan practice, first lead qi to circulate in the conception (*ren mai*, 任脈) and governing vessels (*du mai*, 督脈) to facilitate small circulation (*xiao zhou tian*, 小周天). Then lead the qi to the extremities, skin, bone marrow, and brain for grand circulation (*da zhou tian*, 大周天).

Raise the Spirit of Vitality for Enlightenment. Again, the final goal of Buddhist and Daoist qigong is enlightenment or Buddhahood. To this end, build up and store qi at the real lower dan tian; then lead it up through the thrusting vessel (*chong mai*, 衝脈), spinal cord, to the brain, to nourish the brain and raise the spirit. The goal is to open the third eye. Having lied and cheated to conceal our secrets behind a mask through thousands of years, we humans have closed our third eye. By doing so, we lost the power of telepathy and communion with the spirit of nature. To reopen this third eye, we must be truthful, not hiding anything, and then accumulate qi in the front of the brain.

To raise the spirit to enlightenment, regulate your xin to an extremely calm, clear, and steady state. *Dao Scriptures* (道藏) said, "Xin is the master of the whole body, the commander of a hundred spirits. When calm, wisdom is generated; when acting, confusion originates. Its steadiness and confusion are within the movement and the calmness."[15]

2.2.4 Regulating the Qi (Tiao Qi, 調氣)

The purposes of regulating qi are 1. Producing qi (*sheng qi*, 生氣), 2. Nourishing and protecting qi (*yang qi*, 養氣), 3. Storing qi (xu qi, 蓄氣), and 4. Transporting qi (*xing qi*, 行氣). Next, we will discuss the theory and key practices of these four.

2.2.4.1 Producing Qi (Sheng Qi, 生氣)

There are three ways to produce qi, namely, herbs, breathing, and massage.

Herbs. Qi originates primarily from the biochemical reaction of the food we eat and the oxygen we inhale, which releases energy. Different foods produce different quantity and quality of energy, so herbs have been thoroughly researched in Chinese medical science. Different herbs are used to regulate the body's energy status.

Qi from food and air is called post-heaven qi (*hou tian qi*, 後天氣) or fire qi (*huo qi*, 火氣), because food and air are not pure and clean. The qi generated from them can cause emotional disturbance and physical problems. This is the main cause of fire in our mental and physical bodies.

Abdominal Breathing. Through deep abdominal breathing, oxygen and carbon dioxide are exchanged efficiently, promoting the body's metabolism. The energy from the biochemical reaction is stronger. Deep abdominal breathing also helps convert abdominal fat into qi, increasing the quantity of qi in the body.

This kind of breathing is called pre-heaven breathing (*xian tian hu xi*, 先天呼吸) and the qi produced is called pre-heaven qi (*xian tian qi*, 先天氣), which is clean and pure, able to calm your mind, and make your physical body healthy.

Massaging the Abdomen. The *Muscle/Tendon Changing and Marrow/Brain Washing Classic* describes the correct way to massage the abdomen. Wrong techniques make the body, especially the intestines, too yang, triggering constipation. If qi is increased too rapidly, it can also go up and damage the heart. If you do not know the techniques, you should not attempt to increase qi in this way. Abdominal breathing is much safer than massage. To know more about Muscle/Tendon Changing and Marrow/Brain Washing Qigong, please refer to the book, *Qigong–The Secret of Youth*, published by YMAA Publication Center.

Other than these three methods, you may also strive to maintain your hormone level, original essence, (*yuan jing*, 元精). Hormones act as catalysts in regulating the body's metabolism and expediting biochemical reactions, so qi can be produced smoothly and abundantly.

2.2.4.2 *Protecting and Nourishing Qi (Yang Qi, 養氣)*

Protecting means to preserve and keep, and nourishing means to cultivate and promote. After generating qi, then maintain it and cultivate it to a stronger level. It is like raising a child. After you have generated life, you protect it and raise it so it can grow stronger.

Protect Original Essence. Protect qi by protecting your original essence (*yuan jing*, 元精). A man regulates his sexual activities, abuse of which weakens the kidneys. According to Chinese medicine, this is the primary cause of losing qi for men.

Also, regulate your lifestyle. If you are fatigued, mentally or physically, the consumption of qi increases, so regulate your mental and physical activities. Get enough sleep and rest, and have a regular daily schedule.

Regulate the Breathing. To keep the qi in the body, breathe deeply and softly without holding your breath. Breathing too fast increases the heartbeat, tensing the body and mind, and consuming qi.

But maintaining physical strength requires exercise, during which breathing and heartbeat speed up. The key is knowing when to stop and how much exercise is needed to maintain health. Yang exercise is necessary to maintain physical life, and yin rest is also required to preserve and restore life, through conservation of qi. Both of these are of equal importance.

When you exercise, breathe properly without holding your breath. You need a large quantity of oxygen to convert the glucose into the energy required. Holding the breath too much consumes qi.

Regulate the Xin. Mental fatigue, emotional disturbances in particular, consumes qi. To protect your qi, the most important key is regulating your emotional mind. In a neutral state, qi can stay at its residence without manifesting, so it is preserved and protected. There is a document that emphasizes regulating the mind to preserve qi, which I translate next and offer some commentary.

Steel with One Hundred Words (Lu, Yan)[16]
《百字碑》
（古今圖書集成・博物匯編神異論；呂岩作）

When cultivating qi, do not just talk about preserving it. When calming down the mind, it should be doing without doing. If you know the origins of movement (yang) and stillness (yin), there is nothing for you to ask anyone else. Face the real reality, you must deal with daily affairs, but you should not be infatuated by them. Then your temperament can be steady and self-controlled, and qi will naturally be preserved. Then the elixir can be conceived, and kan and li can interact under control within the kettle. Interaction of yin and yang initiates the repeated cycle, and this will bring a natural derivation of new life, enlightened like thunder. White clouds move upward, and sweet dew sprinkles xu mi (fullness of human virtue). I drink the wine of longevity by myself, how can others know how free and unfettered I am? I sit down to listen to songs by the instrument without strings. I comprehend clearly the pivotal function of natural creation. These sentences offer the ladder to ascend to Heaven (enlightenment).

養氣忘言守，降心為不為。動靜知宗祖，無事更尋誰？
真常須應物，應物要不迷。不迷性自住，性住氣自回。
氣回丹自結，壺中配坎離。陰陽生反復，普化一聲雷。
白雲朝頂上，甘露灑須彌。自飲長生酒，逍遙誰得知？
坐聽無弦曲，明通造化機。都來十二句，端的上天梯。

Cultivating qi is not just about maintaining it. Most important is to regulate your xin (emotional mind). This must be regulated until no more regulating is necessary and it becomes natural. Your mind becomes clear and your judgment neutral and accurate. Whether active or still, you know where the origins are. If you know clearly what is happening, why do you need to ask anyone else? To live in this human world, you deal with necessary affairs, but without being lured by money, glory, dignity, pride, jealousy, power, or other human desires and emotions. If your mind is separated from these temptations, it can be calm and steady. Qi returns to its origin (real lower dan tian), forming the elixir (spiritual embryo). You control life easily through adjusting kan and li. Through kan and li, the yin and yang of your spirit and body is regulated as you wish. Through cultivating yin and yang, when the time is ripe, you open your third eye for enlightenment like a clap of thunder. When this happens, you have no doubt about your life, which will be like pure white clouds floating in the sky and sweet dew upon xu mi (須彌). Xu mi is the Daoist term for the spiritual being in the fullness of human virtue. You live long and enjoy life to the fullest. You communicate with nature like listening to songs without sound, understanding its pivotal functions.

Gather and Exchange Qi with Nature and Partners. Energy from the sun, moon, earth, trees, and any other source of natural energy can nourish the body. By meditating facing the sun at dawn, one absorbs solar energy to enhance the body's qi. Practicing qigong facing the moon a couple of days before a full moon is also a good way of absorbing qi. Orienting a house by coordinating the sun's and the earth's magnetic fields is known as feng shui (風水), wind-water, which determines good energy for living. Using natural energy to nourish your qi is very important in qigong practice.

To harmonize and balance qi, and to nourish one another, many Daoists use partners to exchange qi through meditation or special qigong practices. This is known as dual cultivation (*shuang xiu,* 雙修), which is also described in *Qigong–The Secret of Youth,* and will be further explored in future publications.

2.2.4.3 Storing Qi (Xu Qi, 蓄氣)

After conserving, protecting, and cultivating qi, you must store it in the bio-battery at the real lower dan tian. You lead the qi there and keep it there.

To keep the qi there, you keep your mind there. When your mind strays, you are leading qi away and consuming it. Keeping the mind at this center is called yi shou dan tian (意守丹田), achieved through Embryonic Breathing (Tai Xi, 胎息). There is a document which explains the importance of Embryonic Breathing, which I translate here with commentary. For more on the subject, refer to Master Yang, Jwing Ming's book, *Qigong Meditation–Embryonic Breathing* available from YMAA Publication Center.

Classic of Embryonic Breathing [16,17,18]
《胎息經》

The embryo is conceived from the concealed qi. Qi is developed through (regulating) the breath of the embryo. When qi is present, the body may live. When shen abandons the body and the shape disperses, death follows. Knowing the spirit and qi makes long life possible. Firmly protect the insubstantial emptiness (spiritual embryo) to cultivate spirit and qi. When spirit moves, the qi moves. When spirit stops, the qi stops. For a long life, spirit and qi must coordinate harmoniously with each other. When xin is not infatuated by thoughts coming or going, then spirit and qi will not exit and enter, and will thus remain naturally. To practice intelligently is the true way.

胎從伏氣中結，氣從有胎中息。氣入身來為之生，神去離形為之死。
知神氣可以長生，固守虛無以養神氣。神行則氣行，神住則氣住。若
欲長生，神氣相住。心不動念，無來無去，不出不入，自然常住。勤
而行之，是真道路。

Nobody knows when or by whom this classic was written, but it has been passed down for generations and is considered one of the most important documents about Embryonic Breathing.

The holy embryo (*sheng tai,* 聖胎) or spiritual embryo (*shen tai,* 神胎) is conceived from qi stored at the real lower dan tian. To obtain this concealed qi, practice Embryonic Breathing. Once you have stored it abundantly, your life force becomes strong, bringing you good health and longevity. But to manifest this qi as physical life force, you need a strong spirit, to focus the circulation and manifestation of qi. Without this living spirit, you lose your health and die. To lead a long and healthy life, cultivate your spirit and qi. The first part of the classic explains how to regulate the relationship between physical life, qi, and shen.

Keep your mind firmly at the real lower dan tian, called xu wu (虛無), which means nothingness. Your mind remaining at the real lower dan tian, is the state of wuji (無極, no extremity), the state of no discrimination, or nothingness. Only here can you really be in a neutral state of mind. Clear out emotions and desires. This is described in *Dao De Jing* as, "Approach the nothingness to its extremity, and maintain calmness with sincerity.[19] The mind leads the qi. When actively thinking, you are leading qi away from its residence and consuming it. To store abundant qi, you must conserve, protect, and build it. These three important things are emphasized in internal elixir qigong (*nei dan qigong*, 內丹氣功).

To build up abundant qi, keep your mind at the real lower dan tian, and practice Embryonic Breathing. To manifest qi efficiently for daily life, you need a strong and highly controlled shen. Qi consumption is limited and efficiency high. The key to longevity is to coordinate and harmonize shen and qi. To keep shen pure and strong, calm the xin. Xin is like a monkey, while yi is like a horse (*xin yuan yi ma*, 心猿意馬). To keep the monkey steady, restrain it in 'its cage', the wuji state. This is crucial to success.

2.2.4.4 Transporting Qi (Xing Qi, 行氣)

Having preserved, protected, cultivated, and stored qi, you need to circulate it efficiently.

> *"Use your mind to lead the qi" (yi yi yin qi, 以意引氣). The key to this is "leading" (yin, 引). The mind should not be in the qi, but ahead of it. If your mind pays attention to the qi, it stagnates. If you want to move from where you are standing, your mind must be on the spot you wish to move to. If your mind stays at the place where you are standing, no movement can take place. "The yi should not be on the qi, if on the qi, then stagnant.[20]*

The methods of leading and what you wish to accomplish depend on how extensively and profoundly you grasp the theory, the principles of yin and yang, and the goal of your training. There are five common goals for a qigong practitioner, which vary according to the depth of the training.

Connection of the Yi and Qi. Before you can connect your yi with the qi, you must recognize the existence of the qi originating from the feeling of its existence. Qi is energy that cannot be seen but only felt. You train to establish a sensitive feeling for it. When this feeling focuses on the inner body, it is called gongfu of inner vision (*nei shi gongfu*, 內視功夫).

After this, you establish the connection between the yi and the qi. This feeling is like a piece of rope you hold connected to a cow's nose. Without this rope, you will not be able to lead the qi.

Once you have established this connection, then you must also know how much effort and force you need to lead the cow. Too strong or too weak, the cow will either resist or stay still. This coordination is called harmonization of the yi and qi (yi qi xiang he, 意氣相合).

Leading Qi To or Away From a Specific Spot of the Body. Once you can lead the qi, you lead it from one place to another in the body for different purposes. For healing, you may lead it to a deficient place for qi nourishment (bu, 補). You can also lead stagnant qi away from a specific place for releasing (xie, 洩). If your kidneys are deficient in winter time, you can lead qi to them for nourishment. If you have a joint injury, you can lead qi away to ease the pain and relax the joint to expedite the healing process.

Qigong practitioners also lead qi above the diaphragm to energize and excite the mind and body (yang), and lead it below the diaphragm to cool down (yin). One leads qi to the laogong (P-8, 勞宮) cavities and to the fingertips for healing. Martial artists can use qigong to lead qi to the yongquan (K-1, 湧泉) cavities to establish a firm root for combat.

There are many applications once you can efficiently lead the qi with your yi. The more you practice, the better the results will be. Success depends on your yi, how strong it is, and how much you focus in meditation.

Small Cyclic Heaven Circulation. For a healthy and resilient body, one builds up qi, and then circulates it in the conception and governing vessels (ren, du mai, 任·督脈). This is called small cyclic heaven circulation (xiao zhou tian, 小周天) or simply small circulation. When qi circulation is abundant in these two vessels, the qi in the twelve primary qi channels can be regulated smoothly, which maintains abundant qi supply to the whole body, making it strong and healthy. If you are interested in small cyclic heaven circulation, please refer to the book, *Qigong Meditation–Small Circulation*, published by YMAA Publication Center.[21]

Grand Cyclic Heaven Circulation. Once you have accomplished small cyclic heaven, you have a firm foundation for grand cyclic heaven (da zhou tian, 大周天) practice. This includes A. Twelve primary qi channels grand circulation, B. Martial arts grand circulation, C. Mutual qi exchange grand circulation, and D. Spiritual enlightenment grand circulation.

Since these are such large subjects, I introduce their theory and practice in separate books. Martial arts grand circulation is discussed in the book, *The Essence of Shaolin White Crane*, published by YMAA Publication Center.[22]

Spiritual Enlightenment. Even though spiritual enlightenment practice is part of grand cyclic heaven circulation, due to its profound theory and difficulty in practice, it is discussed separately. It is of more interest to Buddhists and Daoists aiming for Buddhahood or spiritual enlightenment.

In spiritual enlightenment grand cyclic heaven circulation, you practice Embryonic Breathing to store qi at the real lower dan tian, and condition the bio-battery there. Then lead qi up through the spinal cord (chong mai, 衝脈) to energize brain cells and activate their function. When the energy level of the brain reaches a certain level, the qi moves along the spiritual valley (shen gu, 神谷) to re-open the third eye for enlightenment. We will discuss this in more detail in a future book about qigong meditation and spiritual enlightenment.

Jade Pendant Inscription of Transporting Qi[17,18]
《行氣玉佩銘》

When transporting qi, if deep, then accumulate. If qi is accumulated, it can be extended. When extended, it can be sunk downward. If sunk downward, then steady. If steady, then firm. If firm, then able to germinate. Having germinated, it can grow. When growing, it retreats. When retreating, it returns to heaven. The foundation of heaven is the top (upper dan tian) and the foundation of earth is the bottom (real lower dan tian). Following these rules, one may live, otherwise one dies.

行氣，深則蓄，蓄則伸，伸則下，下則定，定則固，固則萌，萌則
長，長則退，退則天。天几春在上，地几春在下，順則生，逆則死。

When circulating qi in the body, deep breathing relaxes the body and calms the mind. Qi circulation can be deep and qi storage abundant. Only then can qi be strong enough to be distributed everywhere in the body. "Transport qi as though through a pearl with a nine-curved hole, even the tiniest place will be reached."[23] The body's metabolism becomes smooth, natural, and healthy. Abundant qi is led down and stored in the real lower dan tian to stabilize and strengthen the life.

Leading and storing qi in the real lower dan tian is the process of Embryonic Breathing (Tai Xi, 胎息). It returns mental and physical life to its origin, in the wuji state (無極). Then new life can germinate and grow. After fulfilling the purpose of qi manifestation, retreat and return to the origin, the real lower dan tian. This process is the way of the heavenly cycle (Dao, 道). Conserving and storing qi at the real lower dan tian, you manifest it efficiently in your life. Having completed the manifestation, you return the qi and conserve it again at the real lower dan tian. Manifesting qi to the maximum depends on how thoroughly you purify your spirit and raise it to govern the qi circulation. The head is the heaven (tian, 天) while the abdomen is the earth (di, 地) in qigong practice. The upper dan tian is the residence of the spirit while the lower dan tian is the residence of qi. Store qi at the real lower dan tian and keep your spirit high and focused at the upper dan tian to achieve longevity.

2.2.5 *Regulating the Spirit (Tiao Shen,* 調神*)*

Here we discuss two important qigong terms, spiritual valley (shen gu, 神谷) and valley spirit (*gu shen,* 谷神). These terms appear in many ancient documents. We then introduce the five keys of training to regulate the shen, followed by two main training keys. Finally we summarize the goals of shen training.

2.2.5.1 *Valley Spirit and Spirit Valley*

In Chapter 6 of the *Dao De Jing* (道德經・六章), it is said, "The valley spirit (*gu shen*) does not die, so it is called *xuan pin*. The key to reaching this xuan pin is the root of heaven and earth. It is very soft and continuous as if it is existing. When it is used, it will not be exhausted."[24]

The spirit (*shen*, 神) resides at the space between the two hemispheres of the brain. It resembles a valley between mountains, trapping energy and generating resonant vibrations that correspond with the energy outside the valley. The shen in this valley is called valley spirit (*gu shen*, 谷神) and the valley is called spiritual valley (*shen gu*, 神谷). The shen residing in this valley governs the energy vibration of the whole body, and thus, the qi status and its manifestation. When this shen is strong, qi manifesting in your life will be strong, and your life will be long and healthy.

Xuan (玄) means original (*yuan*, 元). Pin (牝) refers to female animals and means mothers. Therefore, xuan pin means the origin or root of lives. When the valley spirit is centered (condensed) and functions actively, the life force is strong. Xuan pin (玄牝) is called taiji (太極, grand ultimate) in the *Yi Jing* (*The Book of Changes*). This taiji is the Dao (道) of lives in the great nature. Xuan pin can be summarized as "The root of creation, variation, bearing, and raising of millions of lives. It is the mother of millions of objects in heaven and earth. It is another name for Dao."(25)

The door to reaching this xuan pin is through natural shen (heaven and earth). This is very soft and continuous as though existing, and yet not existing. It cannot be seen, but is felt through cultivation. When used, it will not be exhausted.

To reach this natural shen, you must open your third eye, called tian mu (天目), heaven eye, or yu men (玉門), jade gate, by religious societies, and yintang (m-hn-3, 印堂), seal hall, by medical society. *Wudang's Illustration of Cultivating Truth* (武當修真圖) said, "The place under the mingtang (明堂), (ezhong, m-hn-2,額中), center of forehead, above the midpoint of the line connecting the two eyebrows, where the spiritual light emits, is named heaven eye (*tian mu*, 天目)."[26] It is also mentioned in the document, *Seven Bamboo Slips of the Bamboo Bookcase* (云笈七簽), "The space between the two eyebrows is the jade gate (*yu men*, 玉門) of ni wan (泥丸)."[27] Ni wan (泥丸) is a Daoist term, meaning mud pill, namely the brain, or upper dan tian. The lower center of the spiritual valley (*shen gu*, 神谷) between the two hemispheres of the brain is called ni wan gong (泥丸宮), or Mud Pill Palace (Figures 2-13 and 2-14).

To regulate shen means to cultivate it until it reaches the supernatural divine state. In Daoist society, there is a song, which says, "There is a shen in every human body. There is a supernatural divine light (*ling guang*, 靈光) which can be developed in this shen. This supernatural divine light alone can shine into thousands of valleys. Its Dao of variations is unlimited, spreading millions of ways."[28] Once you cultivate shen to an enlightened level, it can reach everywhere in the universe.

There is a song in Buddhist society, which says, "Do not search far for Buddha since he is in the Spiritual Mountain. Where is the Spiritual Mountain? It is actually in your mind. Everyone should have a pagoda at Spiritual Mountain, under which to cultivate his being."[29] Pagoda (ta, 塔) implies good deeds you have done and the comprehension of nature you have accumulated in spiritual cultivation.

2.2.5.2 Five Trainings of Shen

There are five trainings to regulate shen: 1. Raising the shen (*yang shen*, 養神), 2. Protecting the shen (*shou shen*, 守神), 3. Firming the shen (*gu shen*, 固神), 4. Stabilizing the shen (*ding shen*, 定神), and 5. Focusing the shen (*ning shen*, 凝神). These are called lian shen (練神). Lian (練) means to refine, train, or discipline. There are also two training keys and two purposes of training shen.

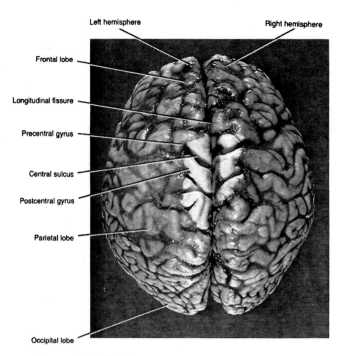

Left hemisphere

Right hemisphere

Frontal lobe

Longitudinal fissure

Precentral gyrus

Central sulcus

Postcentral gyrus

Parietal lobe

Occipital lobe

Figure 2-13. The brain encompasses two hemispheres

Raising the Shen (*Yang Shen,* 養神). Yang (養) means to nourish, promote, or nurse. Yang shen is the main training task for scholars and Buddhists. Shen needs to be nourished with qi. Fire qi from food and air can raise shen easily, but also increases emotional disturbance, leading shen away from its residence. Using yi nourished by water qi to raise your shen is harder, but this shen is stronger and more concentrated than that from fire qi. Adjust xin (yang) and yi (yin) to raise your shen properly so it is raised but not excited and stays at its residence.

Raising the shen correctly is like raising a child. You need great patience and perseverance. One way is to restrain his attention from the seven emotions and six desires. The other is to let him keep this contact with his human nature, yet educate his wisdom to make clear judgments, which is a long process, demanding understanding and patience. Raising shen is not about increasing emotional excitement. This scatters the yi, and shen becomes confused and loses its center. Yang shen builds a strong spiritual center and helps it control your life.

Protecting the Shen (*Shou Shen,* 守神). After raising your shen, keep it at its residence and train it. A child needs to keep his mind with his family instead of straying outside and running wild. Then you can educate him.

Shou (守) means to keep and protect. The training involves keeping shen at its residence, which is much harder than raising it. Shou shen training uses the regulated mind to direct, nurse, watch, and keeps the shen there. It is like keeping your child at home instead of letting him leave home and run wild. Be patient and control your temper, regulating your xin and yi. If you lose your temper, you only

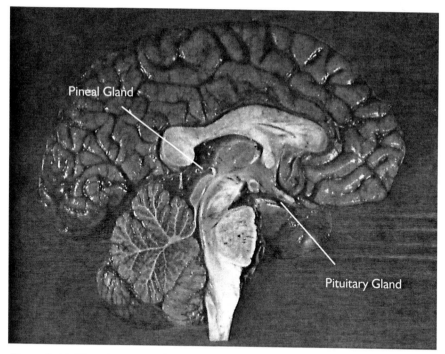

Figure 2-14. The pituitary and pineal glands (Mud Hill Palace) in the spiritual valley

make the child want to leave home again. Once you have regulated your xin and yi, you will be able to keep your shen effectively.

Firming the Shen (*Gu Shen,* 固神). Gu (固) means to coalesce and to firm. After keeping shen at its residence, you firm and coalesce it (*gu shen,* 固神). Gu shen means training shen to stay at its residence willingly. After you control your child in the house, make him want from his heart to stay. Only then will his mind be steady and calm. To reach this, you need more love and patience until he understands the importance of staying home and growing up normally. This third step of shen training is to make the shen willing to stay at its residence in peace, by regulating thoughts and emotions.

Stabilizing the Shen (*Ding Shen,* 定神). Ding shen (定神) means to stabilize and calm the shen. When your child is at peace, he will not be attracted to external distractions. Regulate your shen to calm it, so it is energized but not excited, with the mind peaceful and steady.

Condensing the Shen (*Ning Shen,* 凝神). Ning (凝) means to condense, concentrate, refine, focus, and strengthen. The first four processes, which raise, keep, firm, and stabilize, are the foundations of shen cultivation. After this, you condense and focus your shen into a tiny spot. This is where you train the shen to a higher spiritual state. When focused in a tiny point, it is like a sunbeam focused through a lens: the smaller the point, the stronger the beam.

2.2.5.3 Two Training Keys

Remember, there are two keys in regulating shen: 1. Mutual dependence of shen and breathing (*shen xi xiang yi*, 神息相依), and 2. Mutual harmony of shen and qi (*shen qi xiang he*, 神氣相合).

Mutual Dependence of Shen and Breathing (*Shen Xi Xiang Yi*, 神息相依). After shen has been trained to a high degree, put it to work. The first assignment is coordinating it with your breathing. In qigong training, breathing is considered the strategy. When this is directed by your shen, it obtains optimum results. This strategy is called shen xi xiang yi (神息相依), which means shen and breathing are mutually dependent. Shen xi (神息) means shen breathing. Your shen and breathing become one, and qi is led efficiently. This daunting task requires you to have regulated your body, breathing, and mind.

Mutual Harmony of Shen and Qi (*Shen Qi Xiang He*, 神氣相合). The second shen training key uses shen to direct the circulation and distribution of qi, called shen qi xiang he (神氣相合), shen and qi combine. In battle, the fighting spirit of the soldiers determines their ability to fight and to execute strategy. Shen is the son (zi, 子), while qi is the mother (mu, 母). When mother and son unite in harmony with each other, it is called mu zi xiang he (母子相合), mutual harmony of mother and son.

2.2.5.4 Two Purposes of Regulating the Shen

There are two main purposes of regulating the shen in qigong practice. For secular society, it is to improve health and extend life, but for Buddhists and Daoists, the goal is to reach Buddhahood or enlightenment.

Health and Longevity. Yi is related to shen. When yi is strong and concentrated, shen can be raised high. The most popular and essential purpose of qigong practice is to attain health, using yi to lead the qi (*yi yi yin qi*, 以意引氣). If concentrated yi raises shen, qi circulates smoothly, and the body is healthy. Small circulation meditation increases the qi circulating in the conception and governing vessels, and in the twelve primary qi channels.

Qigong also enhances longevity. It raises the spirit up to a high level, and then uses it to govern the qi (*yi shen yu qi*, 以神馭氣) and to enhance qi circulation in the bone marrow and brain. Qi is compared to soldiers in battle, while shen is their fighting spirit. When the general's spirit is high, the morale of his soldiers is also high, and his orders are carried out effectively. In the same way, qi nourishes the bone marrow and brain. Healthy marrow enhances production of blood cells, promoting metabolism and leading to longevity.

Enlightenment. To spiritual cultivators, the final goal of regulating shen is reaching enlightenment. That means comprehending the meaning of nature and human life, then unifying the human spirit with nature to become as one. This is the final goal of the unification of heaven and man (*tian ren he yi*, 天人合一).

To reach this, you must open the third eye for communication. First, build up abundant qi at the real lower dan tian, which is led up through the thrusting vessel to activate the brain and enhance the resonance of the spiritual valley. When spiritual energy reaches a certain level, the third eye reopens.

To reach this high level of cultivation, first regulate your mind. If it is trapped in emotional bondage, how can you build up your spirit and keep it neutral? Buddhists and Daoists define four steps in spiritual cultivation.

2.2.5.5 *Four Steps to Cultivate Spiritual Enlightenment*

Self-recognition (*Zi Shi,* 自識). First, set your spirit free from emotional bondage; otherwise the spirit stays in the emotional mud of secular society. Once the spirit is free from this bondage, it can reach the neutral state and finally unify with the natural spirit. Self-recognition (*zi shi,* 自識) means observing the heart (*guan xin,* 觀心), that is, observing the initiation of thoughts and emotions to discover your true identity.

Important Script of Similar Contents (同指要抄) said, "All religious styles, throughout generations, all considered observing the xin (*guan xin,* 觀心) as the most important in cultivation."[30]

The Complete Book of Principal Contents of Human Life and Temperament (性命圭旨全書) said, "When learning the Dao, first comprehend your own xin. The deep hidden place of your own xin is the hardest place to find. Once you have found it and no other place can be found, you realize that a secular's xin can be just like a Buddha's."[31] This describes the difficulty of discovering your true self, the one hiding behind the mask. Once you have discovered this hidden xin, you recognize it and cultivate it. This cultivated xin can reach the same level as Buddha.

Self-awareness (*Zi Jue,* 自覺). Having recognized your true identity, ponder deeply and clearly. Discriminate truth from illusion. From discriminating between truth and falsehood, awareness arises. Your mind establishes contact with events and phenomena in your life. The feeling of self-awareness can be profound.

To the Buddhist society, this is the stage where observation is stopped. It is the beginning of regulating the temperament and spirit toward goodness. *Anthology of Daoist Village* (道鄉集) said, "The real meaning of Buddhahood which has been handed down is: observation is stopped. What is observation? It means to place my vision warmly on the ultimate goodness. What is stop? It means to focus my real intention on the ultimate goodness."[32] Buddhist society has three observations (*san guan,* 三觀): 1. Observing emptiness is observing the emptiness of all natural laws and events, 2. Observing falseness is observing the falseness of all natural laws, 3. Observing between is observing the non-emptiness and non-falseness of natural laws, keeping the neutral viewpoint. It also means double observation.[33] Zhi guan (止觀), stop observation, is the way to reach guan zhi (觀止), observation is stopped. Observe and analyze events and occurrences. Once you see through the events in your mind, nothing troubles you. This is the stage of guan zhi reached by cultivating your mind to the stage of ultimate goodness. Pay attention to all goodness, and then nothing bothers you. You are kind, righteous, and gentle, with no inner conflict. You are free from the affinity of emotions and desires.

Extreme calmness and peace within are the key to this self-awareness, reached through practicing Embryonic Breathing (*Tai Xi,* 胎息), as described in the book, *Qigong Meditation–Embryonic Breathing,* published by YMAA Publication Center.

Self-awakening (*Zi Xing*, 自醒) (*Zi Wu*, 自悟). Through Embryonic Breathing, you reach self-awakening. Your mind is clear and allows you to comprehend accurately the truth of your life and nature. This stage is called entering the observation (*ru guan*, 入觀). Entering means to comprehend the observation and the temperament (*wu xing*, 悟性).[34] This is the stage of enlightenment and Buddhahood (*fo*, 佛), called understanding the heart and seeing through the temperament (*ming xin jian xing*, 明心見性). Comprehension is no longer necessary (*liao wu*, 了悟).

How is Buddhahood defined? It means to achieve awareness and wisdom, to awaken through understanding and observation, to awaken through knowing the reasons behind natural laws, and to discriminate them clearly. It is like being awakened from sleep and is called 'awakening through realization'. Comprehend vexations through observation so they are not harmful. It is like observing and sensing 'thieves' (contaminated thoughts) in secular society, so it is called awakening through observation.[35] *Thesis of Buddha Ground* (佛地論) said, "All laws and all manifestations of nature can bloom and be awakened by themselves. We can also bloom and be awakened from emotional bondage, like being awakened from sleep and like the blooming of the lotus flower. This is called Buddha."[36]

To Buddhists, we are born and grow in emotional mud (*chen tu*, 塵土), human matrix. We create dignity, glory, pride, happiness, sadness, jealousy, and desire. We lie and cover our faces with masks, and we all experience significant spiritual pain living in this human matrix. The mud makes us blind and deaf, and nothing is clear in our minds. The conscious mind is active, while the sub-conscious shen is asleep. We are dreaming in the human matrix and not awakening.

Nevertheless, each of us has a lotus seed, our original shen. Through meditation, it buds and grows from deep in the mud. The subconscious mind grows, and after long practice, the lotus flower emerges from the matrix, and you see everything clearly. To awaken your shen, bring all thoughts to your shen center and keep the shen there. This upper dan tian or spiritual mountain (*ling shan*, 靈山), in which there is the spiritual valley (*shen gu*, 神谷), is where the valley spirit (*gu shen*, 谷神) lives.

Remember the song that says, "Do not search far for Buddha since he is in the spiritual mountain. Where is the spiritual mountain? In your mind."[29]

In a state of extreme calmness and emptiness, your mind is clear to comprehend the truth of nature. *The Righteous Rules of Heavenly Immortality: Straight Discussion of Two Qi's Pre-Heaven and Post-Heaven* (天仙正理 · 先天后天二氣直論) said, "Those who apply qi, how do they know it is true pre-heaven practice? When calmness (*jing*, 靜) and emptiness (*xu*, 虛) have reached their extremities, there is no single slight thought involved in consciousness. This is the true pre-heaven practice."[37] Pre-heaven truth (*xian tian zhi zhen*, 先天之真) means the truthful state before birth, where the mind is simple and pure, extremely calm and sincere. However, how do you know you have reached this state in practice: When there is not even the smallest thought existing or initiating in your mind. Your subconscious mind (pre-heaven truthful mind) awakens to activity.

Qigong society classifies the conscious mind as yang, generated by the brain since birth. The subconscious mind is yin and is born with you. The conscious mind and memory are generated from conditioning by the environment and are not truthful. A thick facade covers the falseness of this conscious mind. However, the subconscious mind is truthful, connected with spiritual memory, which is active only when your body is calm and activities of your conscious mind have ceased.

To return to the pre-birth stage, cease physical and mental activity. Then the subconscious mind acts and directs you to the true path of spiritual cultivation.

Freedom from Self-bondage (*Zi Tuo,* 自脫). The last stage of spiritual cultivation is to free yourself from physical, mental, and spiritual bondage. Once you have awakened spiritually, you see clearly who you are and how you want to be. Free yourself from the bondage of the human matrix. In Buddhist terms, the third eye opens. The lotus grows, and the flower emerges from the mud. Your spirit is reunited with the spirit of nature.

Freedom from Material Bondage. Set yourself free from the bondage of your physical body and all material attractions around you. Your body is only recycled material, and beauty is only temporary. Material concerns trigger mental bondage. Take care of this recycled material, protect it and nourish it, but free yourself from attaching to it.

What you need from the material world is enough energy supply for your physical strength, without sinking into the mud of materialism and losing the feeling of your life. Most material things you own will last longer than you will, and you own them only as long as you live. If you pursue material enjoyment, your mind stays focused on materialistic concerns. To set yourself free from material bondage, the first step is to gain enough for comfortable living. (Comfortable can mean a wide range of different levels. Isn't it more accurate to say that you seek to detach yourself from the importance of material objects in your life?) Any extra beyond that entangles you deeper in the mud. To reach profound spiritual cultivation, Buddhists believe you must cultivate a neutral state separate from the emptiness of earth, water, fire, and wind (*si da jie kong,* 四大皆空), the material world. They believe this is crucial to reaching Buddhahood.

Freedom from Mental Bondage. Mental bondage means the thoughts generated from the emotional matrix, and desires for both the mental and material worlds. Again, human suffering is caused by the seven passions and six desires (*qi qing liu yu,* 七情六慾). The seven passions are happiness (*xi,* 喜), anger (*nu,* 怒), sorrow (*ai,* 哀), joy (*le,* 樂), love (*ai,* 愛), hate (*hen,* 恨) and desire (*yu,* 慾). The six desires are the sensory pleasures derived from the eyes, ears, nose, tongue, body, and mind.

We humans, in order to survive in the harsh reality of this world, lie and trick each other. Truth within is hidden behind the mask we wear, decorated with glory, dignity, and honor, which are tools to enslave the souls and bodies of others. Lust for wealth and power has become the common core education for the next generation. A human emotional matrix has been created and all of us suffer within it.

To escape from this matrix, first awaken deep in your heart. With a neutral and open mind, see through the matrix we have created. The truth should always be in your mind, or else the search for the Dao will be in vain.

Ponder the words of Michael Faraday (1791–1867):

The philosopher should be a man willing to listen to every suggestion, but deter-mined to judge for himself. He should not be biased by appearances, have no fa-vorite hypothesis, be of no school, and in doctrine have no master. He should not be a respecter of persons, but of things. Truth should be his primary object. If to these qualities be added industry, he may indeed hope to walk within the veil of the temple of Nature.

Once you have this truth in your mind, you have achieved a peaceful mind, and your spirit can awaken and be cultivated.

Freedom from Spiritual Bondage. You need to be free from mental bondage before setting out to escape from spiritual bondage. The spirit is overshadowed and blinded by traditional religious doctrines based on the emotions of the past.

The various religions bind us in their spiritual religious matrix, created by those considered holy men in the past. The concepts of God, heaven, and hell were created in the human mind and worship was initiated. As time passed, we have been led deeper and deeper away from the truth and trapped in humanly-created spiritual bondage. *Lao Zi*, Chapter 1, said, "Dao, if it can be spoken (described), then it is not the true everlasting Dao. Name, if it can be named, then it is not the true everlasting name."[37] We humans, before really knowing the Dao, have already talked about Dao. Even if we know the true path to search for it, we still cling stubbornly to the old path and dare not change it.

To achieve this true Dao, we must continue to search for it by talking and exchang-ing opinions. Always keep in mind that the Dao we are talking about may not yet be true. Having seen the truth, *we should not be afraid to face it, challenging our old thoughts and beliefs and daring to accept mistakes and to dream about the future.* Science should search for the true Dao, helping us to escape from the traditional religious matrix.

Escape from the traditional matrix and free yourself from spiritual bondage and doctrines. Awaken your subconscious spiritual mind by bringing your mind and spiri-tual feeling to the day you were conceived. From this Daoist principle was derived the theory and techniques of Embryonic Breathing.

To return to the embryonic state, first get rid of the human emotional matrix. Focus the mind on the pineal and pituitary glands at the Mud Pill Palace (*Ni Wan Gong*, 泥丸宫). Where there are brain cells, that is where conscious thought and the human matrix can be created. However, the lower center of the spiritual valley has no brain cells, so no matrix can be generated. Through this center, where the subconscious mind resides, we can resonate or communicate with the natural spirit. By calming the activ-ity of the brain through absence of thought, we can then bring our spiritual awareness to a high level.

For strong resonance between your spirit and the natural spirit, you need strong spiritual energy at this Mud Pill Palace. Store abundant qi at your real lower dan tian (*zhen xia dan tian*, 真下丹田), and lead it up to nourish the Mud Pill Palace, raising spiritual energy up to a high level. Spiritual cultivation is discussed in more detail in the book, *Qigong Meditation–Embryonic Breathing* available from YMAA Publication Center.

Once you bring your spiritual energy to a very high level, you reopen your third eye, called tian yan (天眼), heaven eye by Daoist society and yintang (印堂) m-nh-3, sealed hall, by Chinese medicine. Having reopened the third eye, your spirit can unite with the natural spirit without obstacle. This is the final stage of spiritual cultivation, the unification of heaven and man (*tian ren he yi*, 天人合一).

Notes

1. 真調為無調而自調。

2. 形不正，則氣不順。氣不順，則意不寧。意不寧，則氣散亂。

3. *Qigong Meditation—Embryonic Breathing*, Dr. Yang, Jwing-Ming, YMAA Publication Center, Boston, 2004.

4. *A Study of Anatomic Physiology* (解剖生理學), 李文森編著。華杏出版股份有限公司。Taipei, 1986.

5. 《莊子·大宗師》：〝古之真人，...其息深深。真人之息以踵，眾人之息以喉。〞

6. 《性命圭旨全書·火候》：〝神息者，火候也。〞指文火安神定息，任其自如，謂之神息。即〝不得勤，不得忘者，是皆神息之自然火候之微旨也。〞

7. 《性命圭旨全書·蟄藏氣穴，眾妙歸根》：〝調息要調真息息，煉神須煉不神神。〞

8. 《天仙正理·伏氣直論》：〝古人托名調息者，隨順往來之理而不執滯往來之形，欲合乎似無之呼吸也。〞

9. "Teens' Troubles Tied to Brain," Michael Lasalandra, *Boston Herald*, June 12, 1998.

10. "Inside the Teen Brain," Shannon Brownlee, *U.S. News*, August 9, 1999, pp. 44-54.

11. 《備急千金要方·卷二十七·養性》：〝多思則神殆，多念則志散，多欲則志昏，多事則形勞，多語則氣乏，多笑則臟傷，多愁則心懾，多樂則意溢，多喜則忘錯昏亂，多怒則百脈不定，多好則專迷不理，多惡則憔悴無歡。此十二多不除，則榮衛失度，血氣妄行，喪生之本也。〞

12. 《性命圭旨全書·亨集》：〝身不動而心自安，心不動而神自守。〞

13. 《性命圭旨全書·蟄藏氣穴，眾妙歸根》：〝合真人深深之息，則心息相依，息調心靜。〞

14. 《聽心齋客問》：〝心依著事物已久，一旦離境，不能自立。所以用調息功夫，拴系此心，便心息相依。調字亦不是用意，只是一呼一吸系念耳。至心離境，則無人無我，更無息可調，只綿綿若存，久之，自然純熟。〞

15. 《道藏·坐忘論》：〝夫心者一身之主，百神之帥，靜則生慧，動則生昏，欣迷動靜之中。〞

16. *Chinese Qigong Dictionary* (中國氣功辭典), Lu, Guang-rong (呂光榮), 人民衛生出版社, Beijing, China, 1988.

17. *The Great Completion of Chinese Qigong* (中國氣功大成), Fang, Chun-yang (方春陽), 吉林科學技術出版社, Jilin, China, 1989.

18. *The Complete Book of Nourishing the Life in Chinese Daoist Qigong* (中國道教氣功養生大全), Li, Yuan-guo (李遠國), 四川辭書出版社), Chengdu, Sichuan, China, 1991.

19. 《道德經·十六章》：〝致虛極，守靜篤。〞

20. 意不在氣，在氣則滯。

21. *Qigong Meditation—Small Circulation*, Dr. Yang, Jwing-Ming, YMAA Publication Center, Boston, 2006.

22. *The Essence of Shaolin White Crane*, Dr. Yang, Jwing-Ming, YMAA Publication Center, Boston, 1996.

23. 行氣如九曲珠，無微不到。

24. 《道德經·六章》：〝谷神不死，是謂玄牝。玄牝之門，是謂天地根，綿綿若存，用之不勤。〞

25. 〝指造化生育萬物之根本，亦即天地萬物之母，即道之別稱也。〞

26. 《武當修真圖》：〝明堂下，兩眉連線中點上方。有神光出，而日天目。〞

27. 《云笈七簽》：〝兩眉間為泥丸之玉門。〞

28. 〝人人身中有一神，一神中有一靈光，靈光獨耀超千谷，道化無窮微萬方。〞

29. 〝佛在靈山莫遠求，靈山只在汝心頭。人人有個靈山塔，好向靈山塔下修。〞

30. 《同指要抄》：〝一代教門，皆以觀心為要。〞

31. 《性命圭旨全書·涵養本源，救護命寶》：〝學道先須學自心，自心深處最難尋。若還尋到無尋處，方悟凡心即佛心。〞指覺悟之心。

32. 《道鄉集》：〝佛之真傳，在于觀止。〞〝觀者何？將我目光，溫煦于至善地之義也。〞〝止者何？將我真意止于至善地之義也。〞

33. 〔三觀〕：一·空觀：觀諸法之空諦。二·假觀：觀諸法之假。三·中觀：一觀諸法亦非空，亦非假，即中也。二觀諸法亦空亦假，即是中，謂為雙照之觀。

34. 入觀：觀為觀想之義。入為悟性，即悟真理。

35. 即覺或智之意。如覺悟、覺察、覺知諸法之事理，而了了分明。如睡夢之寤，謂之覺悟。覺察煩惱，使不為害，如世人之覺之為賊者，故云覺察。

36. 《佛地論》：〝于一切法，一切種相，能自開覺，亦開覺一切有情，如睡夢覺醒，如蓮花開，故名佛。〞

37. 《天仙正理·先天后天二氣直論》：〝夫用此氣者，由何以知先天之真也。當靜虛至極時。亦未涉一念覺知，此正真先天之真境界也。〞

38. 老子·第一章：〝道、可道，非、常道；名、可名，非、常名。〞

CHAPTER 3

General Introduction to Taiji Ball Qigong
(太極球氣功之一般介紹)

3.1 Introduction (介紹)

Though the existence of taiji ball qigong has been common knowledge in both Chinese martial arts and laymen societies, its popularity has been limited due to the secrecy of the training techniques. Taiji ball qigong training, in each style, was kept secret and passed down only to trusted students. In martial society, special taiji ball qigong training was considered crucial in bringing martial artists to a much higher level, in both physical condition and with qi's manifestation in battle. Many training methods, especially those that were able to enhance the healthy condition of body, have spread from the martial arts society to laymen society. Now, the most common and popular medical taiji ball qigong training, rotating two ping-pong sized balls in one's palms, has been recognized as one of the most effective ways of improving qi circulation, especially for the lungs and heart. In addition, through this kind of training, the condition of hand arthritis can be remedied effectively (Figure 3-1).

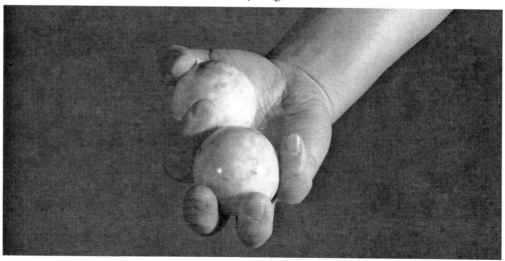

Figure 3-1. Taiji ball movement in hands

Taiji balls (*taiji qiu*, 太極球) used in the martial arts society come in different sizes and are made from a variety of materials. The size can range from as large as a three- to four-foot diameter wooden ball, to, as mentioned earlier, a ping-pong sized ball. The largest wooden balls are hung from the ceiling. The most common sizes for training are from ten inches to one foot in diameter. The balls can range from being made of an expensive blue jade to average cheap rock. Today, the blue jade balls are rare, costing nearly $50,000. The rock taiji balls may be cheap, but are usually quite heavy. This kind of ball training is more commonly practiced in Chinese external martial arts that emphasize physical conditioning more than qi circulation.

For the internal martial art styles, such as Taijiquan (太極拳), Xingyiquan (形意拳), Baguazhang (八卦掌), Liuhebafa (六合八法), Fo Zhang (佛掌) (Buddha palms or Buddha hands), and hu die zhang (蝴蝶掌) (butterfly palm), the balls made from wood are preferred. This is because to these internal styles the quantity of qi built up and also the quality of qi's manifestation are considered the most important in training. With wooden balls, the qi between the palms can be felt and led more easily than with balls made of stone.

The original name of taiji ball qigong training is "yin-yang taiji ball qigong" (*yin-yang taiji qiu qigong*, 陰陽太極球氣功). Although the training methods are different from one style to another, the main training theory and general purposes are the same. We will discuss the training theory in Chapter 4. The general training purposes of taiji ball qigong training are to

- Strengthen the physical torso, especially the spine and lower back.
- Condition the bones, muscles, tendons, and ligaments required for combat.
- Use the mind to lead the qi, improving qi circulation and manifestation. This is the crucial key to enhancing the martial power (*jin*, 勁) required in a battle.
- Build up a higher quantity of qi.

In the next section of this chapter, a brief history of taiji ball qigong will be reviewed. Then, the relationship of taiji ball qigong and health will be discussed in section 3.3. Next, the importance of taiji ball qigong in Chinese martial arts society will be explained in section 3.4. Finally, some suggestions of how to use this book will be offered.

3.2 History of Taiji Ball Qigong (太極球氣功之歷史)

No one knows when and how taiji ball qigong originated. However, logically it can be assumed that when martial artists realized that roundness was the crucial key of neutralizing incoming stiff and square power, they began to search for ways of training this roundness. They looked for an object to help them develop and attain this feeling of roundness. The round objects were adopted. The internal martial styles, compared to external arts, most likely contributed more to the development of taiji ball training, due to the significant emphasis it places on roundness and adhering.

First, let us trace back the origin of internal styles' development in Chinese martial arts history. Available documentation for the time before A.D. 500, reveal that no distinction was made between internal arts and external arts. However, only a short period of time later, the internal arts were developed.

According to the historical record, it is understood that techniques and forms with the same principles as taijiquan were in existence during the Ling dynasty (梁朝) (A.D. 502–557), and were taught by Han, Gong-yue (韓拱月), Cheng, Ling-xi (程靈洗), and Cheng, Bi (程珌). Later, in the Tang dynasty (唐朝) (A.D. 713–905), it was found that Xu, Xuan-ping (許宣平), Li, Dao-zi (李道子), and Yin, Li-heng (殷利亨) were teaching similar martial techniques. They were called the thirty-seven postures (*san shi qi shi*, 三十七勢), post-heaven techniques (*hou tian fa*, 後天法), or small nine heaven (*xiao jiu tian*, 小九天).

If we take a closer look, there is one major event that clearly influenced the change in the training concept of the entire Chinese martial arts society. The shift is attributed to the qigong practice passed down to the Shaolin Temple by an Indian Buddhist priest, Bodhidarma (達摩). According to the books *The Recording of the Shaolin Temple* (*Shao Lin Si Zhi*, 少林寺誌) and *The Complete Art of Shaolin Wushu* (*Shao Lin Wushu Da Quan*, 少林武術大全), Bodhidarma was invited to China, from India, in A.D. 527, during the time of emperor Liang Wu (A.D. 502-557) and emperor Wei Xiao Ming (A.D. 516–528). Before Da Mo passed away in A.D. 536 at the Shaolin Temple, he passed down two important qigong training classics, *Muscle/Tendon Changing Classic* (*Yi Jin Jing*, 易筋經) and *Marrow/Brain Washing Classic* (*Xi Sui Jing*, 洗髓經). The *Yi Jin Jing* taught Shaolin monks how to change, or condition, their physical bodies from weak to strong, while the *Xi Sui Jing* taught the monks how to nourish the brain with qi for enlightenment. The entire concept is based on the simple theory of using the mind to lead the qi to the physical body for strength manifestation or to the brain for spiritual enlightenment. From Da Mo's theory and muscle/tendon change practice, Shaolin monks were able to manifest their martial power to a significantly higher level. This enhancement of power was crucial in battle.

Some martial artists believed that since the mind is the foundation of power, they should train the mind's concentration and focus (internal). When this mind is strongly focused, the qi can be abundantly led for power manifestation with the techniques. This was the beginning of internal styles. While at the same time, many martial artists believed that in order to reach a high level of concentration and focus, it would take many years of meditation practice. In order to survive in a violent society, they should first learn techniques and then gradually enter into the internal side through meditation practice. That is why there is a saying in Chinese martial society, "Internal is from internal to external, and external is from external to internal. Though the paths are opposite, the final goal is the same."[1]

All styles were searching for ways to increase endurance, a crucial key to survival. After generations of practice, they began to realize that in order to conserve energy and physical strength; one must be round and soft. We personally believe that taiji ball qigong, or similar training, existed in almost all the martial styles before the Chinese Song dynasty (宋朝) (A.D. 960–1280), and was kept secret.

Today, taiji ball qigong also has two approaches. One is from internal to external, while the other is from external to internal. The Shaolin Temple in Song Mountain (嵩山) focuses on external training; their taiji balls are made of either rock or wood.

Taijiquan in Wudang Mountain (武當山) has become the leading style of internal training, using balls made of wood.

As mentioned earlier, the size of the ball can differ from one style to another. The small balls, which are commonly used for health, were actually the balls used to strengthen the finder's grabbing power. They were also used to improve one's qi and blood circulation right after iron sand palm (*tie sha zhang*, 鐵砂掌) training, and were also commonly used as a throwing dart weapon (*an qi*, 暗器).

The history of taiji ball training is scarce. One very valuable document is the *Great Dictionary of Chinese Wushu* (中國武術大辭典)[2]. According to the writings of Tang Hao (唐豪) (A.D. 1897–1959), taiji ball qigong training, in taijiquan, was passed down by Liu, De-kuan (劉德寬) (A.D. 1826–1911), and Liu learned it from an unknown, non-taijiquan, martial artist. According to Tang Hao, the biggest ball that could be used was a huge ball made of brass, which was hung from the ceiling. The practice included solo and matching practices.

3.3 Taiji Ball Qigong and Health (太極球氣功與健康)

Since taiji ball qigong is a combination of internal elixir (*nei dan*, 內丹) and external elixir (*wai dan*, 外丹) qigong practice, the health benefits of taiji ball qigong can therefore be divided into two parts, the internal and external side. If you are interested in knowing more about internal elixir and external elixir, please refer to the book, *The Root of Chinese Qigong*, by Dr. Yang, Jwing-Ming, published by YMAA Publication Center.[3]

3.3.1 Internal Benefits

To train the mind to its higher level of concentration and focus. Taiji ball qigong is a soft-moving meditation. Through this meditative training, you will be able to concentrate and focus your mind at a higher level. When this happens, your mental sensitivity will be increased significantly. This will result in a higher level of alertness and awareness. This is a crucial key in improving your mind and body's communication. With this smooth communication, you will be able to see your body's health condition, enabling you to learn how to lead yourself down the right path of a healthier life.

To improve the body's metabolism and also build up an abundant level of qi. Through the correct breathing techniques in taiji ball qigong practice, you will not only able to improve the capacity of your oxygen and carbon dioxide exchange, but you will also be able to build up an abundant level of qi at the lower dan tian (*xia dan tian*, 下丹田). Smooth metabolism is the crucial key in slowing down the aging process. With an abundant level of qi circulating in the body, your immune system will be strong and your life force will be powerful. Without this abundant qi supply, you will unhealthily age.

To learn how to use the mind to lead the qi for its circulation to a smoother level. In order to have your body function healthily, you must also circulate the qi in the body smoothly. In taiji ball qigong, you learn how to use your mind to lead the qi, so that it can circulate smoothly in the body.

To enhance the grand circulation so that the feeling of sensitivity can be significantly increased. One of the taiji ball qigong practices is grand qi circulation. In this practice, you learn how to lead the qi out of the body so that it can be transferable with surrounding objects or live beings. Feeling is a language of the body and mind's communication. Through correct taiji ball qigong training, the qi can be extended beyond the body. This is the crucial key in feeling your opponent in martial arts and also communicating with nature. When this sensitivity is increased, the self-alertness and awareness will be higher.

To heighten the spirit of vitality. The final goal of any qigong practice is spiritual cultivation. When the spirit is high, refined, and regulated, the qi's circulation will be abundant, the mental mind will be strong and firmed, and life can be focused and meaningful. To Buddhist and Daoist qigong practice, the goal has gone even further, aiming for spiritual enlightenment. Taiji ball qigong practice trains the mind to focus. Through this focused mind, the qi can be led efficiently. With the high level of spiritual development, the qi can be led to the brain to nourish the brain cells. This is the crucial key of spiritual enlightenment. If you are interested in knowing more about this brain-washing training, please refer to the book, *Qigong—The Secret of Youth*, published by YMAA Publication Center.[4]

3.3.2 External Benefits

To strengthen the physical body (bones, ligaments, tendons, and muscles). Because of the weight of taiji balls, the movements in taiji ball training strengthen the physical body. The parts of the body in which taiji ball qigong conditions effectively are the bones, ligaments, tendons, and muscles. However, the most known benefit that taiji ball qigong training brings you is the conditioning of your torso, chest, spine, and especially, the lower back.

To establish a firm root, balance, and centering ability, and to strengthen the three major joints of the legs. Another known benefit of taiji ball qigong training is the strengthening of the three joints, the hips, knees, and ankles. With a heavy ball and correct walking, these three joints can be conditioned effectively. This will result in a firm root, good balance, and a feeling of being centered.

To loosen and exercise the joints. When you practice taiji ball qigong, even if there is a heavy ball held in your hands, due to the emphasis of the joints' movements, the joints will be exercised and opened. Heavier balls not only condition the ligaments and tendons, but also enhance the qi's circulation within the joint areas. This can therefore prevent, or even heal, some levels of arthritis. In addition, from this joint exercise, the bone marrow will receive adequate amounts of qi for nourishment so that blood cells can be produced healthily. This is a crucial key to longevity.

To enhance qi circulation in the internal organs. Through the semi-relaxed arm and leg movements, the qi's circulation in the twelve primary qi channels (i.e., meridians) is enhanced. This will result in the gradual conditioning of the internal organs. In addition, according to Chinese qigong theory, due to the required chest movements taiji ball qigong training may not only prevent the development of breast cancer for women, but may also possibly be used to heal it altogether. In addition, due to the hip-joint and leg exercises, taiji ball qigong training can be used in preventing and healing prostate cancer.

To enhance the coordination of the mind, feeling, and body. The most amazing benefit that taiji ball qigong can bring you is coordination and harmonization both internally and externally. The mind, feeling, and body are able to harmonize and coordinate with each other from the inside to outside, mental to physical. This is a crucial key to good health and longevity.

3.4 Taiji Ball Qigong and Martial Arts (太極球氣功與武術)

Using the taiji ball as a tool for martial arts can be very beneficial. From the physical movements, concentration of the mind, and sensitivity of feeling training, taiji ball qigong enhances your fighting skills. Keep in mind that this type of training was required by many different styles of Chinese martial arts as part of their daily regimen. Let's summarize some important martial purposes here.

3.4.1 Purposes of Taiji Ball Qigong training in Chinese martial arts society:

To strengthen and condition the physical body. We know that the body's functions depend on the strength of the bones, ligaments, tendons, and muscles. If any part of the body is weak, the body's coordination and function will be less efficient. Therefore, an effective exercise that allows you to condition from the surface to the deeper areas of the body is crucial. That means you must have an exercise that allows you to condition the shallow places such as the muscles and tendons, while also enabling you to reach deeper to the ligaments and bones. In order to accomplish this, you must be soft, round, and flexible. This allows the tendons and ligaments, located at the joints, to be exercised. Not only that, the exercise must also be able to condition the muscles and bones simultaneously. Taiji ball qigong is able to provide such conditioning.

Let's think about the body's structure. The strength for power manifestation originates from the torso, especially the area of the lower back. Taiji ball qigong specializes in conditioning the torso (spine) and lower back.

To improve the quality of the physical body's structure. Having a strong body structure will provide you with a firm root, center, and balance. In addition to having a strong physical structure, you must also learn to coordinate different parts of the body needed to perform various actions. Without meeting these criteria, the power manifested will be weak and ineffective. In the *Taijiquan Classic*, it is said:

The root is at the feet, (jin or movement is) generated from the legs, mastered (i.e., controlled) by the waist, and manifested (i.e., expressed) from the fingers. From the feet to the legs to the waist, (it) must have an integrated and unified qi. When moving forward or backward, (you can) then catch the opportunity and gain the superior position.

其根在腳，發於腿，主宰於腰，形於手指。由腳而腿而腰，總須完整一氣。向前退後，乃能得機得勢。

If you fail to catch the opportunity and gain the superior position, (your) body will be disordered. To solve this problem, (you) must look to the waist and legs.

有不得機得勢處，身便散亂。其病必於腰腿求之。

If there is a top, there is a bottom; if there is a front, there is a back; if there is a left, there is a right.

有上即有下，有前即有後，有左即有右。

These all refer to body structure. Through time, taiji ball qigong will give you a feel for proper alignment. By knowing this feeling of structure, you will be able to correct postures on your own.

To increase the potential of endurance both physically and mentally. You should understand one important thing. A real battle could last for a few hours, not just a few minutes. You needed good endurance, especially since you would, often as not, be wearing heavy armor. If you did not have endurance, it would not be long until you were killed. It is well known in the Chinese martial community that surviving a long battle did not solely depend on one's power or techniques, but relied more heavily on one's endurance level.

Two keys to improving endurance are knowing how to breathe correctly and how to conserve muscle usage. Knowing how to take in oxygen and expel carbon dioxide efficiently will allow for an abundant supply needed for the body's biochemical reactions or metabolism. In addition, knowing how to cut down muscle usage, you can conserve oxygen in the muscles and reduce acid build up. Without knowing how to breathe correctly, upon manifesting power for either neutralizing or attacking, your power and technique will be weak.

It is important to have a strong and firm spirit when practicing. This is a crucial key to surviving a battle. Losing the morale of fighting, giving up easily, will naturally lead you to be killed. Therefore, the will and self-confidence of surviving must be strong. This mental discipline can only be received from constant taiji ball conditioning practice.

To coordinate actions with correct breathing. In Chinese qigong practice, the body is compared to a battlefield, the breathing is considered as a strategy, the mind is the general, and qi is soldiers, and finally the spirit is the morale of the entire army. From this analogy, you can see that if the breathing is carried out correctly, the qi can be led efficiently.

We cannot deny that when oxygen is abundant, the body's metabolism is smoothly executed. This is crucial when manifesting power. As mentioned before, your metabolism rate plays a huge role in having lasting endurance.

To build an abundant quantity of qi. In order to manifest power on a higher plateau, you must first possess an abundant amount of qi. Without a high quantity of qi, your physical body will not be able to perform to its maximum efficiency. One of the training methods in taiji ball qigong teaches you how to coordinate breathing with the buildup of qi in the lower dan tian (*xia dan tian*, 下丹田).

To learn how to use the mind to lead the qi efficiently and smoothly. This will provide you a quality manifestation of qi. Leading qi efficiently to a specific area of the body is achieved by concentrating and focusing the mind to a higher level. If done correctly, you will be able to use the minimum amount of qi needed to manifest power to its maximum. Conserving the usage of qi is a crucial key to a lasting endurance.

In taiji ball qigong, you learn how to use your mind to lead qi to the four major qi gates of the body, two laogong (勞宮) located at the centers of the palms, and two yongquan (湧泉) cavities, located at the bottoms of the feet. This will provide you with a strong root and the balance of energy needed for power manifestation.

To master the skills required in soft martial styles. In soft martial skills, the capability of listening (*ting*, 聽), adhering (*nian*, 黏), following (*sui*, 隨), connecting (*lian*, 連), coiling (*chan*, 纏), rotating (*zhuan*, 轉), and spiraling (*chan jin*, 纏進 and *luo xuan*, 螺旋) are extremely important. To many internal styles, these skills are the core essences of the arts. Through taiji ball qigong practice, you will be able to learn and master these skills, especially when practicing with a partner.

Notes

1. 『內家由內而外，外家由外而內。其途雖異，其終的則同。』

2. *Great Dictionary of Chinese Wushu* (中國武術大辭典), People's Athletic Publications (人民體育出版社), 1990.

3. *The Root of Chinese Qigong–The Secrets of Qigong Training*, Dr. Yang, Jwing-Ming, YMAA Publication Center, Boston, 1989.

4. *Qigong–The Secret of Youth*, Dr. Yang, Jwing-Ming, YMAA Publication Center, Boston, 1989.

CHAPTER 4
Theory of Taiji Ball Qigong
(太極球氣功之理論)

4.1 Introduction (介紹)

The theoretical foundation of taiji ball qigong is based on the theory and philosophy of taiji (太極). From this theory, practices were developed. In order to understand the root of taiji ball qigong training, you must first understand the meaning of taiji in taiji ball qigong.

In the next section, we will define taiji and summarize important theoretical concepts. In section 4.3, the theory of physical conditioning in taiji ball qigong will be explained. The interpretation of inner qi's cultivation will be given in section 4.4. Section 4.5 will introduce martial arts grand qi circulation. Finally, at the conclusion of this chapter, a list of other benefits, which taiji ball qigong can bring you, will be summarized in section 4.6 and 4.7.

4.2 What is Taiji in Taiji Ball Qigong? (太極球氣功之太極)

4.2.1 About Taiji (太極說)

Changes, "Great Biography" said:

"The ancestor surnamed Bao-Xi had become the king of heaven and earth. (He) looked up to see the phenomenal (changes) of the heavens, looked down to observe the (natural) rules (i.e., patterns) of the earth, watched the (instinctive) behaviors of birds and animals and how they were situated with (i.e., related to) the earth. Near, (he) observed the (changes) of things around him and far, (he) observed the (repeating patterns of) objects, then (he) created the 'eight trigrams.' This was thus used to understand the virtue of the divine (i.e., natural spirit or natural rules) and also thus used to resemble (i.e., classify, pattern, or understand) the behaviors of millions of objects (i.e., lives)." From this, (we) can see that the creation of the 'eight trigrams' was based on the ceaselessly repeating cycles of great nature, following the instinctive behaviors of the million objects (i.e., lives) between heaven and earth.

《易・大傳》曰：「古者包義氏之玉天下也。仰則觀象於天，俯則觀法於地。觀鳥獸之文，與地之宜，近取諸身，遠取諸物。於是始作八卦，所以通神明之德，所以類萬物之情。」由是可知八卦之作乃始於大自然循環不已之理，遵天地萬物之情。

The quotation in this paragraph is from the "Great Biography" section of *The Book of Changes*. Bao-Xi (包羲) was the ancient ruler in China (2852–2737 B.C.). After he observed the cyclical patterns of nature and the instinctive behavior of animals, he created the "eight trigrams" (*bagua*, 八卦). From the eight trigrams, natural cyclical patterns can be classified, traced, and predicted. Since animals and humans are part of nature, the eight trigrams can also be used to interpret an event and predict its possible consequences in the future.

Changes, "Series Diction," said:

(In) changes, there is taiji. This therefore, produces liangyi (i.e., two polarities), Liangyi generates sixiang (i.e., four phases), and sixiang bears bagua (i.e., eight trigrams). (From) bagua, good or bad luck can be defined (i.e., calculated or predicted). (From) good or bad luck, the great accomplishment can be achieved." It again said: "What is liangyi (i.e., two polarities)? (It is) one yin and one yang.

Lao Zi, in Chapter 24, also said:

Dao generates one, one produces two, two yields three, and three yields millions of objects." From this (we) can see that it is due to the natural rules of taiji, that wuji (i.e., no extremity) evolves into yin and yang two polarities. From yin and yang's generation two polarities, the four phases are generated, and subsequently, from yin and yang's generation of the four phases, the eight trigrams are formalized. From this (we) can figure out that "one yin and one yang is called Dao." This also means that the Book of Changes *is the (book which describes) the consistent natural laws that apply to the universe and the human body. From interaction of yin and yang, millions of objects are generated. From the variations of yin and yang, millions of affairs are communicative (i.e., exchangeable). Therefore,* Changes, *Series Diction also said: "To close means kun and to open means qian, one closes and one opens means variations. To and fro exchange from each other ceaselessly means communicative (i.e., exchangeable)." What is kun? It is yin. What is qian? It is yang.*

《易‧系辭》曰：〝易有太極，是生兩儀。兩儀生四象，四象生八卦，八卦定吉凶，吉凶生大業。〞又曰〝兩儀者，一陰一陽也。〞《老子‧四十二章》亦曰：〝道生一，一生二，二生三，三生萬物。〞如是可知，因自然太極之理，無極衍化生為陰陽兩儀。由兩儀之陰陽衍化，四象而生。再由四象陰陽之衍化，八卦而成。由此可推，〝一陰一陽謂之道，〞亦即易經即宇宙人身互古一致之律。由陰陽之交媾，萬物生。由陰陽之變，萬事通。因之，《易‧系辭》又曰：〝闔戶謂之坤，辟戶謂之乾，一闔一辟謂之變，往來不窮謂之通。〞坤者，陰也；乾者，陽也。

Changes, "Series Diction" (易‧系辭), was written by Zhou Wen Wang (周文王), the first ruler of the Zhou dynasty (周朝) (1122–255 B.C.). He wrote an interpretation for *The Book of Changes*. In his book, he clearly pointed out that because of the existence of taiji (太極) (i.e., grand ultimate), there are changes in the universe. Taiji is an invisible force or power which makes the wuji (無極) (i.e., no extremity) divide into two polarities (i.e., yin and yang) and also from two polarities return back to the wuji state.

Moreover, due to the existence of the taiji, two polarities can again be divided into four phases and from four phases into eight trigrams. The explanation of this kind of natural derivation has also been found in Lao Zi's *Dao De Jing* (老子 · 道德經). *Dao De Jing* (道德經) has also commonly been called "Lao Zi" (老子) in Chinese society. Lao Zi explained that due to the existence of Dao, one is created. In addition, one can create two, and then three, and so on, until millions of objects exist. From this, we can see that taiji is the same as Dao. That is why it is said: "What is taiji? It is the Dao" (何謂 太極？道也。).

Furthermore, from yin and yang's mutual interaction and exchange, millions of objects can be differentiated. For example, the soil interacts with water and sunshine to produce growing plants. It is a study of the need of animals to consume other life in order to survive. Finally, animals die and return to the soil. All of these natural cycles are due to the natural exchanges and interaction of yin and yang.

What is wuji? It means the insubstantial emptiness or an infinitesimal point of space, not big or small (i.e., no dimension), no yin or yang. Through taiji's pivotal action, yin and yang two polarities are divided. Thus, the yin-yang symbol is formalized. This symbol can then be again distinguished as yang yin-yang symbol and yin yin-yang symbol depending on how the four phases of yin and yang are demonstrated (e.g., four seasons) through cycling. For example, if we demonstrate it with our right hand, the clockwise direction of cycling is classified as yang symbol while the counterclockwise direction of cycling is classified as yin. However, if we demonstrate it with our left hand, then everything is reversed. This is simply because generally our right hand is classified as yang while left hand is classified as yin.

無極者乃空空虛虛者或為太空之一小微點，無大無小，無陰無陽。由
太極之動機陰陽兩儀因之分別。由之，陰陽圖現。根據陰陽如何運轉
而演化成四象之方向，此陰陽圖可再區分為陽陰陽圖與陰陰陽圖。譬
如我等以右手例，右旋為陽，左旋為陰。然而，如我等以左手為例，
則一切反向矣。亦即左旋為陽，右旋為陰。這是因為一般而言，右手
為陽，左手為陰也。

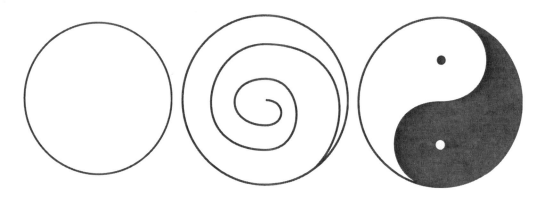

Figure 4-1. Wuji state   Figure 4-2. Taiji state   Figure 4-3. Yin-Yang state (two poles or polarities)

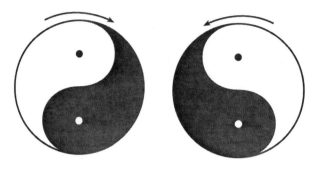

Figure 4-4. Rotations of yin-yang symbol (right hand)

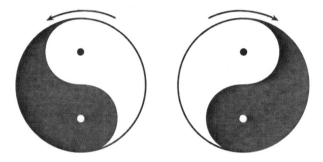

Figure 4-5. Rotations of yin-yang symbol (left hand)

Wuji (無極) is a state of emptiness or simply a single point in space (Figure 4-1). There is no discrimination and there are no polarities (or poles). According to *Yi Jing* (i.e., *Book of Changes*), originally the universe was in a wuji state. Later, due to the pivotal action of taiji (Figure 4-2), two polarities (*liang yi*, 兩儀) (i.e., yin and yang) were discriminated (Figure 4-3). However, we should understand that yin and yang are not definite (or absolute) but relative according to specifically defined rules. From these rules, four phases (*si xiang*, 四象) are again derived. From different perspectives, the yin-yang two polarities can again be divided into yin and yang. For example, if you use your right hand to follow the yin and yang pattern, the clockwise cycling belongs to yang while the counterclockwise cycling belongs to yin (Figure 4-4). Generally speaking, your right hand action is classified as yang and your left hand action is classified as yin. From this rule, the yin-yang cycling will be completely reversed if you use your left hand (Figure 4-5). These general rules are applied in taijiquan and also in other internal styles such as baguazhang.

The description above depicts the yin-yang's derivation in two dimensions. When this yin-yang derivation is manifested in three dimensions, then right spiral to advance forward is classified as yang, while left spiral to withdraw is classified as yin. Similarly, the manifestation of the left hand is reversed. From this, we can see that (if we are) able to comprehend the theory of great nature's yin-yang spiral derivation, then (we) will be able to comprehend the function of the Dao and use this Dao to understand the theory of ceaseless recycling of millions of lives in nature, furthermore, to trace back the origin of our human and physical life. The purpose of learning taiji ball qigong is to aim for the comprehension of taiji and yin-yang so (we) are able to reach the Dao, therefore, (allows us) to protect (our body), strengthen (our body), and enjoy longevity. Furthermore, by nourishing and cultivating (our) human nature, (we are) able to reach the final goal of unification of heaven and human spirit.

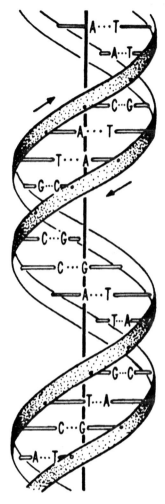

以上所言為陰陽圖在二度空間中之演化。當此
陰陽圖在三度空間演化時，再以右手為例，右
螺旋形而進者為陽，左螺旋形而退者為陰。同
理，左手反之。此為太空中無窮生機變化之
理，萬物賴之而衍生和轉化。因之，能理解此
大自然陰陽螺旋變化之理，即能通乎道機並利
用此道機去瞭解自然萬物生息不已之理，並可
追朔己身性命之來由。習太極球氣功之目的，
乃求此太極陰陽之理解，以臻保身、強身、長
生之道，並由養性、修性晉而達天人合一之地
也。

Figure 4-6. Double helix of DNA

From the above discussion, you can see that there are some specific rules that apply when you manifest the yin-yang polarities into two dimensions. However, we exist in a universe of at least three dimensions. Therefore, the concept of two polarities should be adapted to three dimensions so we can comprehend the natural Dao thoroughly. Once you add the third dimension to the yin and yang symbols, you can see that the energy patterns and derivation are spiral actions. When nature loses its balance, the energy manifests in spirals and millions of lives are influenced, or even created. These manifestations can be seen from galaxies in space, to tornados and other storms, to the formation of seashells, and even the tiny, twisted strands of our DNA (Figure 4-6).

From the above discussion, you can see that when yin-yang is manifested in two dimensions in taiji ball qigong, it is an action of coiling, and when it is acting in three dimensions, it is a spiraling maneuver. If you use your right hand to generate this spiral motion, then the clockwise and forward motion is classified as yang while the counterclockwise and backward motion is classified as yin (Figure 4-7). If you use your left hand, since the left is classified as yin, all directions are reversed (Figure 4-8). This is a method to practice the basic skills in taiji ball qigong for changing from insubstantial to substantial and back again. All action in taiji ball qigong originates from the real

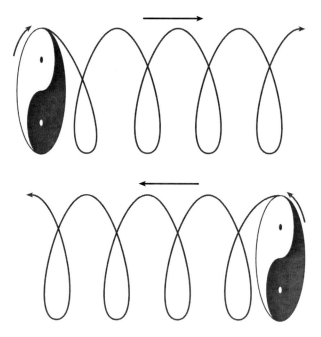

Figure 4-7. Spiral motion (right hand)

dan tian (a point, center of gravity), where the wuji is located. From this wuji center, through taiji (i.e., mind) the qi is led, Yin and yang spiraling actions are initiated, and taiji ball qigong movements are derived.

The creation of taiji ball qigong was based on the above philosophies of taiji and yin-yang. It is believed that from understanding the theory of taiji and yin-yang, we will be able to trace back the origin of our lives. Also, through this understanding, we will be able to train our bodies correctly, maintain the health and strength of our physical and mental bodies, and gain longevity. Since Daoists are monks, the final goal of their spiritual cultivation is to reunite with the natural spirit (*tian ren he yi,* 天人合一) (i.e., the state of wuji). In order to reach this goal, they must cultivate their human nature and nourish it (i.e., discipline their temperament).

4.2.2 *The Meaning of Taiji in Taiji Ball Qigong* (太極在太極球氣功中之義)
Wang, Zong-yue said:

What is taiji? It is generated from wuji, and is a pivotal function of movement and stillness. It is the mother of yin and yang. When it moves it divides. At rest it reunites." *From this, it is known that taiji is not wuji, and is also not yin and yang. Instead an inclination of the natural pivotal function which makes the wuji derive into yin and yang also makes the yin and yang reunite into the state of wuji. This natural pivotal function of movement and stillness is called the 'Dao' or the 'rule' of great nature.*

王宗岳云：「太極者，無極而生，動靜之機，陰陽之母也。動之則分，靜之則合。」由此可知太極並非無極，亦非陰陽，而是自然之機驅使無極演化為陰陽或陰陽復合為無極之勢。此自然動靜之機，即所謂道或大自然之理。

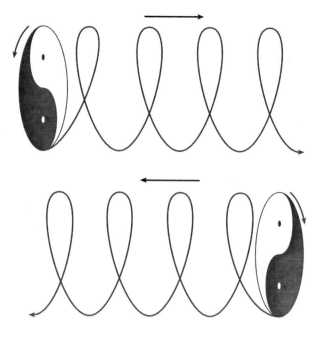

Figure 4-8. Spiral motion (left hand)

Wang, Zong-yue was a renowned taijiquan master who was born in Shan-You, Shanxi Province (山右，山西省), during the Chinese Qing Qian Long period (清乾隆) (A.D. 1736–1796). Taiji (太極) can be translated as "grand ultimate," or "grand extremity," and wuji (無極) is translated as "without ultimate," "without limit," or "no extremity." Wuji can also mean "no opposition." This means wuji is uniform and undifferentiated, a point in space or at the center of your physical, mental, and energetic bodies. For example, at the beginning of the universe, there was no differentiation, and this state was called wuji. Then it began its separation into complementary opposites, called yin (陰) and yang (陽). From the interaction of yin and yang, all things are created and grow.

Even though the theory of taiji (太極) originated from the *Yi Jing* (易經) (*The Book of Changes*) and has been studied and practiced for more than four thousand years in China, its applications in martial arts probably did not begin until several thousand years later. When taiji theory was adopted into the taiji ball qigong training in martial arts society, it significantly improved the health and martial aspect of martial artists. If we wish to understand the real meaning of taiji ball qigong practice, the first task is to comprehend the meaning of taiji.

From Wang, Zong-yue's statement, it is clear that taiji is neither wuji nor yin-yang, but is between them. It is the pivotal force or energy that causes the wuji state to divide into the yin and yang (i.e., two polarities) and also causes the yin-yang to reunite to the state of wuji (Figure 4-9). This natural pivotal force, energy, or function is called "taiji" (太極), "Dao" (道) (i.e., natural way), or "li" (理) (i.e., natural rules) of nature.

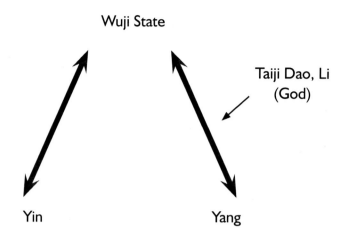

Figure 4-9. The pivotal action of taiji (Dao)

When yin and yang are divided, the two polarities are established. From two polarities, the four phases are generated. From four phases, the eight trigrams (bagua) are produced. Again, from the eight trigrams, sixty-four trigrams are derived, and this pattern continues to divide until unlimited (variations) are produced. Through yin and yang's mutual interaction and correspondence, there are produced thousands of interchanges and millions of derivations, (consequently), millions of objects (i.e., lives) are born. (When) all of this is traced back to its origin there is nothing but the theory of yin and yang. Therefore, those who practice taiji ball qigong must know yin and yang. If (one) wishes to know yin and yang, (he/she) must know the meaning of taiji. If (one) wishes to know the meaning of taiji, (he/she) must first comprehend the Dao and the real meaning of how yin and yang are derived from the wuji state and also how yin and yang return to the wuji state.

陰陽分而兩儀生，由兩儀而生四象，再由四象而生八卦，由八卦再生六十四卦。由此推論，以至無窮。由陰陽之互感互應，千變萬化，萬物衍生。歸其宗，僅陰陽之理而已矣。因此習太極球氣功者，必知陰陽。欲知陰陽，必知太極之義，要知太極之義，必先領悟無極演變至陰陽與陰陽返歸回無極之道與真諦。

Yin and yang, two polarities, originate from wuji through taiji's action or function. From these two polarities, again through taiji's action, four phases are derived. With the same theory, the variations continue until there are unlimited changes in the universe (Figure 4-10). From yin and yang's mutual interaction, millions of lives are born. From this, you can see that all life and all things are produced from the mutual interaction of yin and yang through the mediating function of taiji. Therefore, if you are interested in learning taiji ball qigong, you must understand yin and yang, and their relationship with taiji. Without knowing the theory and the Dao, your taiji ball qigong practice will be limited to the external forms and movements. In this case, you will have lost the real meaning of practicing taiji ball qigong.

Before the action of taiji ball qigong movement, the xin (i.e., emotional mind) is peaceful and the qi is harmonious, the xin and yi (wisdom mind) are at the (real) dan tian and the qi stays in its residence. This is the state of extreme calmness and is the state of wuji. However, when the xin and yi begin to act, the qi's circulation begins, the physical body's movement is thus initiated, and the yin and yang accordingly divides. From this (we) can see that xin and yi are what are called taiji in taiji ball qigong. That means the Dao of taiji ball qigong is the Dao of xin and yi (i.e., minds).

太極球練習起勢在未動之前，心平氣和，心意在丹田，氣守於舍，此極靜之態，是為無極。然者，當心動意動，氣由之引發，身體而動，陰陽始分。由此可知心意在太極球中即所謂太極也。亦即太極球氣功之道即心意之道也。

The wuji state exists inside each of us. It is the state from which all creative impulses grow. Taiji is generated out of wuji and is the mother of yin and yang. Thus, taiji is the cause of the yin and yang division, and is itself neither wuji nor yin and yang, but the cause of the separation of yin and yang. In this sense, it is a part of the divine aspect of the Dao.

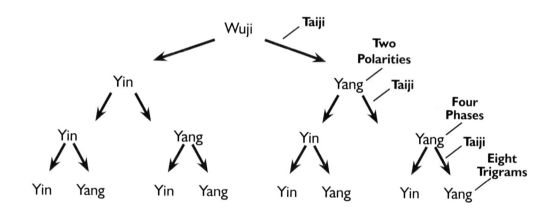

Figure 4-10. The continuous derivations of yin and yang due to taiji's pivotal actions

All objects, ideas, spirits, etc. can be classified as either yin or yang. Taiji ball qigong was created according to this theory. In the beginning posture of the taiji ball qigong practice, the mind is calm and empty, and the weight is evenly distributed on both feet. This state is wuji. When your mind starts to lead the body into the movement, internal (yin) and external (yang) aspects of taiji ball qigong features start to be discriminated. Moreover, the hands and feet are differentiated into insubstantial (yin) and substantial (yang). This is the state of two polarities. Through interaction of substantial (yang) and insubstantial (yin), all of taiji ball qigong moving patterns are generated. From this, you can see that the taiji (i.e., the Dao) in taiji ball qigong is actually the mind. It is the mind that makes the body move and divides the wuji state into yin and yang two polarities. We can conclude from this that taiji ball qigong is actually a qigong practice of the mind (i.e., taiji).

> *Though a human body is bonded between the heaven and the earth, (its) xin and yi are able to reach (anywhere) unlimitedly in the universe without being restricted by time and space. From xin and yi, the yin and yang are initiated and (continue to) move into unlimited variations. This is the theory of millions of divisions and creations of taiji. Therefore, those who practice taiji ball qigong must begin from the (training of) xin and yi.*

人身雖束於天地之間，然心意可達無窮於宇宙，並不為時間、空間所限。由心意，陰陽生而演變分化無窮。此為太極萬象衍生創造之理。因此，學太極氣功者，必須從心意著手。

Though our physical bodies are restricted by our three-dimensional reality, our minds are free to travel and reach anywhere in the universe, or even beyond this universe, unrestricted by time (i.e., the mind is grand ultimate). All human creations, from shovels to airplanes, arose first in our imaginations. From our thoughts, new ideas are created. It is the same for taiji ball qigong. It was created from the mind, and its creation will continue without an end. Since it is an active, living, and creative art, taiji ball qigong is a product of spiritual enlightenment and an understanding of life.

> *Xin (i.e., emotional mind) and yi (i.e., wisdom mind) are contained internally, which belongs to yin. The movements (actions) of taiji ball qigong are manifested externally, which belongs to yang. When the functions of xin and yi are applied to our spiritual feeling, they direct us into the correct Dao of cultivating our human nature through efforts toward strengthening the mind, raise up the spirit to comprehend the real meaning of human life, and from this, further to comprehend the meaning and relationship among humans, between humans and objects around us, and also to search for the truth of nature in heaven and earth. When the function of xin and yi is applied to our physical body, it is the great Dao of cultivating the physical life for self-defense, nourishing the physical life, and strengthening the physical body. This is the foundation for extending our lives and establishing a firm root of health.*

心意者，內含也，陰也。太極球氣功之動作，外顯也，陽也。心意活動於己身之精神內感，即強心、提神、領悟人生之養性正道。由之去瞭解人與人、人與事物關係之真諦並尋求天地自然之真理。心意活動於己身物理之造化，即防身、養生、與強身之修命大道。此為延命立基之本。

As mentioned earlier, xin and yi are the taiji in taiji ball qigong. This internal thinking is yin. When this yin is manifested externally, then yang is demonstrated. When xin and yi are acting on internal spiritual feeling, it serves to cultivate our human temperaments and helps us to understand the meaning of our lives. When xin and yi are acting and manifested externally, it promotes physical health and self-defense.

Therefore, when we practice taiji ball qigong, we should cultivate both our spiritual beings (yin) and train our physical bodies (yang).

Taiji ball qigong originated from the Daoist family. Its ultimate goal is to reach enlightenment and so as to achieve the Dao of unification between heaven and human. Therefore, the final goal of practicing taiji ball qigong is to reach the unified harmonious wuji world (i.e., state) of the heaven and human. From practicing taiji ball qigong, (we are able) to further comprehend the meaning of human life and the universe.

太極球氣功始於道家，其終的在通乎神明以臻天人合一之道。因而習太極球氣功之終的亦即在於天人合一大合諧之無極世界，由習太極球氣功而領悟人生宇宙之理也。

Taiji ball qigong was created in the religious (Daoist) school of qigong. The goal of Daoist cultivation is to reach enlightenment, to unify the human spirit with the natural spirit. This is the wuji harmonious state. To reach this destination, the first step is to appreciate the meaning of life and to understand natural truth.

4.3 Theory of Physical Conditioning (強身之原理)

As explained earlier, taiji ball qigong is able to condition the physical body and change its structure from weak to strong. In addition, it can also increase the quality of endurance of the body. Due to these reasons, taiji ball qigong can be used to enhance fighting capability, and to increase the chance of survival in ancient fighting situations. In this section, we will analyze the theory of how taiji ball qigong can help one to reach these goals. We will discuss this theory by dividing the body into different parts:

4.3.1 Bone Marrow

According to theory of *Muscle/Tendon Changing* and *Brain/Marrow Washing* Qigong (*Yi Jin Jing, Xi Sui Jing*, 易筋經、洗髓經), the qi enters the bone marrow through the joint areas. Whenever the joints are moving, qi will build to a higher potential of storage. When the body relaxes, the qi accumulated will either be dissipated outward through the skin or enter into the bone marrow to nourish it. Since taiji ball qigong focuses on joint exercises, and through the correct breathing technique, the qi can be led inward to the bone marrow effectively. This is the crucial key of slowing aging. If you are interested in knowing more about Muscle/Tendon Changing and Brain/Marrow Washing Qigong, please refer to the book, *Qigong–The Secret of Youth*, published by YMAA Publication Center.

4.3.2 Bone

It is known that the bone is constructed of piezoelectric material.[1] Whenever there is a pressure generated in the bones, there is some electricity (i.e., qi) generated and circulated. This electric circulation is the crucial key of maintaining the bone density and keeping it strong. When you practice taiji ball qigong, due to the constant circular motion or rotation of the heavy ball, the muscles, tendons, and ligaments are constantly stretched and contracted. This generates pressure on the bones and improves the qi's circulation. In addition, due to the low walking stepping, you also condition the legs' physical strength. Naturally, this will also increase the bone density and strength.

4.3.3 Ligaments, Muscles, and Tendons

From practicing the special patterns or routines designed in taiji ball qigong, the entire body's ligaments, muscles, and tendons can be conditioned. At the beginning, a beginner will start with a light ball. When the body has reached a stronger stage, the ball will be exchanged for heavier ones. Through this weight change, the entire body's strength will gradually improve. The entire body's framework can be strengthened.

4.3.4 Internal Organs

Through taiji ball qigong training, the quantity of the qi will be built up and the quality of qi's circulation and manifestation will be improved. When the qi's circulation is abundant and smooth, the internal organs will be conditioned.

4.4 Theory of Inner Qi's Cultivation (內氣培養之理論)

The internal side of taiji ball qigong training includes building up an abundant level of qi in the real lower dan tian (真下丹田) and establishing an efficient way of leading and manifesting the qi. In other words, it emphasizes the quantity of qi and also the quality of qi's manifestation or circulation. However, in order to understand the theory and the practices of these subjects, you must first understand the most fundamental qi structure or two polarities of a human body. We can then discuss how to produce more qi and how to **store** it to an abundant level. Finally, we will review the theory and training methods of qi's manifestation.

4.4.1 Theory of Two Polarities in a Human Body (Ren Shen Liang Yi, 人身兩儀論)

According to Chinese qigong practice, it has been understood that we have a two-pole system, which constitutes a human central energy line. These two polarities, one yin and one yang, synchronize and harmonize with each other. They are just like the polarities of a magnet that cannot be separated. One of the polarities, the upper dan tian (*shang dan tian*, 上丹田), is located at the brain while the other, the real lower dan tian (*zhen xia dan tian*, 真下丹田), is located at the center of gravity (i.e., physical center) area where the human guts (the second brain) are located. The real lower dan tian is the North Pole and it stores qi and supplies it for the functioning of the entire body. The upper dan tian is the South Pole that directs and governs the quality of qi manifestation.

These two polarities are connected by the thrusting vessel (*chong mai*, 衝脈) (i.e., spinal cord), which is constructed of highly conductive tissue. Physically, there are two polarities; however, in function, since these two polarities correspond with each other simultaneously, it is one. Since the construction of our body is influenced by the natural energy, the construction of our body's qi system should also be influenced by the yin-yang theory of nature. Therefore, we should be able to compare our body with the taiji yin-yang symbol.

If you observe the taiji yin-yang symbol closely, you can see that there is a hidden yang fountain (*yang quan*, 陽泉) in the center of the yin water while there is a

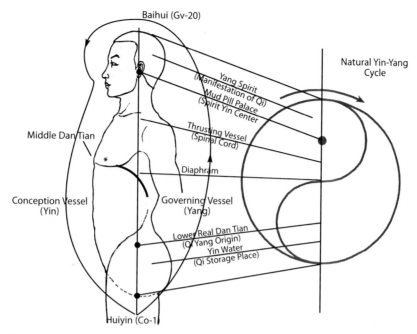

Figure 4-11. The body's yin and yang, and the two polarity centers

concealed yin spirit (*yin shen*, 陰神) in the center of the yang spirit. In fact, in qigong Embryonic Breathing training, you train these two polarity centers of hidden yang and concealed yin. For example, if you are able to keep your mind at the center of the hidden yang in the yin water, the qi at the real lower dan tian will continue to be stored and preserved. It is just like a spring of a fountain that is able to produce water continuously. Not only that, but if you also know how to keep the spirit condensed at its center (concealed yin), then the quality of qi manifestation will reach a higher level of efficiency.

These two concealed polarities, one at the center of the head (Mud Pill Palace) (*ni wan gong*, 泥丸宮) and the other at the center of the gut, though they are two, they function as one. If you are able to keep your mind at these two poles, the spirit and the qi will stay in their residences. This process is called "embracing singularity" (*bao yi*, 抱一).

Here, we would like to compare and summarize the natural taiji yin-yang symbol with the body's yin and yang energy structure. From this comparison, you can easily see through many things that may inspire your qigong pondering and practice. As mentioned earlier, since a human body is a part of nature, qi manifestation in this body should be able to be interpreted by the natural yin-yang symbol (Figure 4-11).

1. The qi circulation along the conception and governing vessels (*ren and du mai*, 任・督脈) is reversed from the natural yin-yang cycle so the yin and yang in the body can be balanced from natural yin and yang. Please refer to the book *Qigong Meditation: Small Circulation Meditation* available from YMAA Publication Center for further discussion.

2. Shen (神) (i.e., spirit) is generally considered as yang. That is why the term "yang shen" (陽神) (yang spirit) is commonly used in Chinese qigong documents. Shen is the general who controls the manifestation of the qi. When shen is high, the qi can be controlled and manifested efficiently and effectively. That means once you are able to raise your shen to a higher level, your vital force will be enhanced. Normally, the raising up of the shen takes place through the baihui (Gv-20, 百會), which is located at the top of the yin-yang symbol, the place of extreme yang. Baihui means "hundred meetings" and implies the meeting place of the entire body's qi. That means it is the pivotal controlling point of the entire body's energy. The baihui is considered as the most yang place of the entire human body.

3. The area located in the real lower dan tian, where it is able to store qi to an abundant level, is called "qi ocean" (*qihai*, 氣海). The qi stored in the real lower dan tian is thus called "yin shui" (陰水), which means "yin water" (Figure 4-12). Huiyin (Co-1, 會陰) (i.e., perineum) is considered as the most yin place in a human body. Huiyin is also commonly called "haidi" (海底) and means "sea bottom." This is because qi is analogous to water, with the large and small intestines as the ocean or qi residence (*qi she*, 氣舍), which is able to store the water (qi). When the qi stays at its residence, the physical body will be calm and peaceful. However, when the qi is led away from its residence for manifestation, then the mind and body will be excited, and the shen will be divergent. In this way, the qi is consumed. The way of maintaining calmness of the mind (and shen) and the physical body is to lead the qi downward. For example, when you are excited, your breathing is shallow and fast, and your body is tensed. In this case, calm your mind, inhale deeply and use your mind to lead the qi downward to the abdominal area, and then exhale while relaxing your mind and physical body. When

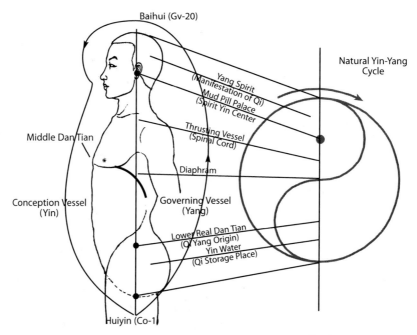

Figure 4-12. The real lower dan tian is called *yin shui* (陰水).

this happens, the body's mental and physical tension will disappear gradually. This is one of the crucial keys to lowering high blood pressure in qigong practice. On the contrary, if you lead the qi upward to the brain, you will be excited and more tensed. Naturally, the blood pressure could also be raised.

4. The body's two polarities, yin and yang, are connected by the thrusting vessel (*chong mai*, 衝脈) (spinal cord). The "spirit yin center" (*shen shi*, 神室) located at the Mud Pill Palace (*ni wan gong*, 泥丸宮) (the site of the pineal and pituitary glands) in the yang spirit (*yang shen*, 陽神) (the brain or upper dan tian), controls and restrains the yang shen's manifestation. This spirit yin center is just like a steering wheel that is able to control the status of the shen's actions. If the shen can stay at this center, then it can be focused and centered. If the shen is away from this center, then it is scattered. When this happens, even if the shen is high, it is not focused. In order to bring the shen to this yin center, first your mind must be calmed. To keep your mind calm, you must avoid any emotional disturbance and desires. This is one of the main focal points in qigong Embryonic Breathing.

The lower site of the two polarities is at the real lower dan tian located at the center of the large and small intestines (second brain). This area acts as a bio-battery, which is able to store the qi (bioelectricity). It is in this area that the food essence is absorbed and converted into energy (qi). In order to keep the qi at its residence, you must also learn how to keep your mind at the qi yang origin (real lower dan tian or center of gravity). Here the qi can be preserved and stored to an abundant level (yang).

5. The real lower dan tian, the bio-battery, produces and stores the qi, and is thus able to increase the quantity of the qi and supply it to the body and brain for their function. However, the upper dan tian center (spirit yin center) controls the quality of the qi's manifestation (Figure 4-13). From the

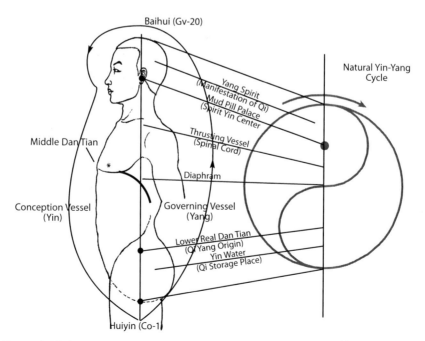

Figure 4-13. Upper dan tian center or spirit yin center (*shen shi*, 神室).

girdle vessel (extreme yang vessel) and thrusting vessel (extreme yin vessel), it forms a "spiritual cultivation triangle" (Figure 4-14). The more abundant the storage of qi (strong guardian qi), the higher the shen can be raised. The base of the triangle represents physical life, while the height of the centerline represents spiritual life. When you have abundant qi (i.e., strong and healthy physical life) and a high level of spiritual cultivation, the heaven eye (*tian yan*, 天眼) (i.e., the third eye) can be re-opened.

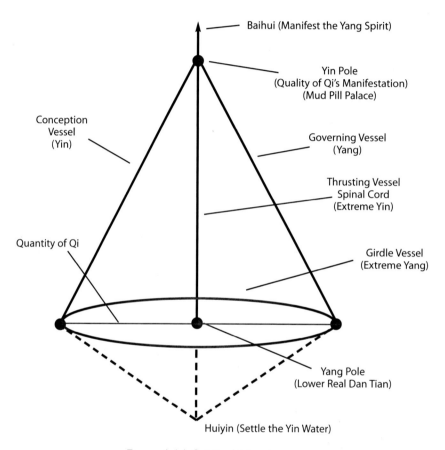

Figure 4-14. Spiritual triangle

Amazingly, the above theory of two polarities in humans has matched a scientific discovery made in 1996. According to an article in *The New York Times*, a human being has two brains.[2,3] One brain is in the head, and the other is in the gut (i.e., the digestive system). Though these two brains are separated physically, through the connection of the spinal cord (high electrically conductive tissue) (thrusting vessel, 衝脈), they actually function as one (Figure 4-15).

This article explains that the upper brain is able to think and has memory. It is able to store data, utilizing electrochemical charges. The lower brain has memory, but does not have the capability of thought. This discovery offers confirmation of the Chinese

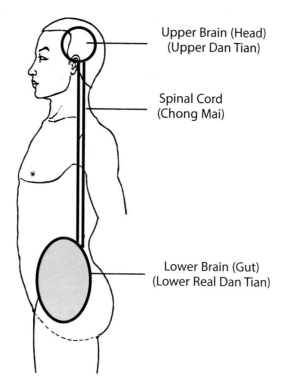

Upper Brain (Head)
(Upper Dan Tian)

Spinal Cord
(Chong Mai)

Lower Brain (Gut)
(Lower Real Dan Tian)

Figure 4-15. Two polarities (brains) of a human body

belief that the real lower dan tian (large and small intestines) is able to store qi, while the upper dan tian governs thinking and directs the qi. Theoretically speaking, if the upper brain is able to think, then it should be able to generate an electromotive force (EMF) while the lower brain should have a large capacity for storing the charge. In other words, the lower brain is the human battery in which the life force resides. Once the brain has generated a thought (EMF), the charge will immediately be directed from the lower brain, through the spinal cord and nervous system to the desired area in order to activate the physical body for function.[4]

According to Ohm's Law in Physics,

$$\Delta V = I R$$

Where ΔV is potential difference or EMF, I is current, and R is resistance.[5]

From this formula, we can see that if R is a constant, then the higher the potential, or EMF, the stronger will be the current that is generated. If we assume that the resistance of our body remains constant, then the more we are able to concentrate (higher EMF), the stronger the qi flow will be. This parallels the Chinese qigong concept that **the more you concentrate, the stronger the qi can be led.** From Chinese qigong, higher levels of concentration can be trained through still meditation. In addition, if we assume the EMF to be constant, that means the mind's concentration remains the same. Then, the lower the R (resistance), the higher the current flow will be. According to past qigong experiences, the more you are relaxed (i.e., lower resistance), the more qi (current) can flow.

Next, we would like to discuss the conditioning of the bio-battery (real lower dan tian), which is followed by methods of increasing qi quantity.

4.4.2 Conditioning the Bio-battery (Real Lower Dan Tian) (Zhen Xia Dan Tian Zhi Gai Liang, 真下丹田之改良)

From the ancient classics, *Muscle/Tendon Changing* and *Marrow/Brain Washing* Qigong (*Yi Jin Jing, Xi Sui Jing*, 易筋經,洗髓經), it is recognized that the most efficient way of conditioning this bio-battery (false and real lower dan tians) is through massage and stimulation. Massage gets rid of the fat hidden within so the circulation can be smoother, and stimulation will condition the sensitivity of the nerves in the area so they are able to handle and store a larger quantity of qi. The entire conditioning process is long and needs a great deal of training and patience. You must understand the theory behind the conditioning clearly. It is impossible to explain the entire conditioning process here. If you wish to know more about this training, please refer to the book *Qigong–The Secret of Youth*, available from YMAA Publication Center.

4.4.3 Increase the Quantity of Qi (Qi Liang Zhi Jia Qiang, 氣量之加強)

We have already discussed the methods of how to increase the quantity of qi to its abundant level in Chapter 2. We will now briefly summarize these methods. Please review Chapter 2 for detail.

There are various ways of producing extra qi at the lower dan tian. For example, you may use herbs to increase the quantity of qi in the body. You may also use massage methods to convert the fat at the lower dan tian area into qi. You may also use the abdomen's up-and-down movements with the coordination of breathing.

When using herbs, you must find the herbal stores that have all the ingredients required. However, it is not easy to find these herbs other than in Asia (i.e., Taiwan, Hong Kong, and China). Even then, some special ingredients may not be available because they are seldom requested. The cost of the herbs can be very high.

If you use massage methods, you will need a massage partner. In addition, both of you must know the correct massage techniques and also how to regulate the power used at each step of the process. If you use breathing techniques, you must also know the how and why, so your practice can be effective without causing problems. If you wish to know more about using the herbal prescriptions and massage methods to increase the quantity of qi, please refer to the book *Qigong–The Secret of Youth*, available from YMAA Publication Center.

In Chapter 2, we discussed two known breathing methods that can be used to increase the quantity of qi in your body. These are two methods that were commonly used by Buddhist and Daoist monks in the past. As long as you practice patiently and know the theory, with these two methods you will be able to convert the fat stored at the abdominal area into the extra qi in your body. The theories of these two breathing methods have been introduced in previous chapters. They are normal abdominal breathing (*zheng fu hu xi*, 正腹呼吸) (Buddhist breathing) or reverse abdominal breathing (*fan, ni fu hu xi*, 反 · 逆腹呼吸) (Daoist breathing).

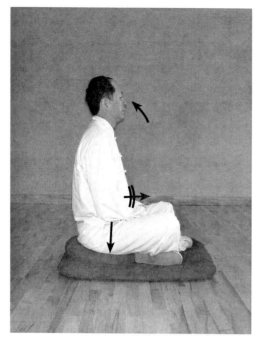

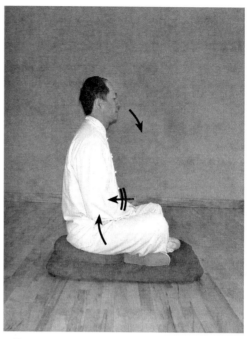

Figure 4-16. Normal Abdominal Breathing (Inhalation)

Figure 4-17. Normal Abdominal Breathing (Exhalation)

Normal Abdominal Breathing (Buddhist Breathing) (*Zheng Fu Hu Xi,* 正腹呼吸) (*Fo Jia Hu Xi,* 佛家呼吸). In normal abdominal breathing, when you inhale, the abdomen is gently pushed out, and when you exhale, the abdomen is withdrawn (Figures 4-16 and 4-17). In order to fill up the qi to an abundant level in the lower abdominal area, (elixir furnace or elixir field) (丹爐；丹田), when you inhale, you should also gently push out your huiyin (Co-1) cavity (or perineum), and when you exhale, you hold it up gently. When you do so, you are converting the food essence (fat) into qi through the abdominal movements. Not only that, through the movements of the abdomen and the huiyin cavity the original essence (*yuan jing,* 元精) (hormone) in the pancreas (islets of Langerhans) and gonads (sex glands) will also be produced. Remember, you should not tense the huiyin during either inhalation or exhalation, unless you are doing some special training such as hard qigong.

After you have practiced for a few weeks, you will start to experience some warm feeling and even some trembling at the abdominal area. This signals the increase of the qi in this area.

As a beginner, you should practice normal abdominal breathing for at least six months until your mind is able to control the muscles around the abdominal area efficiently. This kind of breathing is relaxing and natural and so will not cause any troublesome tension at the stomach area.

Reverse Abdominal Breathing (Daoist Breathing) (*Fan Fu Hu Xi,* 反腹呼吸) (*Ni Fu Hu Xi,* 逆腹呼吸) (*Dao Jia Hu Xi,* 道家呼吸). After you have practiced normal abdominal breathing for at least six months, then you may proceed to reverse abdominal breathing. In reverse abdominal breathing, when you inhale, the abdomen

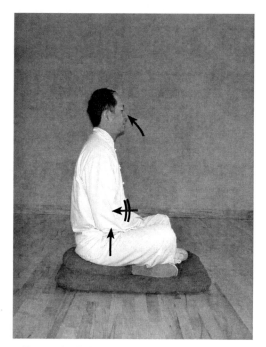
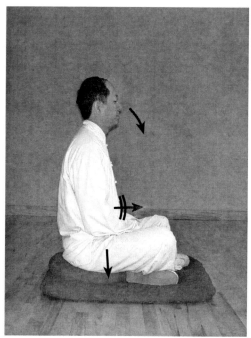

Figure 4-18. Reverse Abdominal Breathing (Inhalation)

Figure 4-19. Reverse Abdominal Breathing (Exhalation)

is gently pulled inward, and when you exhale, the abdomen is gently pushed outward (Figures 4-18 and 4-19). Again, the coordination of the huiyin (Co-1) cavity (perineum) is very important. The huiyin cavity is a major gate that regulates the four yin vessels and therefore controls the qi status of the body. Traditionally, a master would not reveal this secret of huiyin control to any student until he was completely trusted by the master. Again, you should not tense the huiyin area during either inhalation or exhalation unless you are doing some special training such as hard qigong.

Often, a qigong or martial arts beginner encounters the problem of tightness in the abdominal area. The reason for this is that in reverse abdominal breathing, when you inhale, the diaphragm is pulling downward while the abdominal area is withdrawing. This can generate tension in the stomach area. To reduce this problem, you must already have mastered the skill of normal abdominal breathing and be able to control the abdominal muscles efficiently, or you may start on a small scale with reverse abdominal breathing; and only once you can control the abdominal muscles efficiently, should you then increase to a larger scale of abdominal movement. Naturally, this will take time. If you experience any tension, gently massage the abdominal area to disperse any stagnant energy.

4.4.4 Improving Quality of Qi's Manifestation

Next, we would like to discuss how the quality of qi's circulation or manifestation can be improved. First, we should recognize thatfrom Chinese martial art history, it was not until the fifth century that Chinese internal styles were developed, recognized, and practiced.

The most influential person in this practice was the Indian monk Da Mo (達摩). Da Mo, whose last name was Sardili (沙地利) and who was also known as Bodhidarma, was once the prince of a small tribe in southern India. He was of the Mahayana school of Buddhism and was considered by many to have been a bodhisattva, or an enlightened being, who had renounced nirvana in order to save others. From the fragments of historical records, it is believed that he was born about A.D. 483.

Da Mo was invited to China to preach by the Liang Wu emperor (梁武帝). He arrived in Canton, China, in A.D. 527 during the reign of the Wei Xiao Ming emperor (魏孝明帝) (A.D. 16–528) or the Liang Wu emperor (梁武帝) (A.D. 02–557). When the emperor decided he did not like Da Mo's Buddhist theory, the monk withdrew to the Shaolin Temple. When Da Mo arrived, he saw that the priests were weak and sickly, so he shut himself away to ponder the problem. When he emerged after nine years of seclusion, he wrote two classics: *Muscle/Tendon Changing Classic* (*Yi Jin Jing*, 易筋經) and *Marrow/Brain Washing Classic* (*Xi Sui Jing*, 洗髓經).

The *Yi Jin Jing* taught the priests how to build their qi to an abundant level and use it to improve health and change their physical bodies from weak to strong. After the priests practiced the *Yi Jin Jing* exercises, they found that not only did they improve their health,but they also greatly increased their strength. When this training was integrated into the martial arts forms, it increased the effectiveness of their martial techniques. This change marked one more step in the growth of the Chinese martial arts: martial arts qigong.

The *Xi Sui Jing* taught the priests how to use qi to clean their bone marrow and strengthen their immune systems, as well as how to nourish and energize the brain, helping them to attain Buddhahood. The *Xi Sui Jing* was difficult to understand and practice because the training methods were passed down secretly to very few disciples in each generation. Da Mo died in the Shaolin Temple in A.D. 536 and was buried on Xiong Er Mountain (熊耳山). If you are interested in knowing more about *Yi Jin Jing* and *Xi Sui Jing*, please refer to the book, *Qigong–The Secret of Youth*, published by YMAA Publication Center.

From Da Mo's muscle/tendon changing theory, it has been understood that in order to condition your physical body to a higher level, you must "use the mind to lead the qi and from qi's manifestation, the power and strength are initiated and conditioned." Therefore:

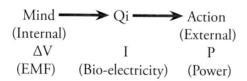

From this, you can see that in order to manifest your qi to a higher efficiency, you must know how to regulate your mind to a higher concentration. It has been experienced and understood that meditation is the way to reach this goal.

This theory had divided Chinese martial training into two major fields. One was from internal to external (i.e., internal styles) and one was from external to internal (i.e., external styles). The internal stylists believed that in order to improve the efficiency of fighting power, they should begin with internal mind training. However, the external stylists believed that they must first learn defensive techniques to survive, and then gradually enter into internal mind conditioning. In Chinese martial arts society, there is a proverb: "Internal styles from internal to external, external styles from external to internal. Though the paths are different, both reach the same goal."[6]

Let's review Ohm's Law.

$$\Delta V = I\,R \qquad\qquad P = I^2 R$$

ΔV: Potential Difference or EMF
I: Current
R: Resistance
P: Power

In order to increase the power of qi's manifestation, we must have an abundant and smooth qi circulation. Since I (i.e., current) is proportional to ΔV (i.e., mind), it is understood that if the mind is stronger and more focused, the qi's circulation will be more fluent and abundant. Not only that, the power will be significantly increased since power is proportional to I2. From the formula, it can also be seen that since I is in reverse proportion to R (i.e., resistance), then if we are able to reduce R, the circulation of I can also be improved significantly. The way of reducing R is relaxation of the physical body.

Therefore, the quality of qi's manifestation depends on how the mind can be focused and also how deep the physical body can be relaxed. To know more about how to regulate your mind, please refer to the book *Qigong Meditation–Embryonic Breathing*. To learn how to relax your physical body, please refer to the book *The Root of Chinese Qigong*. Both are available from YMAA Publication Center. The result of this mind training is to make the mind more focused and this will result in the increased sensitivity. This means the entire body's awareness and alertness will be increased. This is the crucial key of surviving in a battle.

4.5 Martial Grand Qi Circulation (武學大周天)

To apply the taiji ball qigong into martial arts and health effectively, a practitioner should learn and understand martial grand qi circulation. If he does not apply this circulation technique into the taiji ball qigong practice, the qi led will be weak. Naturally, the manifestation of qi will not be as strong as well. This martial grand qi circulation training was commonly kept as top secret in all Chinese martial styles. If the opponent knew this secret, he would have the same advantage in manifesting his fighting power to its maximum.

Grand qi circulation (*da zhou tian*, 大周天) is an advanced qigong qi circulation practice. From this practice, a practitioner learns how to exchange the qi with surrounding objects. These objects can be common non-living objects, such as the air, ground, or taiji ball. They can also be of things alive such as trees, grass, animals, or humans. In this section, we will only discuss the theory and techniques, which are applied in martial arts grand circulation. If you are interested in knowing more about this subject, please refer to my book *Qigong Meditation–Grand Circulation*, available from YMAA Publication Center.

Taiji ball qigong adopts martial grand qi circulation techniques. This is because taiji ball qigong was created and developed in martial arts society in which the original purpose of the training was to improve fighting capability. From taiji ball grand qi circulation training, a practitioner is able to communicate and exchange his qi with the ball and also with a partner through the ball.

To understand martial grand circulation, you should understand the concepts of a human's two polarities connected by the thrusting vessel (*chong mai*, 衝脈) (i.e., spinal cord), and you should also know the body's seven pairs of corresponding gates (*qi dui xue*, 七對穴).

4.5.1 Seven Pairs of Corresponding Qi Gates (Qi Dui Xue, 七對穴)

The human body has seven major pairs of corresponding qi gates from which its qi structure is constituted: 1. huiyin (Co-1, 會陰) and baihui (Gv-20, 百會); 2. yintang (m-hn-3, 印堂) and qiangjian (Gv-17, 強間) [or naohu (Gv-18, 腦戶)]; 3. renzhong (Gv-26, 人中) and fengfu (Gv-16, 風府); 4. tiantu (Co-22, 天突) and dazhui (Gv-14, 大椎); 5. jiuwei (Co-15, 鳩尾) and lingtai (Gv-10, 靈臺); 6. yinjiao (Co-7, 陰交) and mingmen (Gv-4, 命門); and 7. longmen (m-ca-24, 龍門) [or xiayin (下陰)] and changqiang (Gv-1, 長強) [or weilu (尾閭)]. Among these seven, the two pairs that are the most important are huiyin (yin) and baihui (yang), and yinjiao (yin) and mingmen (yang). Huiyin is connected to baihui through the thrusting vessel, which establishes the central balance of qi distribution in the body. Yinjiao is also connected to mingmen through the thrusting vessel and joins the conception vessel in the front and the governing vessel in the back, providing front and rear qi balance to the body. These four are the main qi gates (Figure 4-20).

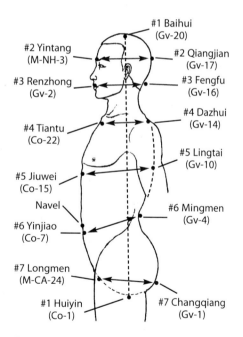

Figure 4-20. Seven pairs of corresponding gates

Tiantu controls vocal vibrations and generates the sounds of hen (哼, *yin*) and ha (哈, *yang*) for manifestation of qi. It is a gate of expression, and its energy is balanced with yintang, where the spirit resides. When spirit is high in yintang, the energy manifested is strong, and alertness and awareness are high. Jiuwei and lingtai connect to the heart (emotional mind) and offer a strong driving force to elevate the spirit. These four minor gates control manifestation of qi in the body. So the eight gates are defined. If you wish to know more about qi gates, please refer to the book, *Qigong Meditation–Small Circulation*, available from YMAA Publication Center.

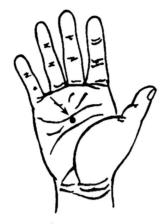

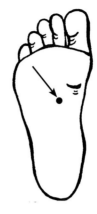

Figure 4-21. The laogong (P-8) cavity

Figure 4-22. The yongquan (K-1) cavity

4.5.2 *Four Gates Breathing Grand Circulation* (四心呼吸大周天靜坐)

The purpose of Four Gates Breathing is to lead qi from the real lower dan tian to the four gates. Two of these gates, called laogong (P-8, 勞宮), which means labor's palace, belong to the pericardium channel and are located at the center of each palm (Figure 4-21). The other two gates are called yongquan (K-1, 湧泉), which means gushing spring. They belong to the kidney channel and are located at the front center of the soles (Figure 4-22).

These four cavities are the main gates which regulate the qi level of the heart and kidneys. When qi flows smoothly to them, the body is healthy, and great power is generated in the limbs. Four gates meditation is emphasized in Chinese martial arts, especially in the internal arts. It has been discussed at length in the YMAA books *The Essence of Taiji Qigong* and *The Essence of Shaolin White Crane.*

4.5.3 *Spiritual Breathing (Shen Xi,* 神息)

Spiritual breathing is also called Fifth Gate Breathing (*Di Wu Xin Hu Xi,* 第五心呼吸), baihui breathing (*baihui hu xi,* 百會呼吸), or upper dan tian breathing (*shang dan tian hu xi,* 上丹田呼吸). It means to breathe through the third eye and is crucial in opening the third eye for enlightenment.

Reaching the level of spiritual breathing presupposes regulating your body, breathing, mind, and qi, and now the spirit. Your qigong practice and the search for spiritual enlightenment have reached the final stage and are approaching maturity. According to *The Complete Book of Principal Contents of Life and Human Nature* (性命圭旨全書), "What is spiritual breathing? It means the maturity of cultivation."[7] That means cultivating the interaction of kan and li has reached the stage of regulating without regulating, and all the cultivations have become natural. We will discuss this subject further in the forthcoming books on the subjects of qigong meditation and spiritual enlightenment.

4.5.4 *Five Gates Breathing* (五心息)

Five Gates Breathing means that, after (you have) regulated the Four Gates Breathing to the point that regulating is unnecessary, then (you) add the fifth gate's breathing. The first possible fifth gate is the baihui. The baihui cavity connects to the huiyin through the chong mai (i.e., thrusting vessel). The chong mai is what is called the spinal cord and is made of electrically highly conductive material. Therefore, though the baihui and the huiyin are located in two different places, their functions are connected and act as one. The huiyin is the most yin place in the entire body, while the baihui is the residence of the yang-shen (i.e., yang spirit) and is the most yang place in the entire body. The huiyin is the yin meeting place of the four yin vesselsconception, thrusting, yin heel, and yin linking vessels and is the key controlling gate of the entire body's yin and yang. To qi practitioners, it is the secret gate for leading qi. When the huiyin is held upward, the huiyin gate is closed and the body's qi is condensed inward into the bone marrow, the spirit is converged and the qi is gathered, the entire body turns yin, and consequently, the jin is stored. Conversely, when the huiyin is pushed out, the huiyin gate is opened, qi is released from the four yin vessels, the yang spirit is raised up, the entire body turns yang, and consequently, the jin is emitted. One stores and one emits; this is the key cycle of the internal jin's storing and emitting.

五心息者，在四心息調至不調而自調之境地時，即加添第五心之息。第五心者，百會也。百會由衝脈相通於會陰。衝脈者，脊髓神經也，特高之電導體也。因而百會與會陰雖於上下兩處，其作用唯一己矣。會陰為陰為全身最陰之所，百會為陽為陽神顯陽之地，亦是全身最陽之處。會陰者，四陰脈，任、衝、陰蹻、陰維脈交會之所，是全身陰陽控制之關，是練氣者引氣之竅門。會陰上提，會陰鎖，氣內斂入骨髓，神凝氣聚，全身趨陰，勁由之而蓄。反之，會陰下推，會陰開，氣由四陰脈外放，陽神上提，全身趨陽，勁由之而發。一蓄一發，此為內勁蓄發關要之鑰。

The Fifth Gate Breathing is the most important key to the jin's manifestation. The yi and the qi of this gate are balanced with the other four gates, and when the yi and qi are strong in this gate, the yi and qi of the other four gates will also be strong. Naturally, the jin's manifestation will be powerful.

The baihui (Gv-20, 百會) is the residence of the shen, and the huiyin (Co-1, 會陰) is the storage place of water. The shen is yang while water is yin. That is why the shen is commonly called yang shen (陽神) while the huiyin (Co-1, 會陰) is called sea bottom (*haidi*, 海底) (Figure 4-23). The huiyin is the place that connects the real dan tian and the four yin vessels and thus stores the qi, while the shen is the place that governs the effectiveness of the qi's manifestation. In fact, these two cavities are the two poles of the body's central energy through the spinal cord. When this central energy is strong, the body's vital force is strong. Naturally, the jin manifested will be powerful and precise.

According to Chinese medicine, huiyin means "yin meeting" and is the gate that controls the qi's storage or release from the four yin vessels. When the huiyin is pushing out, the qi in the four yin vessels is released, and when this cavity is held upward, the qi is preserved. This implies that when you store your jin, you are holding this

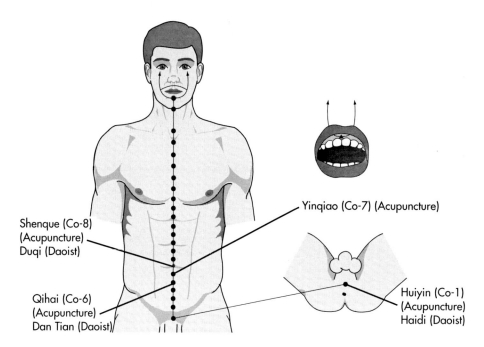

Figure 4-23. Course of the governing vessel (du mai)

cavity upward while inhaling and when you emit your jin, you are pushing this cavity outward while exhaling.

Wŭ, Yu-xiang said:

(Throughout your) entire body, your mind is on the spirit of vitality (jing shen), not on the qi. (If concentrated) on the qi, then stagnant." This is the Fifth Gate Breathing. Spirit (i.e., shen) is the master of the qi's circulation. When the spirit is high, the qi's circulation is natural, strong, and smooth. When the spirit is low, then the qi is stagnant, weak, and hard to circulate. This is the secret key to jin manifestation.

武禹襄云；〝全身意在精神，不在氣，在氣則滯。〞此即意第五心之呼吸也。神為氣行之主宰，神高，氣行自然沛而順，神低，氣滯弱而難行。此為勁發之訣竅也。

When the entire body's concentration is on the spirit, the spirit can be high and the qi can be led effectively. However, if the yi is on the qi, then your mind is not ahead of the qi and so not leading the qi, and the qi will be stagnant. This will cause the power to stagnate during expression. The key to leading the qi efficiently is to develop a sense of enemy. This means that you have an imaginary opponent. When your mind is on your opponent, your yi will lead the qi there for jin manifestation. The strength of your qi depends on the strength of your yi. However, the strength of your yi depends on your fighting spirit and morale. When this spirit is high, your alertness and awareness will also be high. Naturally, the qi can be directed efficiently.

4.5.5 *Grand Transportation Gong (Zhou Tian Mai Yun Gong,* 周天邁運功)

Grand transportation gong is a practice in which a martial artist learns how to use the mind to lead the qi, following the spine upward (i.e., governing vessel) to the shen-zhu (Gv-12,身柱) or dazhui (Gv-14,大椎) cavity. It is then divided and spread to the arms for jin manifestation (Figure 4-24). In order to balance the qi leading upward, another flow of qi is also led downward to the bottoms of the feet for rooting.

Theoretically, there are two gates that connect to the real lower dan tian (i.e., bio-battery). One is on the front, called yinjiao (Co-7, 陰交), and the other is on the back between vertebrae l2 and l3, called mingmen (Gv-4, 命門). Normally, the qi exits from yinjiao and distributes the qi to the entire body through the conception and governing vessels (*ren, du mai,* 任、督脈), and the twelve meridians (*shi er jing,* 十二經). However, Chinese martial artists discovered that if they were able to lead more qi from the real lower dan tian through the mingmen to enter the governing vessel, they would have extra qi to support the manifestation of power. This discovery marked a huge step of progress in Chinese martial arts qigong practice.

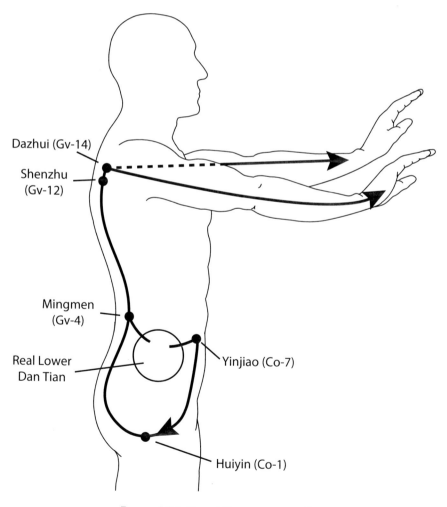

Figure 4-24. Grand Transportation Gong

In the application, when you inhale, first you lead the qi from the real lower dan tian, through the yinjiao, and then downward to the huiyin, and finally upward to meet the extra qi led from real lower dan tian to the mingmen and join the upward movement of qi. When the qi has reached to shenzhu or dazhui cavity, you exhale and divide the qi into two paths, entering the arms for manifestation (Figure 4-25). When you exhale, you also lead a flow of qi from the real lower dan tian downward to reach the bottom of your feet (Figure 4-26).

Alternatively, you may also lead the qi from the real lower dan tian to the huiyin while exhaling. Then, you inhale and lead the qi upward following the governing vessel to meet the extra qi led out from the real lower dan tian through the mingmen. Finally, you follow the same paths as described earlier and lead qi to the arms and feet (Figure 4-27).

When you practice taiji ball qigong, you are also using this grand circulation. You must practice until the entire process of using the mind to lead the qi has become natural and a habit. This is the internal side of martial arts practice in all Chinese martial arts styles.

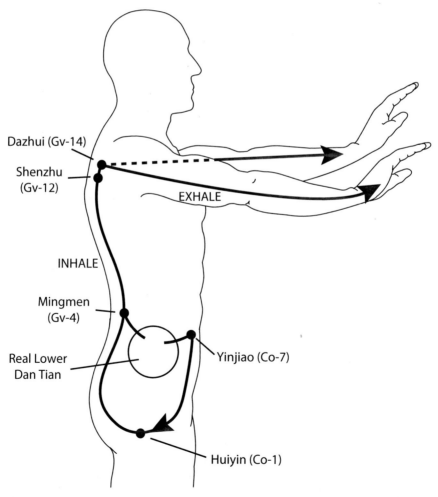

Figure 4-25. Procedure of inhaling and exhaling in Grand Transportation Gong.

4.6 Other Benefits (其他益處)

In addition to the above benefits that taiji ball qigong is able to bring you, there are other benefits:

1. Practicing taiji ball qigong will increase your awareness and alertness due to the sensitivity built up in the training. From this high awareness and alertness, your mind focus can be enhanced.

2. Practicing taiji ball qigong can improve the coordination of your mental center and physical center; consequently, your balance, centering, and rooting can be enhanced.

3. Practicing taiji ball qigong is able to increase the softness and flexibility of physical movements, especially the three joints of the legs, the crucial key of establishing rooting in soft Chinese martial arts styles, such as Taijiquan (太極拳) and Liuhebafa (六合八法).

4. It has been well-recognized that through taiji ball qigong training, many spine problems such as lower back pain and joint problems such as arthritis

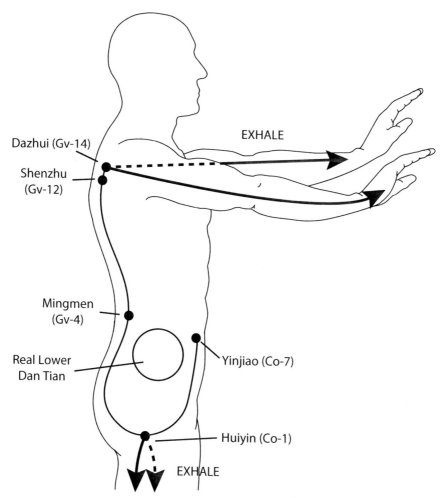

Figure 4-26. Additional qi lead from the real lower dan tian downward to reach.

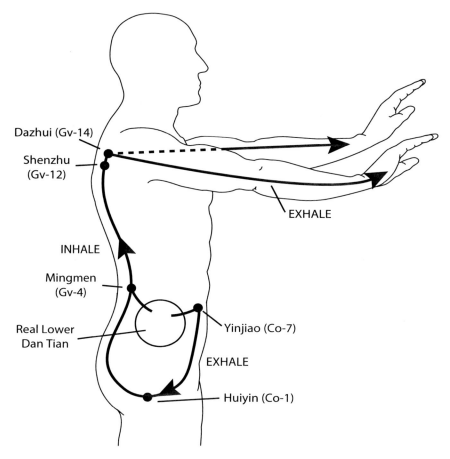

Figure 4-27. Alternative breathing method while leading qi in Grand Transportation Gong.

can be prevented and healed.

5. From practicing taiji ball qigong with partners, you are able to establish a healthier social lifestyle through exchanging ideas, qi, and skills with others.

4.7 Conclusions (結論)

Though taiji ball qigong theory is simple, its practice provides the potential for reaching a high level of skill. Through this theory, countless variations of patterns can be generated. From these variations, unlimited applications, both in health and martial arts, can be derived. taiji ball qigong is an art and therefore, it is developed through deep feeling. Only those who have reached a deeper feeling are able to be creative. The theory is the root while the patterns and applications are branches and flowers. Therefore, understanding the theory will help you establish this foundation and root of the practice.

Notes

1. *The Body Electric*, Robert O. Becker, M.D. and Gary Selden, Quill, William Morrow, New York, 1985.

2. "Complex and Hidden Brain in the gut makes stomachaches and butterflies," by Sandra Blakeslee, *The New York Times*, Science, January 23, 1996.

3. *The Second Brain: The Scientific Basis of Gut Instinct and a Groundbreaking New Understanding of Nervous Disorders of the Stomach and Intestine*, Michael D. Gershon, New York, Harper Collins Publications, 1998.

4. *Fundamentals of Physics*, Holliday and Resnick, John Wiley & Sons, Inc., 1972, pp. 512-514.

5. *Fundamentals of Physics*, Holliday and Resnick, John Wiley & Sons, Inc., 1972, pp. 512-514.

6. 內家由內而外，外家由外而內。其途雖異，其的則同。

7. 《性命圭旨全書‧火候》：〝神息者，火候也。〞指文火安神定息，任其自如，謂之神息。即〝不得勤，不得息者，是皆神息之自然火候之微旨也。〞

Taiji Ball Qigong Training

(太極球氣功之練習)

5.1 Introduction (介紹)

Taiji ball qigong is a mixture of internal gong (*nei gong*, 內功) and external gong (*wai gong*, 外功). The internal gong includes the development of the feeling between the physical body and qi and also learning how to use the mind to lead the qi efficiently. Feeling is a language that allows your mind and body to communicate. If you are able to develop a high level of sensitivity, your alertness and awareness will be higher than others. Naturally, your mind will also be able to sense the problem of physical body's tightness and qi's stagnation. This implies the mind will be able to manipulate the qi's circulation effectively. From this, you can see that your mind is the key of the entire practice. In qigong practice, the mind is just like a general who is in charge of the strategies and actions. It is also through this mind and sensitive feeling that your mind is able to regulate the body (i.e., battlefield), the breathing (i.e., strategy), and lead the qi (i.e., soldiers) effectively and efficiently.

Once you have all of these important internal elements, you can then manifest them into external actions. When the action is manifested, it is the coordination and harmonization of the external (*wai gong*) and internal (*nei gong*). **Effective manifestation requires coordinating and harmonizing the external (*wai gong*) and internal (*nei gong*) into an action.**

In this chapter, we will first introduce the basic taiji ball qigong training. The contents and procedures training will be reviewed in next section. Section 5.3 will discuss warm-up procedures used to begin the training while section 5.4 will discuss the internal training of taiji ball qigong. Finally, we will introduce the external side of training in Sections 5.5 and 5.6.

5.2 Taiji Ball Qigong Training Contents and Procedures (太極球氣功練習之 內含與程序)

Before you begin practicing taiji ball qigong, you should have some clear ideas about the practice, for example, how to choose a good taiji ball, what are the contents of taiji ball qigong, and what are the correct practicing procedures. In this section, we will summarize important points related to these subjects.

LECTURE
ABOUT
TAIJI BALLS

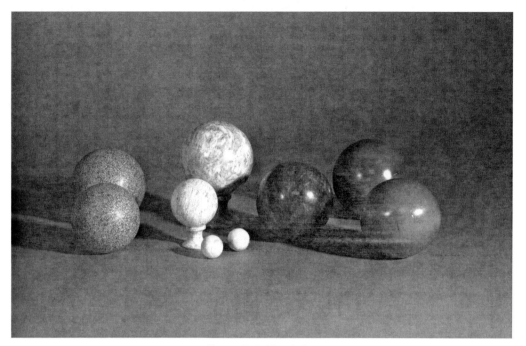

Figure 5-1. Taiji balls

5.2.1 Choosing the Balls

Material. The material used for making the ball should be natural. The best material for the ball is either wood or jade. A plastic bowling ball should not be used because it is too heavy for any beginner and not qi conductive. Also, a basketball is not a good choice because it is made from rubber. Basically, wooden balls are lighter and the qi led by the mind can penetrate through more easily. Wooden balls are commonly used by internal martial artists who consider qi development to be more important than that of physical strength (Figure 5-1). However, to external martial artists, the physical conditioning is considered more important than qi development. Therefore, the balls made by rock are often used (Figure 5-2). Actually, the best material for physical conditioning is jade due to its copper content. Unfortunately, jade is too expensive for most martial arts practitioners. Naturally, if a rock taiji ball is used, though a practitioner is able to build up a strong physical body, the development of qi will be difficult because it is more difficult for qi to penetrate through a ball made from rock. In addition, due to the resulting physical tension, it is more difficult to circulate or lead qi.

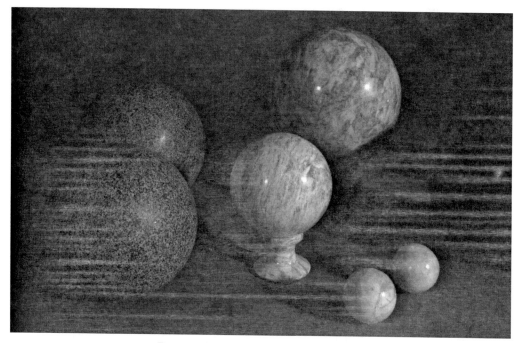

Figure 5-2. Granite and marble taiji balls

For a beginner, a wooden ball made with a single solid piece of wood is highly recommended. The material can be redwood or oak. Those balls constructed by gluing a couple pieces together are not as good as those made from a single piece since the glue will create a barrier for qi's circulation. Though a taiji ball made from a single piece of wood is more expensive, it is worth it because you can use for your entire life.

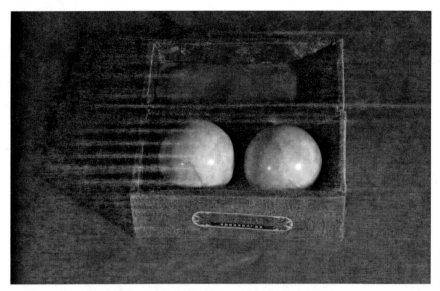

Figure 5-3. Taiji balls used for the hands

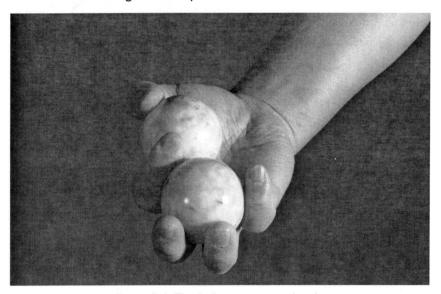

Figure 5-4. Taiji ball movement in hands

Sizes. The sizes of balls are varied. They can be the same size as a ping-pong ball (Figure 5-3). These kinds of taiji balls are commonly used in Chinese medical society to improve the qi's circulation in the hands, especially for healing arthritis in the hand. Normally, two balls are used at the same time. Through circling and rolling the balls, the qi at hands can be developed and then circulated (Figure 5-4).

The biggest ball ever documented is approximately one meter in diameter. The ball is very heavy and hanging from the ceiling. This kind of large ball is very rarely seen today. It was used in Wudang Mountain (武當山).

For a beginner, we highly recommend a wooden ball, 10-12 inches in diameter with the weight of 4-8 pounds. There are some wooden balls that are hollow at the center available in the market. They are very light and suitable for beginners to use to learn the pattern, but for long-term goals of the training, they are not as good as a solid wooden ball.

5.2.2 Training Rules

Light to heavy. The first rule is to prevent injury. Injuries are commonly caused by training with balls that are too heavy and by practicing with them too long.

Few to many. When you practice the routine patterns, begin with only a few repetitions. Only if you feel comfortable the next day should you increase the number of repetitions. You must proceed gradually since your body cannot be conditioned in one day. You must proceed slowly and gradually so the body can be conditioned gradually and safely.

Simple to difficult. You should begin with the simple patterns. Generally speaking, the simple routine patterns are the ones that can condition the body most effectively. Only when the physical foundation is established and feeling of control has been increased should you try more difficult challenges.

Mind-qi-body coordination and harmonization. If you wish to train both internal gong and external gong in taiji ball qigong, you must learn how to establish a fluent and smooth communication between your mind, qi, and body. Without this coordination, the effectiveness of the training will be shallow. You must practice until you reach the stage of "regulating of no regulating" (*wu tian er tiao*, 無調而調). Only then can your mind, qi, and body be in harmony.

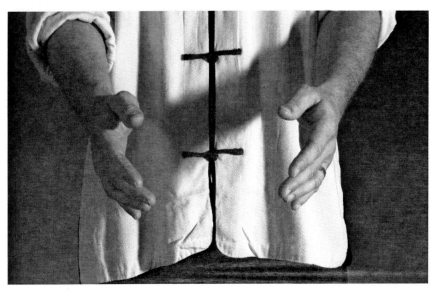

Figure 5-5

5.2.3 *Three Steps of Practice*

5.2.3.1 *Internal–Conditioning Qi Body (Without the Ball)*

FOLLOW ALONG

TAIJI BALL QIGONG CIRCLE PRACTICE

In this first step of practice, there is no physical ball. Place your hands, palms facing each other, about 10 inches apart. You may immediately feel a qi ball being constructed between the palms (Figure 5-5). This round qi field is established from the center of the palms, laogong cavity (P-8, 勞宮), and fingers. If you cannot feel this qi ball, do not worry. Your feeling will become more sensitive as you train. You might like to try this experiment: ask a partner to form the qi ball between his/her palms. Then, move your hand down at the center from top to the bottom (Figures 5-6 and 5-7). Most people can feel the qi established between the palms this way.

The purposes of this no-ball practice for a beginner are
- to establish a communication between the mind and the qi. If you have a physical ball, your arms will tense and the qi will be stagnant. In this case, it will be harder for any beginner to feel the qi.
- to become familiar with the training routines or patterns. Without a physical ball, the practice can last longer and this allows you to learn and familiarize yourself with the patterns.

The most important part of taiji ball qigong practice is the conditioning of the torso. If you have a heavy ball in your hands, your torso will tense and this will prevent you from moving your vertebra from section to section.

When you have a physical ball in your hands, you will pay more attention to the ball and the moving patterns of the arms instead of the torso and chest. Without the correct spine and chest movements, all taiji ball qigong conditioning will stay at the surface level.

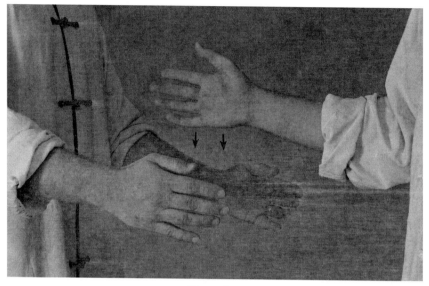

Figure 5-6

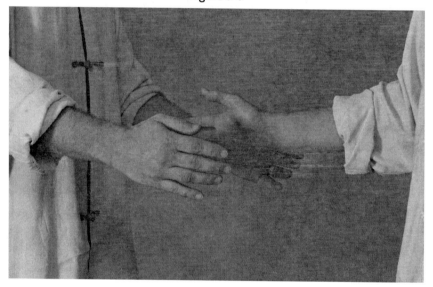

Figure 5-7

5.2.3.2 External–Conditioning Physical Body (With Ball)

Once you have established the feeling of correct spine and chest movements, the mind, qi and body communication, as well as familiarization of the routines, then you can step into the practice with a ball in your hands. As mentioned earlier, you should begin with a light ball, and then gradually increase the weight of the ball. You want to condition from as deep as to the bone marrow, bones, and ligaments to as shallow as the tendons, muscles, and skin. In order to keep qi in good circulation, the physical body cannot be too tense. If you proceed gradually and slowly, you will see the progress of your physical body in a few months. The most beneficial product of this practice is a strengthening of your immune system. This is due to the expansion of the guardian qi (*wei qi*, 衛氣) generated from practice. Another amazing benefit of this practice is the improvement of the bone density. Remember, our bones are constructed of piezo-electric material.[1] That means if there is pressure applied to the bone, there is electricity circulating in the bone. Through this circulation, the bones can be conditioned.

5.2.3.3 Unification of Internal and External (Without Ball)

After you have conditioned your physical body and qi body, you will enter the third stage of the taiji ball qigong practice. In this stage, there is no ball necessary. Both the qi body and physical body have been conditioned. Now you need to learn how to lead the qi to the bone marrow to nourish the marrow and establish stronger marrow qi (*sui qi*, 髓氣). Marrow is the factory of blood production. When the marrow is healthy, the immune system will be enhanced and the body's qi and nutrients will be transported efficiently and smoothly. This is also the basis of the secret of longevity as understood in Chinese Marrow Washing Qigong practice.[2] The most amazing part of this stage of practice is when you relax the muscles and tendons, you can reach a very high level of qi circulation.

In addition, you are learning how to lead the qi to the muscles and to the skin to enhance the guardian qi (*wei qi*, 衛氣). Through this enhancement, the immune system can again be boosted to an even higher level. However, to a martial artist, the main purpose of this training is not just for the immune system; it is also for jin (勁) (martial power) manifestation. If the qi can be led efficiently and effectively by the mind to the muscles and tendons required for a fight, the power manifested can be very high, which allows you to optimally manipulate your abilities.

5.2.4 Training Theory

5.2.4.1 Internal Gong (Nei Gong, 內功)

Internal gong includes five training elements: regulating the body, breathing, mind, qi, and spirit. We will discuss these five individually.

Regulating the Body (*Tiao Shen*, 調身). You are not just learning the moving patterns. The moving patterns are external. The internal communication that allows the body to relax to its profound state is internal. Without this deep relaxation, the qi cannot reach deep to the bone marrow or to the surface to enhance the guardian qi.

Regulating the Breathing (*Tiao Xi*, 調息). After you have regulated the body to its profound level, then begin to coordinate the breathing. Breathing is considered a strategy in qigong practice. With correct breathing techniques, the qi can be led by the mind efficiently.

Regulating the Mind (*Tiao Xin,* 調心). After you have regulated your body and breathing to their harmonious state, train to bring your mind to a high state of concentration, alertness, and awareness. In qigong practice, the mind can be compared to a general. When a general has a clear mind, rational judgment, and quick and precise response to the situation, the strategy will be effective and the soldiers (qi) can be controlled efficiently.

Regulating the Qi (*Tiao Qi,* 調氣). Once you have regulated your body, breathing, and mind, qi will be led effectively. Then you must train to increase the quantity of qi through correct abdominal methods.

Regulating the Spirit (*Tiao Shen,* 調神). Spirit is like the morale of the army. When the spirit is raised, the fighting units can be powerful and effective in carrying out their orders.

5.2.4.2 *External Gong (Wai Gong,* 外功)

Solo Practice

Without Object. There are 48 basic patterns of taiji ball qigong. These patterns can be divided into two main categories, vertical and horizontal. The vertical category is again divided into forward and backward. The horizontal category is further divided into clockwise and counterclockwise. This results in four major subgroups. Each subgroup includes four possible actions: stationary, rocking, stepping, and bagua stepping.

With Object. On the table: During the period of training with the 48 basic patterns, you may also practice with the ball on a table. Because the table supports the weight of the ball, it does not completely focus on the conditioning of the torso or joints. This training emphasizes increasing the sensitivity of hands.

On a book or a plate: Rotate and roll the ball along a plate edge. This exercise will develop the feeling of finding and maintaining contact with the center of another object. This will help you to develop the feeling of attachment to your opponent's physical center. This is a crucial key of destroying an opponent's balance in taiji pushing hands practice.

Against a wall: This is another example of a practice method. Roll the ball up and down a wall. Because the ball is heavy, you must know how to adhere to the ball with adequate power. If there is too much force applied to the ball, the ball cannot be moved smoothly and easily. Too little force and the ball will fall. You can also practice rolling the ball horizontally along the wall and in circles.

Against a point: The big challenge of this practice is to rotate the ball on a tiny tip.

With a Partner

Double hands. In order to improve your feeling of opponent, you should practice with a partner. When the opponent's force is coming strong, you should not resist. Instead, you should lead it and neutralize it so you can create an advantageous situation for your counterattack. Listening and following is the key of this neutralizing practice.

Single hand. After you have practiced with two hands with a partner, then you may practice with a single hand. That means you and your opponent each touch the ball with one hand. Both of you must employ a high level of listening and following skills; otherwise, the ball will fall.

Seizing the ball: The final stage in taiji ball qigong training is to seize the ball from your partner. You may use circling, rotating, and wrap-coiling techniques to take the ball away from opponent. You should not use force. Naturally, it is not easy to reach the profound level of this practice.

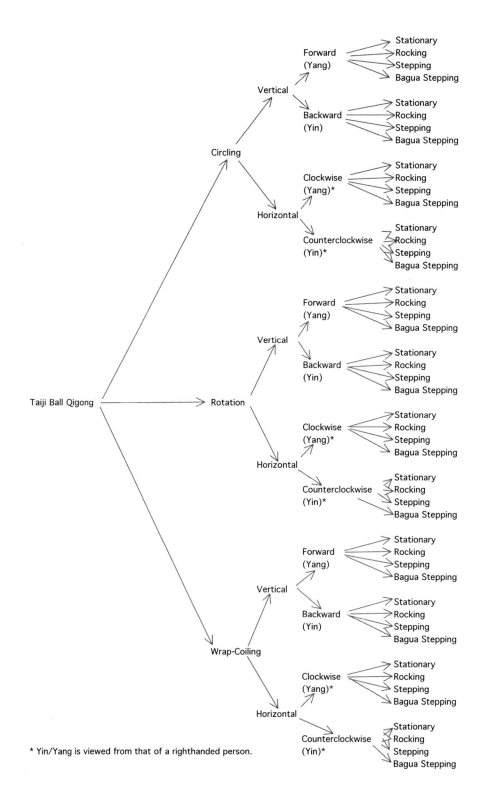

* Yin/Yang is viewed from that of a righthanded person.

Taiji Ball Qigong Yin-Yang Training–Single

The above applications only offer you some examples. Once you have learned and practiced to a proficient level, you will see many other possible applications. Remember the basic patterns are limited but the applications can be unlimited. It is just like dancing the waltz; although the basic three-step pattern is simple, the variations which can be developed are many.

5.3 Warm-Up (軟身)

In this section, we will introduce some basic warm-up and stretching exercises. With these preparations, your body will be ready for taiji ball training. In fact, these physical preparations are highly recommended for any and all external exercises. They are designed to prepare the body for more strenuous activity.

5.3.1 Loosening (Song Jie, 鬆節)

These movements are designed to loosen the muscles and tendons in the areas surrounding the joints. The movements will also assist the synovial fluids to lubricate the joints.

To begin, stand with your feet shoulder width apart and parallel. Raise your hands in front of your body approximately chest height and shake your wrists back and forth as well as up and down (Figure 5-8).

Once you have warmed up your wrists for approximately 30 seconds, drop your arms to the sides. Loosen the joints in your arms from your shoulders to your fingertips by gently moving your arms in the shoulder sockets. Your elbows will flap gently as will your hands.

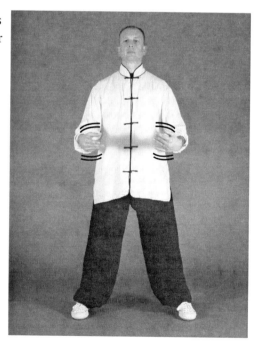

Figure 5-8

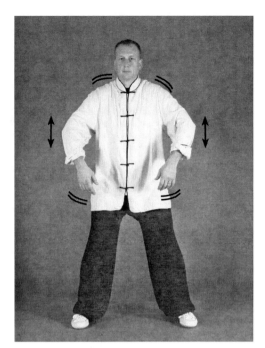

Figure 5-9

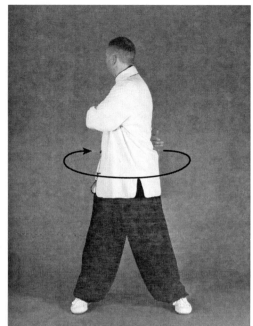

Figure 5-10

Next, bounce gently to loosen the shoulder joints (Figure 5-9). At the same time, you should make small circles with your arms to focus on loosening the elbow joints. Bounce your body without allowing the feet to rise off the ground. It should only be enough to get the shoulders to move in an up-and-down motion

Now that you have warmed up your wrists, elbows, and shoulders, move on to the waist area. Rotate your hips in both directions. This hip movement will cause your arms to swing. (Figures 5-10, 5-11, and 5-12). The twisting action will help loosen the whole torso. Repeat this action for at least 12 repetitions.

In the next warm-up exercise, move your torso in a downward arcing motion, starting to your right, sweeping down toward your left side and then lifting your torso and moving toward your right side to complete the counterclockwise cycle. (Figures 5-13 and 5-14). Repeat this for at least 12 repetitions; then change the direction of the movement and repeat this action for an additional 12 repetitions.

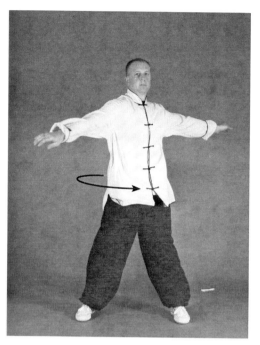

Figure 5-11

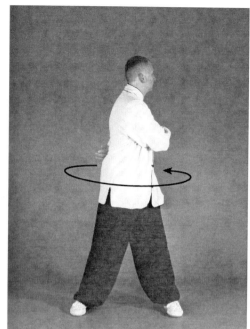

Figure 5-12

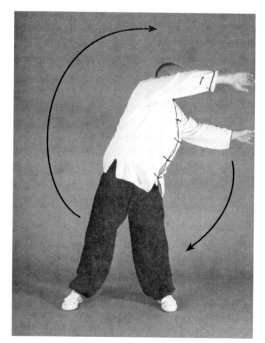

Figure 5-13

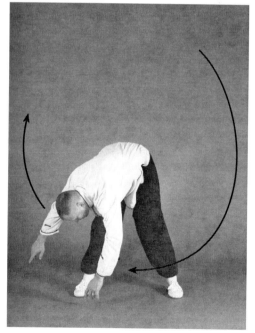

Figure 5-14

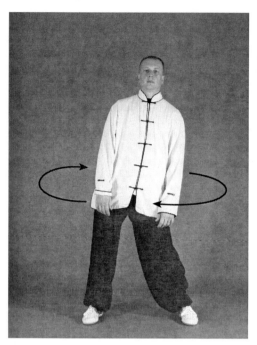

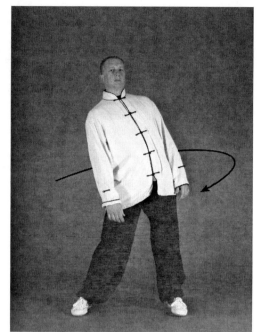

Figure 5-15   Figure 5-16

Make large gentle circles with your hips. Your hips should trace a circle parallel to the ground. Your arms should drop naturally to your sides and move only as a result of your hip action. After completing 12 repetitions change the direction and repeat for an additional 12 repetitions.

Continue your warm-ups by focusing on the lower torso. Circle your hips in a counterclockwise direction (Figures 5-15 and 5-16). Next, bend your knees and place your hands lightly on them. Circle your knees counterclockwise (Figure 5-17). Repeat for 12 repetitions, and then change to the opposite direction for 12 more.

Finally, warm up the ankle joints. Transfer your weight to one leg. Place the nonweighted leg slightly behind you with only the balls of your feet on the floor (Figure 5-18). Circle the ankles in one direction for 12 repetitions, and then 12 repetitions in the opposite direction. Switch to the opposite ankle and repeat the same action as before. If desired, you may also include a gentle circular movement with the thigh. This will provide an additional rotation to the joint of the thighbone in the hip socket.

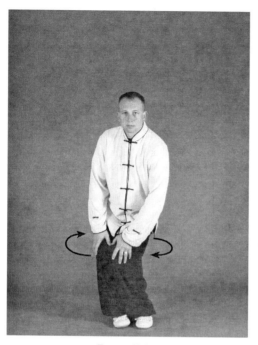

Figure 5-17

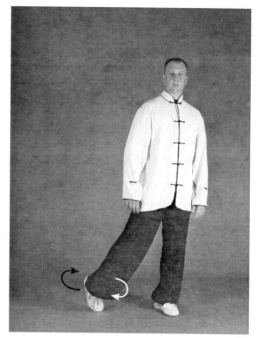

Figure 5-18

5.3.2 Stretching (Ba Jin, 拔筋)

After you have warmed up your joints, you should stretch the muscles in your body. If you stretch your body correctly, you will be able increase your muscular flexibility and joint range of motion. In addition, you can stimulate the cells into an excited state thus improving qi and blood flow. This is the key to maintaining a healthy physical body. Remember your muscles, tendons, and ligaments are like rubber bands. If stretched too fast and too far, they will tear. A good stretch should feel comfortable and stimulating. For each static pose you perform, we are recommending 20 seconds minimum to stretch or lengthen the muscles you are working on. Generally speaking, stretching beyond 6 seconds allows the Golgi tendon organs to send the necessary signal to the central nervous system allowing the muscle to relax and stretch. If at any time you feel this is too much, it is best to back off to a point where you feel comfortable. If necessary, shorten the time of the stretch and work your way up to the 20 seconds. Remember to listen to your body. The purpose of a good stretch is to allow the muscle to extend to its optimal length and this will not occur if you are not relaxed. Most important of all of these exercises is to remember to breathe throughout the movements.

Start by stretching the torso, then the outer limbs. The torso contains major muscles that control our trunk and also surround our internal organs. If our torso is tense, the whole body will be tense and as a result our internal organs will be compressed. In addition, there will be stagnation of qi circulation in the organs and body. Therefore, prior to any qigong practice, you should stretch the muscles of the torso and the limbs. The best qigong practices remove qi stagnation and maintain smooth qi circulation in the internal organs.

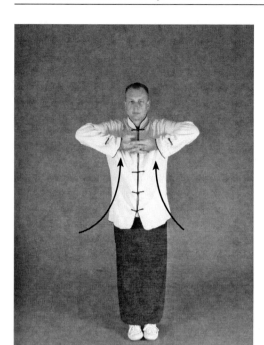 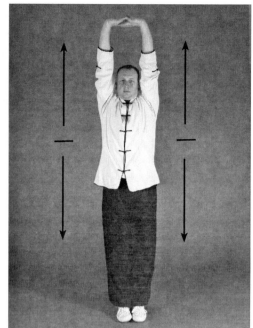

Figure 5-19   Figure 5-20

To start, stand with your feet together and interlock your fingers. Inhale while raising your hands in front of your body. As your hands pass your head, begin to exhale and continue to raise your interlocked hands up above your body, rotating your hands so the palms face toward the ceiling (Figures 5-19 and 5-20). Imagine your feet pushing into the ground and your hands pushing into the air. This action will open up your triple burner (*san jiao*, 三焦) (i.e., torso).

The triple burner is one of the yang organs in Chinese medicine and divides the torso into three sections: chest, stomach, and lower abdomen. The function of the triple burner involves the combustion, digestion, and excretion of the food the body uses for energy. Lifting your arms above your head will assist the triple burner by opening or expanding these three sections and allowing the qi in the area to flow more freely. Slightly tuck in your pelvis to assist in the stretch and do not allow the body to arch backward. Your arms should be as straight and parallel to each other as possible, while keeping your shoulders and chest relaxed. Remain in this position for 20 seconds, gently adjusting the body and arms to reach their optimal extension.

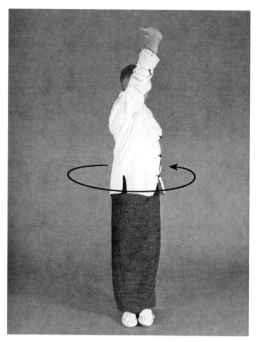

Figure 5-21

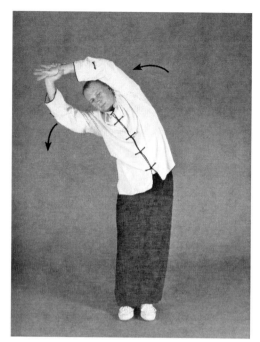

Figure 5-22

Next, twist the torso toward your left side as far around as is comfortable for you (Figure 5-21). Hold the position for 20 seconds; then relax back to the neutral position. (*Important note:* While you are in the twisted position, DO NOT hold your breath. The twisting action creates different pressures on the lungs. Breathing deeply in the varied positions allows different parts of the lungs to reach excited states.) Next, twist your body as far around as you can to the right side. Hold this position for 20 seconds, and then relax back to the neutral position. Repeat this procedure for both sides; however, when you reach your maximum stretching point, keep your chin tucked in, twist your head, and look back behind you are far as you can. This will provide an additional stretch of the spine up through the cervical area.

Once you have twisted the body twice to each side, face forward, and bend the upper body to one side. As you tilt to one side, grasp the wrist of the opposite hand and pull gently (Figure 5-22). Hold this stretch for 20 seconds; then change to the opposite side. To check your posture, you can perform this stretch while standing against a wall. Try to keep your back flat against the wall throughout the stretch. Again, remember to breathe deeply.

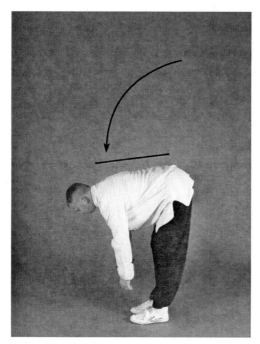

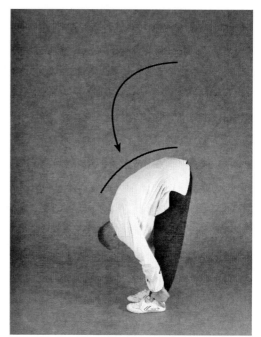

Figure 5-23   Figure 5-24

Next, come back to the center and bend over reaching down in front of your body as far as you can (Figure 5-23). Initially, keep your legs and back straight. Concentrate on stretching the hamstring and calf muscles.

After 20 seconds, gently relax the back and allow it to curve naturally (Figure 5-24). This will change the focal point of stretching to the lower lumbar section. It is also good to turn or twist the waist side to side. (*Important note:* If you have lower back problems, be especially careful when stretching the lower lumbar section.)

After 20 seconds, squat down. Try to keep your feet flat on the ground throughout the stretch and focus on the Achilles tendon (Figure 5-25). If you have problems squatting with your feet together, try squatting with your feet farther apart. If squatting with your feet close together is easy for you, try placing your hands behind your back. Hold this position for 20 seconds.

Next, while in the seated position, rise up on your toes (Figure 5-26). This will focus on the muscles, tendons, and ligaments on the bottoms of your feet (Figure 5-27).

5.3.3 *Spinal Qigong Warm-Up (Ji Zhui Ruan Shen,* 脊椎軟身*)*

Now that you have warmed up your joints and stretched out your body, it is time to exercise the spine and trunk muscles. The torso is supported by the spine and trunk muscles. These muscles are constantly being stressed from the time you get up until you go to bed at night. Performing these exercises on a daily basis will assist in relieving the tension of these muscles. In any martial art, it is important to recognize what is known as the six bows (*liu gong,* 六弓) of the body, which are used for the manifestation of power, or jin. These bows occur in the two arms, two legs, the spine, and the chest.

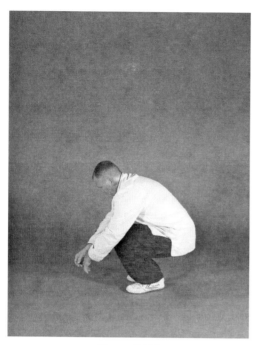

Figure 5-25

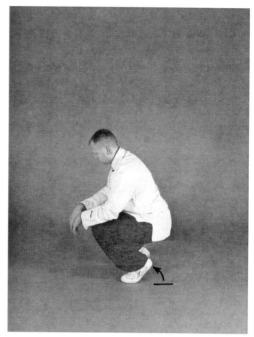

Figure 5-26

First layer

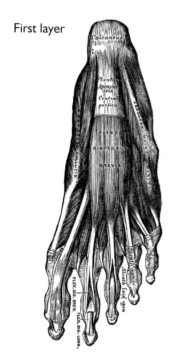

Second layer

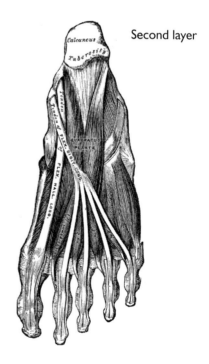

Figure 5-27. Muscles, tendons, and ligaments located in the bottom of the foot.

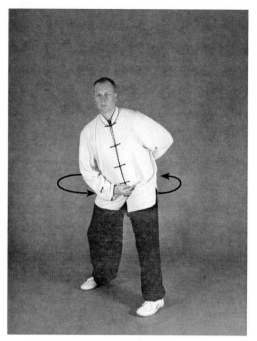

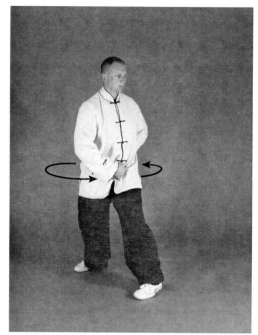

Figure 5-28   Figure 5-29

1. Circle the Waist Horizontally (*Pin Yuan Nui Yao,* 平圓扭腰)

The first movement of the spinal motion is circling the waist horizontally. This exercise will help you regain conscious control of the muscles in the lumbar section of the back and the abdominal muscles. Loosening this area will also help you lead your qi from the lower dan tian.

To practice this movement, stand with your feet approximately shoulder width apart, knees slightly bent. Begin to circle the waist on a horizontal plane. Try to keep your knees in alignment with the direction of your toes. Your upper body should not initiate the circles (Figure 5-28). Start with small circles; then gradually make them larger. Reaching the desired size, repeat the movements for 12 repetitions.

Next, slowly turn the upper body as far as you comfortably can to the left for an additional 12 repetitions. Do the same to the right side. (Figures 5-29 and 5-30). The twisting action will assist in loosening up the waist area when practicing the horizontal movements of taiji ball. Return to facing forward and reduce the size of the circles until reaching your original position. Reverse the direction of the circles and repeat the exercise. At first, your muscles may be tense. Through time you will be able to relax and focus on the flow of qi in the area. The ultimate goal is to have strong qi flow with minimal physical movement, thus enhancing the presence of qi in the girdle vessel.

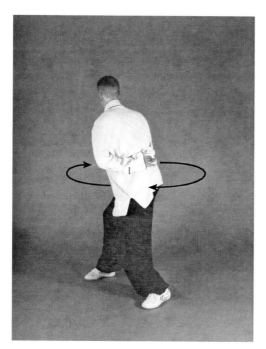

Figure 5-30

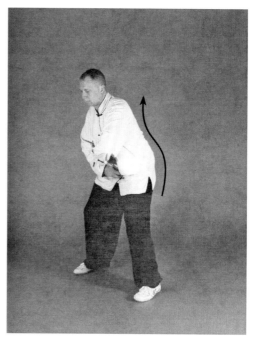

Figure 5-31

2. Waving the Spine and Massage the Internal Organs (Ji Zhui Bo Dong, Nei Zang An Mo, 脊椎波動、內臟按摩)

The next exercise is similar to the last except the movement is now vertical. Place one hand on your dan tian and the other hand above it with the thumb on the solar plexus (Figure 5-31). Now gently create a wave-like motion from your lumbar section and dan tian area up the spine to the midsection of your body approximately in the diaphragm area. Allow the motion to flow back down again as well. In addition to moving the spine, you are massaging the internal organs. Repeat this exercise for 12 repetitions.

Now twist your waist to one side while continuing to vertically move the spine. Remember to stay centered, do not rock back and forth, and do not lean too far forward. Wave the spine to one direction for 12 repetitions; then change the direction to the other side for an additional 12 repetitions.

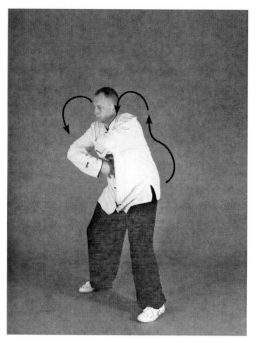

Figure 5-32

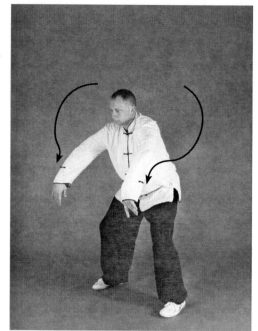

Figure 5-33

3. Thrust the Chest and Arc the Chest (*Ting Xiong Gong Bei,* 挺胸拱背)

Next, extend the motion up into your chest. To assist in this movement, place one hand farther up in front of your sternum while leaving the other hand in front of your abdomen (Figure 5-32). Begin to inhale and start your wave-like motion up the spine. Roll the shoulders back while inhaling, then forward while exhaling. Your elbows should make large vertical circles following the action of opening and closing the chest. Each time you move, try to feel the movement flow in your spine, vertebra by vertebra. This exercise will help loosen up the chest as well as improve the qi circulation in the lungs. Repeat this action for 12 repetitions.

4. White Crane Waves its Wings (*Bai He Dou Chi,* 白鶴抖翅)

Now, extend the motion out into your arms and fingers. As the movement flows through the shoulders, elbows, wrists, and fingers, allow both arms to extend out in front of you (Figure 5-33). Repeat this action for 12 repetitions.

Finally, retract one hand back to your waist area while the other one remains out in front of you. This time generate the wave-like motion as before; then twist the waist and redirect the arm accordingly (Figures 5-34 and 5-35). Repeat for 12 repetitions, and then repeat the action for the opposite arm.

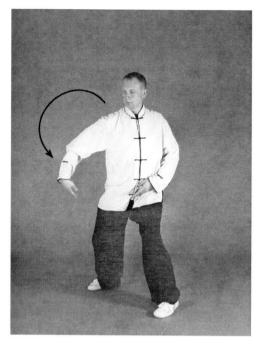

Figure 5-34

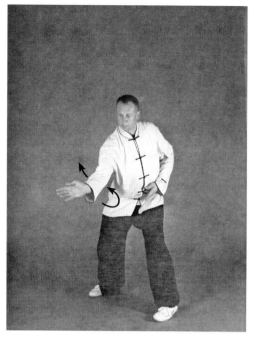

Figure 5-35

5.4 Internal Training (內功)–Breathing Exercises

The following section will highlight some fundamental techniques required for nei gong. Nei gong is also known as internal gongfu. Internal gong focuses on regulating the body, breathing, mind, qi, and spirit. The theory is briefly explained in Chapter 2 and Chapter 4. It is impossible to cover all of this training in this section. If you are interested in all of this training, please refer to the books *The Root of Chinese Qigong*, *The Essence of Taiji Qigong*, and *Qigong Meditation–Embryonic Breathing*, by Dr. Yang, Jwing-Ming, published by YMAA Publication Center.

First, we will focus on exercises for regulating the breathing that allows you to build up the quantity of qi to an abundant level and subsequently circulate the accumulated qi. Practice these exercises in the order that they are presented. Become comfortable and proficient in one technique before moving on to the next.

LECTURE
INTERNAL
FOUNDATION

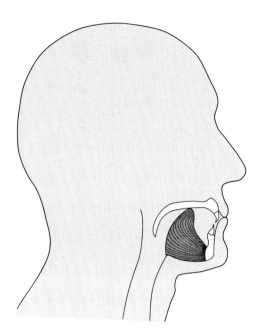

Figure 5-36. Tongue position

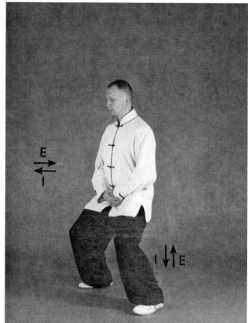

Figure 5-37

5.4.1 Normal Abdominal Breathing (Zheng Fu Hu Xi, 正腹呼吸)

Stand with both hands touching the lower dan tian lightly. This light touch can help you feel the movement of the abdominal muscles and thus increasing the communication level between your mind and the lower dan tian. The tip of your tongue should touch the palate of your month to connect the yin conception and yang governing vessels (Figure 5-36).

Inhale deeply through the nose while gently pushing your abdominal muscles out and huiyin (Co-1, perineum) down. As you exhale, draw your abdomen inward and pull the huiyin cavity upward gently (Figure 5-37).

You should practice this method of breathing until your mind is able to control the abdominal muscles effectively and efficiently. Only then can this area remain relaxed and allow the qi to circulate freely. Allow a minimum of 6 months of training this type of breathing to allow the body to adjust to the conditioning; then proceed on to the next form of breathing exercises.

5.4.2 *Reverse Abdominal Breathing (Fan Fu Hu Xi, Ni Fu Hu Xi,* 反腹呼吸 · 逆腹呼吸)

Once again, stand with both hands touching the lower dan tian and the tongue touching the palate of the mouth. When you inhale, draw in your abdomen and pull up your huiyin cavity. When you exhale, push the abdomen out and huiyin cavity down gently (Figure 5-38). Practicing reverse abdominal breathing may cause some tension in the dan tian. If that happens, stop using this method of breathing and return to normal abdominal breathing. You may also gently massage the abdomen to relieve the tension. As long as abdominal area is relaxed, you should not have a problem.

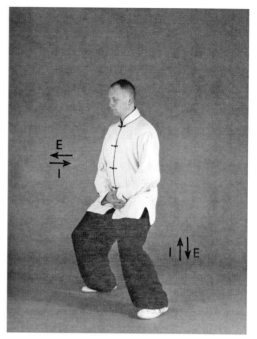

Figure 5-38

5.4.3 *Wuji Breathing (Wuji Hu Xi,* 無極呼吸)

This breathing is also called "Embryonic Breathing" (*Tai Xi,* 胎息). In this practice, you keep your mind at the center of gravity that is also recognized as the real lower dan tian (*zhen xia dan tian,* 真下丹田). When you practice, use reverse abdominal breathing. The only difference is when you inhale, you are also pulling the muscles on the lower back inward, and when you exhale, you are pushing them out. This will help you locate the center of gravity. This breathing helps you lead the qi to the real dan tian and store it to a higher level. If you wish to know more about Embryonic Breathing, please refer to the book *Qigong Meditation–Embryonic Breathing,* published by YMAA Publication Center.

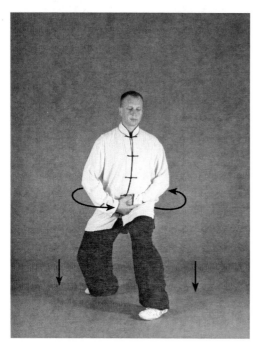

Figure 5-39

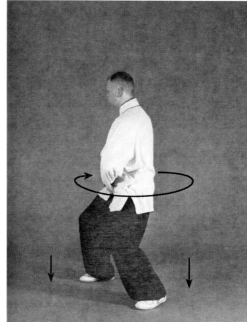

Figure 5-40

5.4.4 *Yongquan Breathing (Yongquan Hu Xi,* 湧泉呼吸*)*

Yongquan breathing is also called "sole breathing" (*zhong xi,* 踵息). It was described in the book, *Zhuang Zi* (莊子), around the fourth century B.C. It is called yongquan xi (湧泉息) (yongquan breathing) in Daoist society.

In this breathing exercise, stand with your legs open to about shoulder width apart. Again, the hands touch the abdominal area and the tongue touches the palate of mouth gently. First, inhale and lead the qi to the real lower dan tian. Next, exhale, squat down slightly and imagine you are pushing the feet downward. Through this image of pushing, you are using your mind to lead the qi down through the yongquan cavity. When you imagine pushing the feet downward, your mind should aim at least six inches under the feet so that qi does not get trapped. A variation of this exercise is to twist your torso to one side as you squat and exhale. On the next breath, twist your torso to the opposite side (Figures 5-39 and 5-40). This will increase the stretching of the tendons and ligaments in the ankles, knees, and hips resulting in a strengthening of the joints. If you practice this correctly, you may feel the hot or warm feeling caused by qi accumulation at the bottom of your feet in just a few minutes. To remove the qi accumulated, simply raise your heels and then your toes, alternately, a couple times after you have finished practicing.

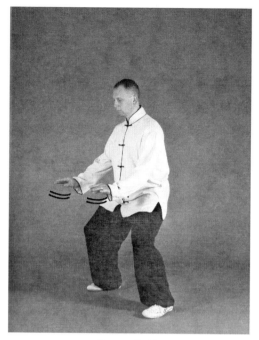

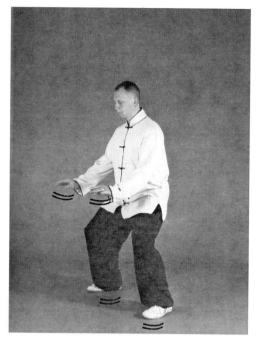

Figure 5-41   Figure 5-42

5.4.5 *Laogong Breathing (Laogong Hu Xi,* 勞宮呼吸*)*

In laogong breathing, use your mind to lead the qi to the laogong cavity located at the center of your palms. Again, stand with legs opened as wide as your shoulders. The hands touch the abdominal area and the tongue touches the palate of mouth gently. Use Embryonic Breathing. First, inhale and lead the qi to the real dan tian. Next, exhale and imagine you are pushing your hands downward without moving your hands. Through this pushing image, you are using your mind to lead qi through the laogong cavities. When you imagine you are pushing your hands downward, your mind should aim at least six inches beyond the palms (Figure 5-41). If you practice correctly, in just a few minutes you may feel some sensations, a tingling or static feeling at the palms.

5.4.6 *Four Gates Breathing (Si Xin Hu Xi,* 四心呼吸*)*

This breathing is a combination of yongquan and laogong breathing. The posture remains the same as in the previous two exercises. As you inhale, use your mind to lead qi to the real dan tian. As you exhale, gently squat downward and imagine you are pushing both your hands and feet downward (Figure 5-42).

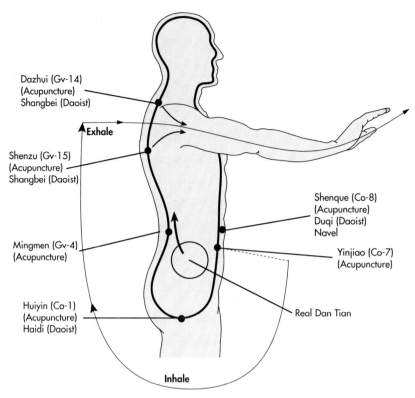

Dazhui (Gv-14)
(Acupuncture)
Shangbei (Daoist)

Exhale

Shenzu (Gv-15)
(Acupuncture)
Shangbei (Daoist)

Shenque (Co-8)
(Acupuncture)
Duqi (Daoist)
Navel

Mingmen (Gv-4)
(Acupuncture)

Yinjiao (Co-7)
(Acupuncture)

Huiyin (Co-1)
(Acupuncture)
Haidi (Daoist)

Real Dan Tian

Inhale

Figure 5-43

5.4.7 Martial Grand Circulation Breathing (Wuxue Da Zhou Tian Hu Xi, 武學大周天呼吸)

In this breathing technique you are leading the qi into the governing vessel through the mingmen (Gv-4,命門) cavity in addition to the normal qi circulation path, which passes from the real dan tian to the conception vessel through the abdomen-yinjiao (Co-7,陰交) cavity. This will increase the supply of qi to the small circulation path and enhance the power of physical manifestation.

When you practice, stand with your legs opened about a shoulders' width apart. Allow both arms to relax along the sides of the body. When you inhale, lead the qi from the real dan tian, downward through yinjiao, pass the huiyin, and then lead the qi upward. When the qi reaches the

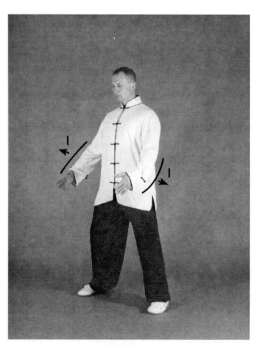

Figure 5-44

mingmen cavity, gently push back the lower back to open the mingmen cavity and lead the qi out to combine with the qi from the front. This qi is then led upward to dazhui (Gv-14, 大椎) (Figure 5-43). When you exhale, lead the qi outward through the arms while also leading it from the real dan tian downward to the bottom of your feet. When you have reached a deeper level of taiji ball qigong training, use Martial Grand Circulation Breathing.

5.4.8 Taiji Ball Breathing (Taiji Qiu Hu Xi, 太極球呼吸)

In this breathing, apply the Martial Grand Circulation Breathing into the taiji ball practice. (Follow the steps described in the previous section.) In addition, hold both of your hands in front of your lower dan tian with palms facing each other. When you inhale, draw the abdomen inward, and the huiyin is moving upward

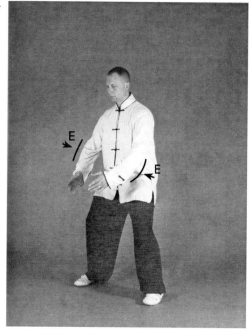

Figure 5-45

(i.e., internal ball is condensing), while the palms spread apart (i.e., external ball is expanding) (Figure 5-44).

Then exhale to expand the internal ball while pressing your both palms toward each other (Figure 5-45).

After you have practiced for a few minutes, you may begin to feel an invisible qi ball forming between the palms. The longer you practice, the stronger the qi can be felt. This is a basic foundation of taiji ball internal gong training. Eventually, you will apply this kind of breathing through the entire taiji ball qigong practice.

5.5 External Training (外功)–Fundamental Stances

5.5.1 Fundamental Stances (Ji Ben Zhuang Bu, 基本庄步)

In this section we will describe the fundamental techniques required for wai gong (外功) training. Wai gong is also known as external gongfu. External gong focuses on regulating the body, breathing, mind, qi, and spirit. We will first introduce some basic stances that are needed for taiji ball qigong training. Once you have become familiar with these stances, you should begin training your taiji ball exercises. These will be described beginning in section 5.6.

The fundamental stances we have selected are part of eight stances (ba shi, 八勢) common to all styles of martial arts. They are necessary to build a physical foundation for stability and movement. While familiarizing yourself with the stances, you may ignore the position of the hands.

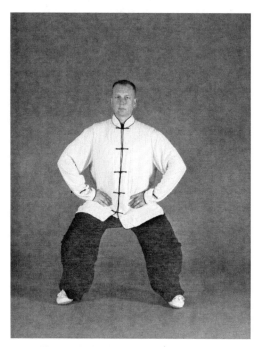

Figure 5-46. Horse stance (ma bu)

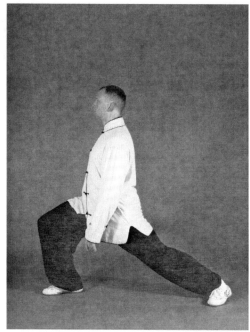

Figure 5-47. Mountain climbing stance or bow and arrow stance (deng shan bu, gong jian bu)

Horse Stance (*Ma Bu,* 馬步). The horse stance is commonly used as a transition between techniques and forms. To assume this stance, first place the feet parallel, slightly wider than your shoulder width. Next, slightly bend the knees and sink your weight into your feet. The torso should be upright, natural, centered, and relaxed. The knees should extend no farther than the tip of your toes. Both feet must remain flat. In order to avoid straining the sides of the knees, the knees must always line up in the direction of the toes. Depending on your training intent and your physical ability, you may train with your knees bent so that the angle between the back of the thighs and calves create a 90-degree angle. Beginners should not train in this low stance until their leg muscles are sufficiently strengthened. Always proceed gradually in order to avoid injury (Figure 5-46).

Mountain Climbing Stance or Bow and Arrow Stance (*Deng Shan Bu, Gong Jian Bu,* 登山步、弓箭步). This stance is used when rocking as well as stepping. First, place one leg forward and distribute your weight so 60 to 70 percent of your weight is on your forward leg (Figure 5-47). The toe of the forward leg is pointing 15 degrees inward, Make sure that the knee does not extend over the toe and that the lower leg is perpendicular to the feet. The knee of the rear leg must be slightly bent in this stance. Again, to avoid injury, make sure your knee aligns with the direction of the toes. Keep the torso naturally upright.

Sitting on Crossed Leg Stance (*Zou Pan Bu,* 坐盤步). This stance is commonly used for forward movement. First, assume a ma bu stance (Figure 5-48) or deng shan bu stance.

Second, turn the body and the right foot on the heel up to 90 degrees clockwise

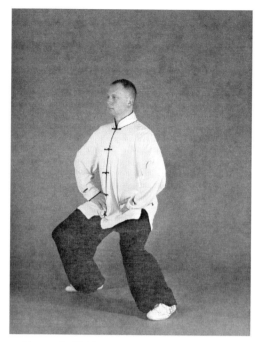

Figure 5-48. Sitting on crossed leg stance (zou pan bu)

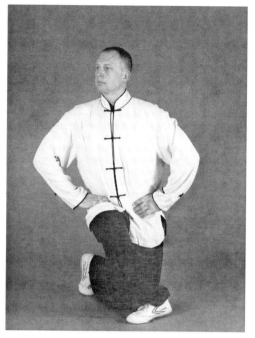

Figure 5-49. Sitting on crossed leg stance (zou pan bu)

while releasing the left heel so you can pivot on the left toe (Figure 5-49).

The same can be done to the left side. Turn the body and the left foot on the heel 90 degrees counterclockwise, and pivot on the right foot on the toes. Approximately 90 percent of your weight moves into your forward foot.

Four-Six Stance (*Si Liu Bu,* 四六步). This stance is also commonly used in the rocking and stepping patterns. In weight distribution, it is exactly the opposite of mountain climbing stance; the front leg supports 40 percent of the weight and the rear leg supports 60 percent (Figure 5-50). The rear leg is bent, with the knee and toes turned outward, while the front leg is held loose, slightly bent, and relaxed.

There are other fundamental stances that will not be explained here. If you wish to explore these further, please re-fer to *Taijiquan—Classical Yang Style,* by Dr. Yang, Jwing-Ming, published by YMAA Publication Center.

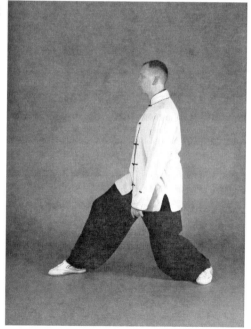

Figure 5-50. Four-six stance (si liu bu)

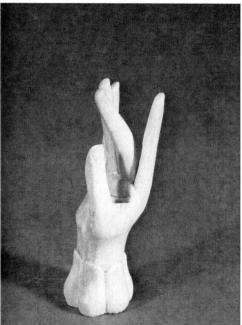

Figure 5-51. Wa shou

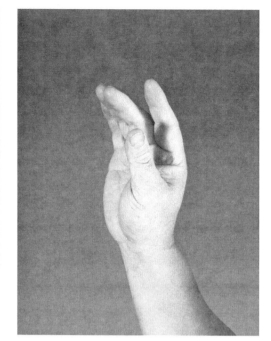

Figure 5-52. Wa shou

5.6 External Training (外功)–Exercises

5.6.1 Introduction to Taiji Ball Qigong Training (Taiji Qiu Qigong Lian Xi, 太極球氣功練習)

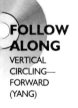

FOLLOW ALONG

VERTICAL CIRCLING— FORWARD (YANG)

The following exercises will provide you with the basic foundation of taiji ball training. They are to be performed solo and then with a partner. Each pattern will be discussed as if you had a ball in hand. The placement of the hands on the ball is as follows: allow each palm to touch the ball with the pinkie finger and index finger slightly raised off the ball. This posture of the hand resembles what is known as taiji palm or tile hand (*wa shou*, 瓦手) (Figures 5-51 and 5-52). This will slightly restrict the flow of qi to these fingers and allow an increase in flow to the middle finger and laogong cavity. This hand posture is also useful, in martial art, for attacking and controlling an opponent/partner. With the fingers loosely extended, the jin, or martial force, is able to reach the palms and exit easily for attack. When controlling an opponent's movements, the hand is often cupped with the fingers wrapping over the individual's joint areas allowing better communication through the hands between you and the opponent.

Each of the following patterns will be described in the following manner. First, we will start with circling, then follow with rotating and wrap-coiling. Second, they will be described as a yang pattern while stationary, rocking, stepping, and finally using bagua stepping. This will be followed by the yin pattern, which will also be described while stationary, rocking, stepping, and bagua stepping. We will also include the yin-yang exchange, vertically, horizontally, and mixed, or freestyle.

All the patterns begin with a small internal circle produced by the dan tian. This movement will follow up the spine, out along the arms, and end with the ball. Each time the pattern completes a revolution, your body will continue to increase the size of the motion and gradually spiral outward until you reach your maximum range of motion. The maximum range of motion is the point at which your arms are extended in front of your body as far as you can without locking the elbows. Also, do not allow your arms to rise above your head. In both situations, you will tense the muscles and trap the flow of qi, defeating the purpose of the training exercise. After the select number of repetitions, each motion should gradually get smaller and smaller until you are back to the center, or starting point.

5.6.2 Circling (Rao Quan, 繞圈)

The first pattern is known as circling. Within this pattern are four different methods to complete the circle. Two are related to a vertical plane and two are related to a horizontal plane. The motion forward over the top of the circle is considered yang forward circling while the motion backward over the top of the circle is considered yin backward circling. When you are circling horizontally in a clockwise motion it is considered yang clockwise circling and circling horizontally in a counterclockwise motion is considered yin counterclockwise circling.

For each set of exercises, we suggest 12 repetitions as a minimum number to adequately condition the body, breath, mind, qi, and spirit. As described earlier, you should first practice each exercise without a ball in order to allow sufficient time for your body to adapt to the movements. The next step would be to include the ball in the training exercise. Remember that an important part of the training is improving your ability to communicate with your own body. **Listen to your body.** If you feel you cannot complete the exercise using the number of repetitions suggested, you may elect to reduce the number of repetitions. Pick a number of repetitions and increase them gradually as you practice. The increase of repetitions should be done only if your body feels strong enough to do so.

5.6.2.1 Vertical Circling (Chui Zhi Rao Quan, 垂直繞圈)

Vertical circling refers to a vertical plane that extends out from the center of your body. It is also known as the median, or midsagittal plane, which divides the body into the symmetrical left and right sides. Imagine you are carrying a large bass drum like the ones used in a marching band. Basically, you will be tracing the outline of the drum. Your pattern begins at the center of the circle and gradually spirals out until reaching your maximum range of motion. After you have completed your number of repetitions, you will gradually decrease the size of the circles until you arrive back at the center of the circle.

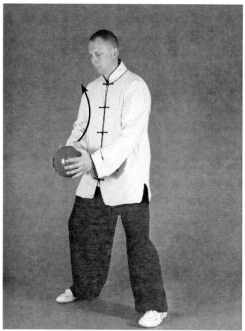

Figure 5-53

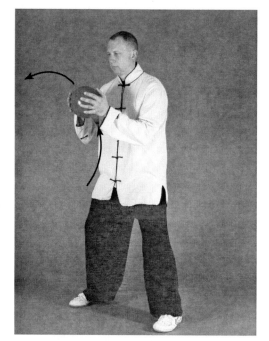

Figure 5-54

Yang Circling (*Yang Rao,* 陽繞)–Vertical

I. Stationary (*Ding Bu,* 定步)

The first stage of the vertical circling pattern is a yang, or forward pattern, while stationary. Stand in ma bu, feet parallel approximately shoulder width apart, knees slightly bent. Lightly cradle the ball between your hands and hold it in front of your dan tian (Figure 5-53).

Take a moment to lead your qi to your dan tian using a few deep breaths. To begin circling, inhale and initiate the movement of the ball from your dan tian. As the movement continues up your spine and into your arms, draw in your chest and move the ball up toward your body (Figure 5-54).

Keep the wrists relaxed while moving the ball. Reaching the top of the circle, allow the chest to open up and exhale while extending the arms outward (Figure 5-55).

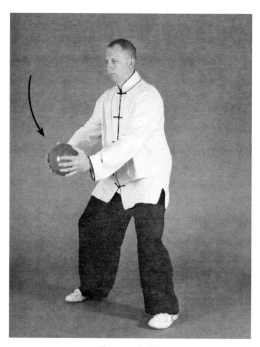

Figure 5-55

Allow the wrists to settle and the chest to begin closing as the ball begins to return to the original position (Figure 5-56).

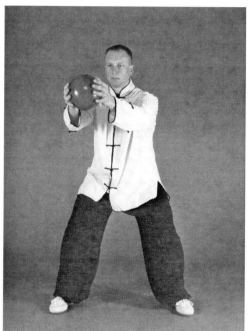

Figure 5-56

Gradually increase the size of the circling with each repetition until you have reached the maximum range of motion desired. The maximum size or diameter of your circle will depend on you. It should be large enough to allow your arms to extend fully out in front of your body without locking the elbows and no higher than your eyes. Throughout the motion, you should remember to keep your tailbone tucked in slightly and your head held upright, inhaling as you bring the ball toward you and exhaling as the ball moves away from you. The following diagram will assist you with your breathing patterns as well as your chest movements:

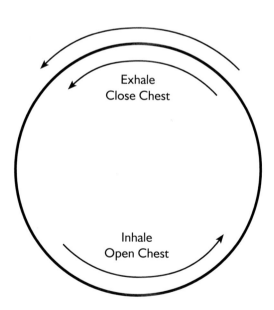

Diagram 1. Breathing and chest movements for yang vertical circling.

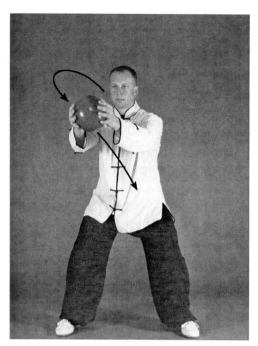

Figure 5-57

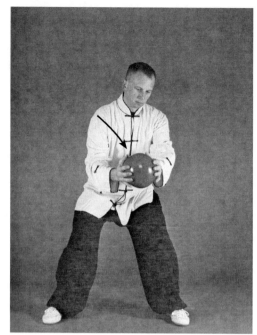

Figure 5-58

Once you have built up a smooth circular motion with the correct coordination of spine and chest movements, you should circle the ball vertically, moving it no more than the width of your shoulders. The ball should now follow a path from one shoulder diagonally down to the opposite hip (Figures 5-57 and 5-58).

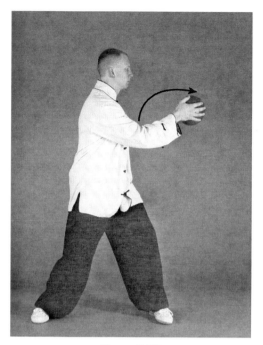

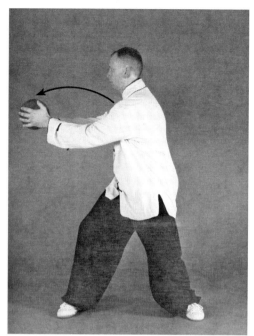

Figure 5-59   Figure 5-60

The next stage of this vertical exercise is to twist your torso as far as you comfortably can, both to the left and right while vertically circling (Figures 5-59 and 5-60).

As with the initial circling exercise, you may also circle the ball diagonally from one shoulder to the opposite hip. Practicing this exercise with your upper torso twisted in either direction allows you to condition your joints, ligaments, tendons, and muscles on different angles. In ancient times, this training was necessary for those who often fought while on horseback.

Repeat each stage of this circling action for at least 12 repetitions; then you should turn back to face forward and gradually reduce the circling pattern until you have spiraled back to your center.

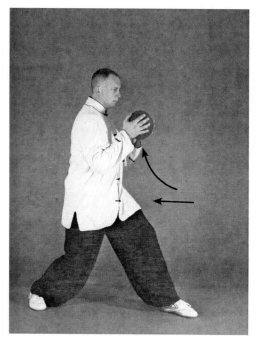

Figure 5-61

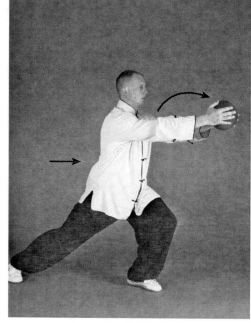

Figure 5-62

2. Rocking (*Qian Hou Dong,* 前後動)

The next stage of this pattern is to perform it while rocking. Rocking is the initial stage of stepping and teaches you to connect the rooting of the feet with the rest of the body.

To begin the rocking pattern, start in the ma bu stance with the taiji ball held in front of your dan tian. From this position, step into your si liu bu stance. Place either foot forward first. Practice on both sides.

To start circling, inhale while rocking slightly aft. Arch your back slightly, and draw the ball downward and in toward your body. Reaching the most aft position, begin to exhale and start your forward motion while moving the ball over the top of the circle and forward. Settle the wrists, close the chest and allow the ball to return to the original position, completing the circle (Figures 5-61, 5-62 and 5-63).

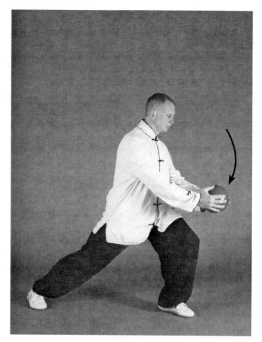

Figure 5-63

Once again initiate the pattern with small circles; then gradually increase to larger circles. The ball will appear to spiral outward when observed from the side. You should

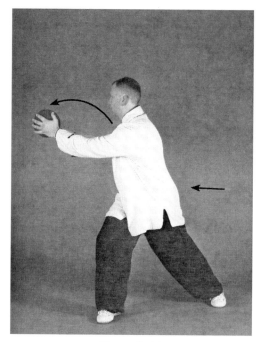

Figure 5-64

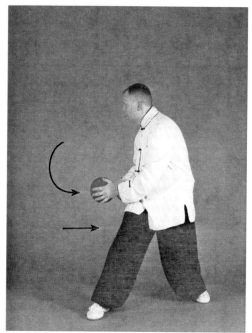

Figure 5-65

note that the initialization of movement now starts with the feet and continues up through the body ending with the ball.

Next, vertically circle the ball, as you did in the stationary exercise, diagonally from one shoulder to the opposite hip while rocking. Once you become comfortable with this movement, increase your range of motion by twisting your waist to the left and right while rocking (Figures 5-64 and 5-65). After a minimum of 12 repetitions, return to the center and continue to decrease the circles until you reach your original starting position.

Step back into your ma bu stance, and then step into the si liu bu stance with the opposite foot forward. Repeat the pattern for an additional 12 repetitions for each section. To complete this exercise, return to the center, reduce the pattern to the original position, and step back into ma bu.

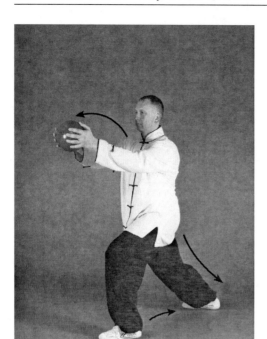

Figure 5-66

3. Straight Line Stepping (*Zhi Xian Xing Bu*, 直線行步)

The next step is to vertically circle the taiji ball while stepping. Stepping is simply a continuation of rocking. Instead of remaining in a fixed area, continue the motion forward or backward as desired. This can be done using two methods: 1) Use momentum to move forward or backward. 2) Use a balance technique of stepping. This is where the ball moves forward while you simultaneously slide your foot backward (Figure 5-66).

Although you may step to different angles using either method described, in this section we are moving linearly. In either technique, you may take more than one step in either direction.

Start in a ma bu stance, step into si liu bu, with either foot forward. Hold the taiji ball in front of your dan tian. Begin to vertically circle the ball in a yang direction as described in the rocking pattern. Continue this action until you have reached your maximum range of motion.

To step forward, begin from the most aft position in rocking. You will be transitioning from inhaling to exhaling and your chest movements will be moving from opening to closing. The path of the ball will be rising up in front of your body.

Initiate the forward momentum by pushing off your aft foot, and allow the energy to flow up your rear leg into the waist. Turn both your waist and forward foot out slightly and begin to shift your weight forward. From this point, the energy will transfer from the waist through the arms and into the ball. This will cause the ball to flow over the top of the circle. As you extend your arms, the ball will pull the body forward.

Slide the aft foot forward and set it down so you are in a si liu bu stance with the

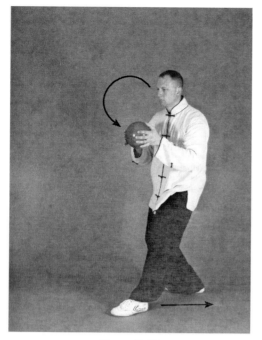

Figure 5-67

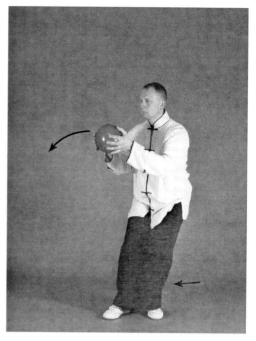

Figure 5-68

opposite leg forward (Figures 5-67, 5-68, and 5-69). The taiji ball will now be circling down and away from your body. This allows the transfer of energy back down through the body and into the forward foot. Continue stepping until you have traveled as far as you can in your practice area.

To step backward, initiate the movement from your most forward position of rocking. You will now be transitioning from exhaling to inhaling and your chest will be moving from closing to opening.

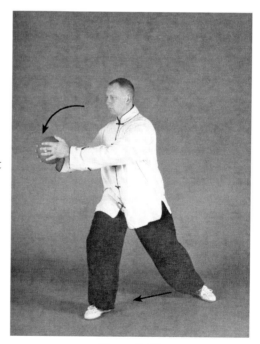

Figure 5-69

Initiate the momentum by pushing off the forward foot and shift your weight to the aft foot (Figure 5-70). Your body will now pull the ball through the bottom of the circle and aft. Slide your forward foot aft and place it down, toes pointed 45 degrees away from your centerline. You will now be in a si liu bu stance with the other leg forward. The forward foot should be readjusted so the toes are pointed in slightly toward your centerline.

To step back farther, simply rock forward; then push off the forward foot again creating the same momentum as before. Continue this stepping pattern until you have reached the original starting area; then decrease the circling pattern back to the center and step up into your beginning stance.

You can then practice taking more than one step at a time forward and or backward while circling the ball. Depending on the

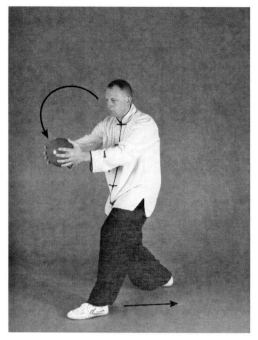

Figure 5-70

size of your circle and the speed, you may find you can take two or possibly three steps per one circle. It is also acceptable to combine your forward and backward stepping at any time.

The next phase of stepping is known as balance stepping. In this exercise, you will remain in the same space. The ball will travel back toward your body while your rear leg slides up to the other leg. You may then elect to shift your weight onto this foot or remain weighted on the original foot. The ball will then continue forward on its pattern while you slide the non-weighted foot back. When performed correctly, the ball and aft leg will correspondingly move together and separate simultaneously.

To begin, step into si liu bu. Start the vertical circling pattern in a yang direction while rocking and increase the size of the pattern to your maximum range of motion. From your most forward position in rocking, slide your aft foot forward while simultaneously circling the ball back toward your body. Place the foot down next to the other one and shift your weight onto it. Continue with the circling action of the ball and slide the opposite foot back as the ball moves forward. You will end this movement in the most forward position of rocking with the opposite foot aft.

Practice this exercise until you can do it smoothly. You may also elect to slide back the same foot you slid forward by not shifting the weight onto it. When you are comfortable with stepping using either method, you should try different combinations of momentum and balance stepping. You may also elect to step on angles when practicing the balance method of stepping.

4. Bagua Stepping (*Bagua Xing Bu,* 八卦行步**)**

The next exercise of this section is to perform the vertical circling while using bagua stepping. Bagua stepping is used in the Chinese martial art style, baguazhang. This style is based on the theory of the bagua whose source was the *I Ching (Book of Changes)*. The bagua practitioners imagine the eight trigrams of the *I Ching* are placed on the ground in a circle. They then step around this circle while moving the arms in various postures and directions derived for self-defense training. For our exercises, you will step in the circular fashion of the bagua practioner while practicing the vertical circling pattern. This will place more emphasis on the joints in the legs as well as increase the twisting action placed on the spine. To learn more about baguazhang, please refer to the book, *Baguazhang–Emei Baguazhang* by Master Liang, Shou-yu, Dr.

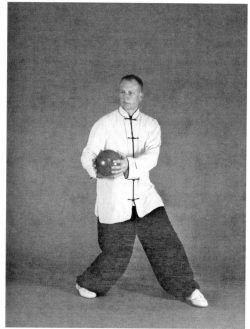

Figure 5-71

Yang, Jwing-Ming, and Mr. Wu, Wen-ching, available at YMAA Publication Center.

To perform this pattern while bagua stepping, you will need to find an area where you are able to walk around in a complete circle without any obstructions. In our case, the path will begin by moving clockwise around the circle.

Start in the ma bu stance with the taiji ball lightly cradled between your hands. Step into your si liu bu stance, left leg forward. Twist your body to the right so you are facing toward the center. The ball will vertically circle toward the center of your intended path (Figure 5-71). The movements of the chest and breathing will be the same as the previous exercise while stepping forward and backward.

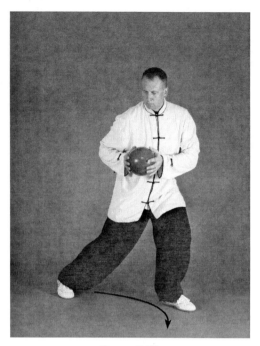

Figure 5-72

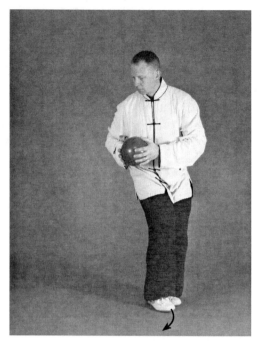

Figure 5-73

To move forward, the motion begins with a push off the back foot and follows through to the ball. The chest will be open in the aft position, and the chest will be closed in the forward position. Inhale while in the aft position and exhale while moving forward (Figures 5-72, 5-73, and 5-74). In this stepping your upper body is twisted toward the center of your circular path. Continue this pattern until you have completed 12 circles in one direction.

If you are familiar with and proficient in bagua stepping, then you may go ahead and change the direction of your path. If not, decrease your vertical circling back to the original position and step back into ma bu. From there, you can step into a si liu bu stance, right leg forward, and repeat the exercise while bagua stepping in a circle, in the opposite direction.

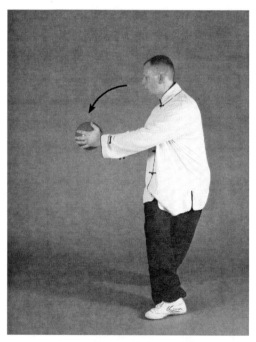

Figure 5-74

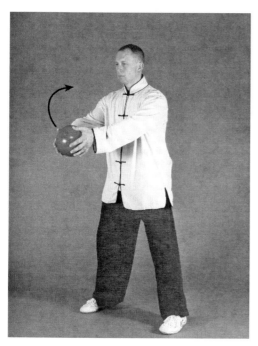

Figure 5-75

Yin Circling (*Yin Rao,* 陰繞)

1. Stationary (*Ding Bu,* 定步)

The next pattern is known as yin vertical circling, or backward circling. It is the same as the yang pattern only the movement is done in the reverse direction. Remember to start with small circles; then gradually transition to larger ones.

Once again stand in the ma bu stance with your feet parallel, shoulder width apart, knees slightly bent, and your hands cradling the ball in front of your dan tian. Take a few deep breaths while leading your qi to the dan tian. Once again, initiate the movement from the dan tian, up the spine and out through the arms to the ball. Slowly inhale while raising the ball upward and toward you (Figure 5-75).

FOLLOW ALONG
VERTICAL CIRCLING—BACKWARD (YIN)

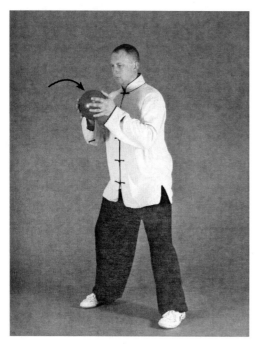

Figure 5-76

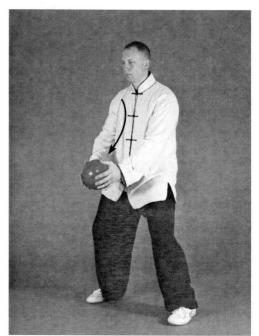

Figure 5-77

Draw in the chest and redirect the path of the ball down (Figure 5-76).

Allow the ball to continue its circular path down and away from you while opening the chest and exhaling (Figure 5-77).

Do not push the ball so low that it causes your wrists to bend too much and results in restriction of the flow of qi (Figure 5-78).

Once you have become comfortable with this movement, alter the direction of your yin circle slightly by circling the ball diagonally from one shoulder to the opposite hip. This exercise should be followed by twisting the waist both to the left and right while practicing the same pattern (Figures 5-79 and 5-80). Repeat each section of this exercise for at least 12 repetitions; then return to the center and decrease the circling pattern until you have reached back to the original starting position.

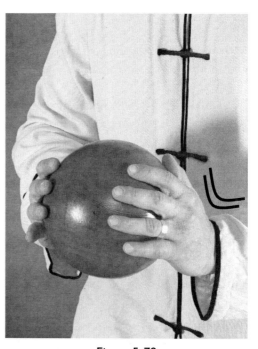

Figure 5-78

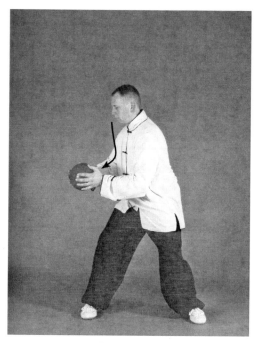
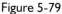

Figure 5-79

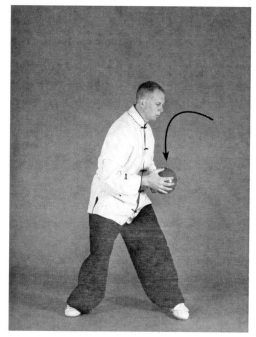

Figure 5-80

2. Rocking (*Qian Hou Dong,* 前後動)

Next, practice yin vertical circling while rocking.

To start this exercise, place the ball in front of your dan tian while standing in ma bu. Step into si liu bu with either leg forward and breathe deeply while leading your qi down into the dan tian. Begin to rock forward into deng shan bu by pushing off the aft foot. Allow this movement to continue up through the body, out through the arms, and into the ball. Rocking forward, raise the ball, exhale, and open the chest. Do not tense the wrist while raising the ball. Instead, allow the weight of the ball to pull upon the hands. (Figure 5-81).

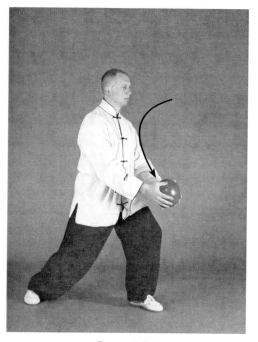

Figure 5-81

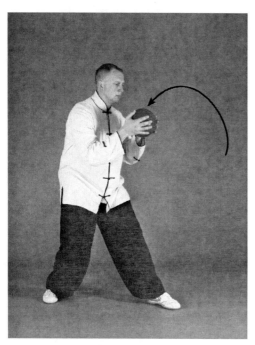

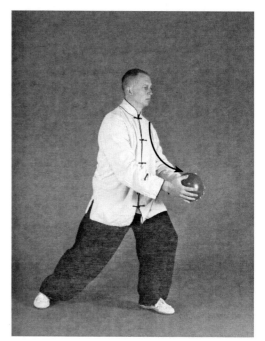

Figure 5-82   Figure 5-83

After you reach your desired position rocking forward, change to rocking aft. The taiji ball will continue its circular movement over the top, toward the body, and down. The chest should begin to close as the ball is drawn toward you and you complete your inhalation (Figure 5-82). At this time, your body will have reached the desired aft position.

Begin the forward rocking motion. Begin to open the chest and start exhaling. Allow the ball to continue its descent; then settle your wrists as it moves away from the body, returning to the original starting point (Figure 5-83).

Repeat the pattern, gradually increasing its size upon completion of each circle. Once you have reached the desired range of motion, continue for 12 repetitions.

Next, you should practice the diagonal movement as well as the twisting of the waist as described in the previous exercises. Complete each section for 12 complete repetitions; then return to the center and gradually spiral the movements back to your original starting position located by your dan tian. Finally, step back into the ma bu stance.

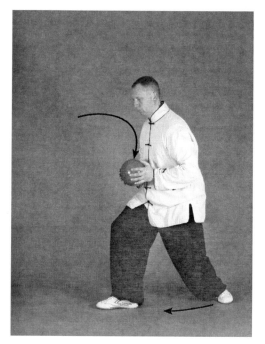

Figure 5-84

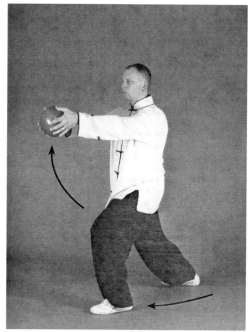

Figure 5-85

3. Straight Line Stepping (*Zhi Xian Xing Bu,* 直線行步)

The next exercise incorporates stepping in a linear direction while moving the ball in a yin vertical circling pattern. This also should be done using both the momentum and balance methods of stepping as explained in the yang circling section.

Start in ma bu with the ball cradled in front of your dan tian. Step into the si liu bu stance with either foot forward and begin your normal rocking pattern as previously described. Once you have reached your maximum range of motion you may begin the stepping exercise. To step forward, start from the most aft position in rocking. Begin to exhale and open your chest. Turn the forward foot out slightly, and then push off the aft foot. (Figure 5-84).

Shift your weight forward, lift the aft foot, and slide it out in front of you. From this position, your ball will now be ascending on the far side of the circle (Figure 5-85). Continue to step linearly while vertically circling the ball in a yin direction until you have reached the end of your practice area.

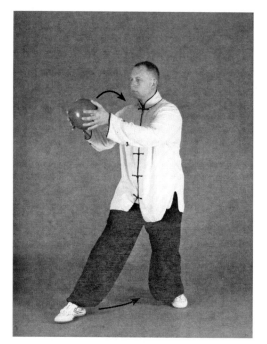

Figure 5-86

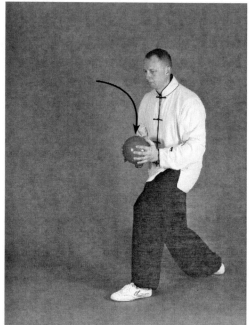

Figure 5-87

This is an opportune moment to begin to practice stepping backward. Begin from the most forward position of your yin circle. Push off the forward foot and draw the ball over the top of the circle toward you (Figures 5-86 and 5-87).

Continue to step backward until you have returned to your original starting point. Next, you should practice stepping using the balance method of stepping. This will be done the same as described for the yang circling; only this time the ball will be traveling in the opposite direction.

You should continue to practice stepping back and forth across your practice area until you are comfortable in doing so. This should include taking more than one step at a time, forward and backward.

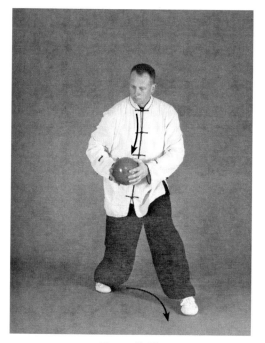

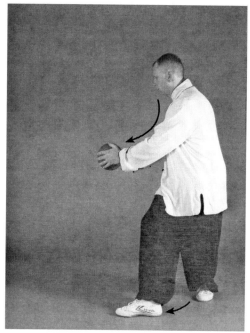

Figure 5-88   Figure 5-89

4. Bagua Stepping (*Bagua Xing Bu,* 八卦行步**)**

Finally, you should perform the same movement as above but using the yin vertical circling pattern. The difference here will be that you will move forward while the ball's path is traveling outbound on the bottom of the circle, and you will move backward while the ball travels inbound over the top of its circle (Figures 5-88, 5-89). Due to its similarity to the previous bagua stepping exercise, we will not describe the pattern in full detail here. Be sure to step around for at least 12 full circles for both sides.

Yin-Yang Exchange Circling (*Yin-Yang Hu Huan,* 陰陽互換)

In the following section, we will describe the yin-yang exchange while using the circling pattern. First, we will describe the exchange of the pattern itself; then we will explain how to change the direction you are facing while circling, followed by stepping and bagua stepping.

At this stage, you have done your circling patterns both in yin and yang directions. This was done by stopping the existing pattern, then restarting the pattern in the opposite direction. Now, we will change the direction of the ball through a continuous flow.

1. Stationary (*Ding Bu,* 定步)

To start, stand in ma bu and begin your stationary vertical circling pattern in a yang direction. Once you have reached your maximum range of motion, continue for a few repetitions.

Now we will change the direction of the pattern to yin. Picture the infinity symbol or the figure '8'. As the ball travels over the top of its circle and downward, begin to draw the ball through the center of the circle toward you (Figure 5-90). Viewed from your left side, your movement will appear to form the top of the letter 'S'. Once the ball reaches the center of the circle, you can change the direction of the pattern from yang to yin. The center of this circle is known as the wuji point.

To further illustrate this, imagine the curve of the taiji yin-yang symbol (Diagram 2). The ball passes through the center of the symbol. The outer section is representative of your initial circle and the curved line through the center is your transition area. Now look at the center of the "S" curve. This is the place of no extremity known as the wuji. This is the point where the taiji begins to divide into yin and yang. It is at this point that you can begin to change directions. To do this, you must pass through this center.

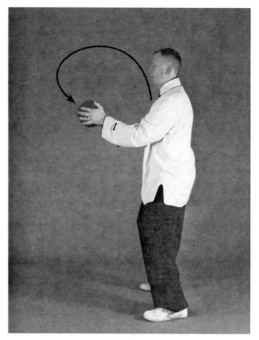

Figure 5-90

Allow the ball to continue its path down toward your body, then outward and up, following the path of the yin pattern (Figure 5-91). As you practice this exercise, your chest movement and breathing pattern will be as follows. Exhale and close the chest as the ball moves away from you in the yang section of the circle. Drawing the ball through the center, begin to inhale and continue to close the chest. The ball will now continue to the bottom part of your new yin circle, and you may resume the normal breathing and chest movements of the yin circling pattern. Continue this yin pattern for a few repetitions before attempting to switch back to yang.

To switch to the yang pattern, begin from the bottom of the yin circling pattern. Allow

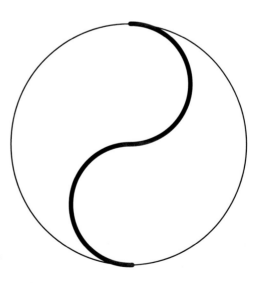

Diagram 2. 'S' curve of yin-yang symbol.

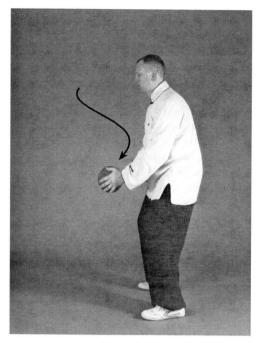

Figure 5-91

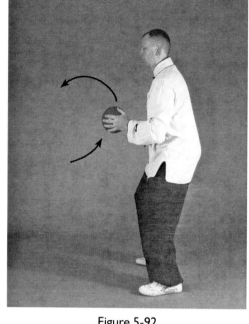

Figure 5-92

the ball to rise up slightly; then draw it toward you, once again pulling it through the center of the circle. As it reaches the center of the circle, change the pattern back to the yang pattern (Figures 5-92 and 5-93).

The ball will continue to rise up close to you and upon reaching the original size of the circle begin its path over the top of the original yang pattern. On this exchange, you are exhaling while opening the chest. While you draw the ball in toward you, begin to inhale while allowing the chest to continue to open. Once the exchange is complete, you may resume the normal chest and breathing patterns of the yang pattern. Practice this exchange back and forth between yin and yang until you can execute the exchange smoothly without interruption. Occasionally skip the exchange to practice circling in the same direction.

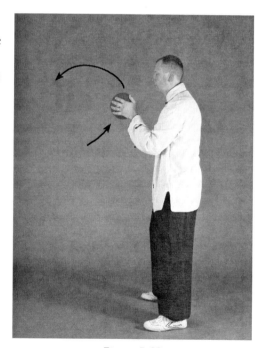

Figure 5-93

As you become more comfortable with the exchange, try to change the patterns at different sections of the circle. You may begin to experience the three dimensionality of the circling patterns.

2. Rocking (*Qian Hou Dong*, 前後動)

Next, practice exchanging between yin and yang while rocking, as well as changing the direction you are facing using this yin-yang exchange. The circling patterns are the same as the ones used in ma bu stance; therefore, we will only describe how to change the direction to which you are facing. We will first use the vertical circle pattern in a rocking motion.

Step into your si liu bu stance and begin your vertical circling pattern in a yang direction. Once you have reached your maximum range of motion, complete a few repetitions before performing the exchange to the other side.

To turn and face the opposite side, initiate the movement as the ball descends at the far end of the yang circle. This will coincide with your body being forward in the rocking position, your breathing transitioning from exhaling to inhaling, and your

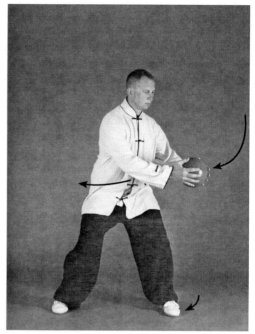

Figure 5-94

chest beginning to close. As your ball descends, begin to rock aft while pulling the ball toward you just as you did in the original rocking exercise. In this situation, however, you should be rocking aft while simultaneously turning the forward foot in toward your body and inhaling (Figure 5-94).

Twist the waist to redirect the ball, and turn the opposite foot out. Begin exhaling, and allow the ball to continue on its path waist height to the opposite side. You should now be facing 180 degrees in the opposite direction in a si liu bu stance with the ball moving out into the new circle.

From this position move into your deng san bu stance while moving the ball forward and upward on the far end of the circle and then back down toward your body on its yin circling path. Continue this yin circling pattern while rocking for a few repetitions; then change your direction using the same yin-yang exchange used to reach this side. Once you have changed back to your original position, change your pattern to the yang circling pattern, and then change the direction you are facing while maintaining the yang vertical circling pattern.

You will notice that in both cases, it will not be necessary to move the ball into the center of each circle when changing the directions. Instead, you are using your body as the center, or wuji point. This will allow you to remain rooted throughout the maneuver and also be able to change to either a yang or yin circle when changing directions. Continue to practice this exercise until you are able to change directions as well as perform exchanges consistently and fluidly.

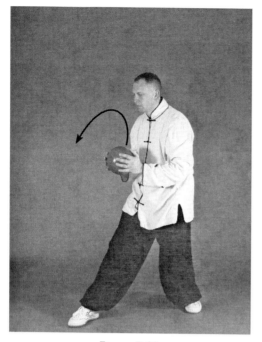

Figure 5-95

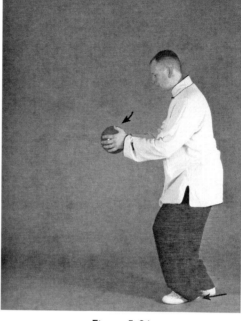

Figure 5-96

3. Straight Line Stepping (*Zhi Xian Xing Bu,* 直線行步)

The next stage of yin-yang exchanging is to practice it while stepping linearly. You may use the momentum or balance method of stepping. To begin the momentum stepping exercise, step into your si liu bu stance with the ball in front of your dan tian. Start your vertical circling pattern in a yang direction while rocking until you have reached your maximum range of motion.

To change from yang to yin, begin from your most aft position. Push off the rear foot and begin to step forward just as you have in the normal stepping exercise. The chest will be transitioning from open to close and your breathing will be changing from inhaling to exhaling. As the body shifts forward, allow the ball to travel through the center of the circle and continue down to the far lower end of your circle (Figures

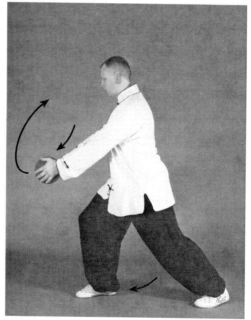

Figure 5-97

5-95, 5-96, and 5-97). With the proper timing, you should end with your desired foot forward and the ball will now be down and far forward, circling in the yin direction.

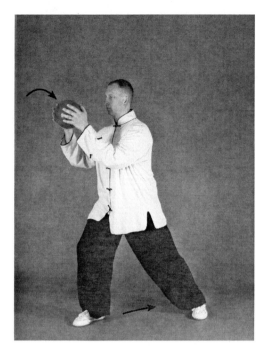

Figure 5-98

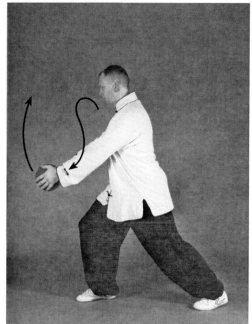

Figure 5-99

To change back to a yang direction while stepping, simply repeat the procedure as before, allowing the ball to drop down through the center of the circle. Although you may exchange between yin and yang anywhere in the circle, it is best to initially perform the exchange with the ball traveling forward and down through the center of the circle while stepping. This will allow the body to remain rooted. As you become more comfortable, you may try the exchange from different sections of the circle. Of course, one rule will remain. The exchange will have to be initiated from the most aft position of stepping when moving forward. This means the ball will be closest to you in the circling pattern. Continue to practice this exercise until you have traveled to the end of your practice area.

To perform the same exchange while stepping backward, you will initially execute it as you did when performing your normal backward stepping pattern. In this exercise, you push off your forward foot, allow the ball to travel from the far end of the circle down through the center, and arrive at the lower end of the circle close to your body (Figure 5-98). Using this technique, continue to perform your exchanging while stepping backward until you have returned to your original position in your practice area.

Next, practice the exchange while using the balance method of stepping. While circling the ball in a yang direction, begin to step forward as you were previously. Allow the ball to pass once again through the center of the pattern for the exchange. This time you will slide one foot back as the ball passes the central wuji point and begins its forward motion in the opposite direction (Figure 5-99).

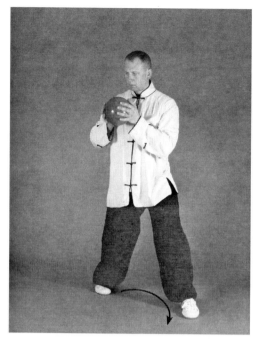

Figure 5-100

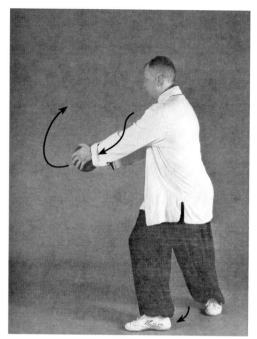

Figure 5-101

This may also be done for moving backward as well. Continue to practice this exercise until you are able to perform the yin-yang exchange smoothly for each situation described here in this section. To finish the exercise, reduce the size of your pattern back to your starting position and step back into ma bu.

4. Bagua Stepping (*Bagua Xing Bu,* 八卦行步)

The final stage of this exercise is to perform the exchange while bagua stepping. Step into a si liu bu stance with your left leg forward and twist your waist until you are facing the center of the circle you will be walking around. With the ball in front of your dan tian, start your vertical circling in a yang direction while rocking until you have reached your maximum range of motion. The stepping for this exercise will remain the same as described in the previous bagua stepping sections. To change from yang to yin, allow the ball to flow from the higher end of the circle down through the center, and end at the lower end of the circle (Figures 5-100 and 5-101). This will allow you to stay rooted throughout your stepping until you have become more comfortable with this exercise.

Continue to practice this exchange until you are comfortable stepping both forward and backward while exchanging between yang and yin. Just as you have done in the regular bagua exercise, you should practice exchanging while stepping both to the right and left.

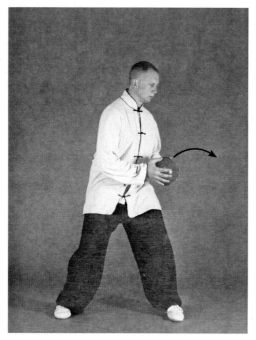

Figure 5-102

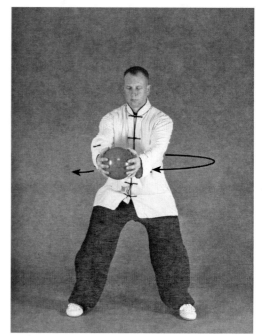

Figure 5-103

FOLLOW ALONG
HORIZONTAL CIRCLING—CLOCKWISE (YANG)

5.6.2.2 Horizontal Circling (Shui Ping Rao Quan, 水平繞圈)

The next pattern is known as horizontal circling. This motion involves moving your ball in a circular path on a transverse or horizontal plane. It will help you focus on the basics of utilizing the hips and shoulders as one unit as well as increase the strength and flexibility in the ankles, knees, and hip joints. This increase in flexibility will in turn change the shape of your pattern from a circle to more of an oval.

As we have mentioned earlier, circling horizontally in a clockwise manner is considered a yang pattern, and circling horizontally in a counterclockwise pattern in known as a yin pattern when viewed from a right-handed person. (When considering the direction of your pattern, it follows the principles of the yin-yang symbol training. With your right hand circling clockwise, you are performing a yang circle. If you use your left hand and circle it clockwise, it is considered a yin circle. When both hands are on the ball, you will consider it yin or yang based on your dominant hand.)

Yang Circling (*Yang Rao,* 陽繞)

1. Stationary (*Ding Bu,* 定步)

Start in ma bu stance while lightly cradling the ball between your hands. Initiate the horizontal circling by inhaling, twisting your waist slightly to the left, arching your back, and moving the ball slightly on an inward circular path (Figure 5-102).

Reaching your desired position to the left, initiate a right turn by twisting at the waist. The ball should now be on its outbound path and beginning to move to the right with the body. At this stage, the chest should now be opening and you should be exhaling (Figure 5-103).

When you pass through the centered ma bu stance, start to inhale, draw the ball back toward the body, and begin to close your chest. Reaching the desired position to the right, continue your circling motion back to the left pulling the ball along its circular path close to your body. Once again, on passing the central area, begin exhaling, move the ball outward, and start to expand your chest. Continue this movement back and forth, allowing the ball to spiral outward making a large circle. The maximum range of motion on the horizontal plane is the point your arms are fully, yet comfortably extended on the forward section of the circle. Use caution when the ball is extended out in front of you because there is a tendency to allow the upper body to lean over.

As you become more comfortable with this exercise, be sure to circle the ball horizontally at different heights. The highest level should be no higher than shoulder height. Continue this pattern for at least 12 repetitions; then slowly and gradually decrease the pattern until it has reached back to the center.

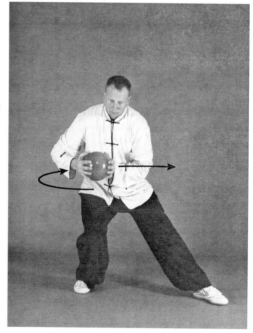

Figure 5-104

2. Rocking (*Qian Hou Dong,* 前後動)

The next pattern to practice is circling while rocking. This exercise will allow you to focus more on the twisting action in the joints of your ankles, knees, and hip joints or kua, all while rocking forward and backward. You will also notice the circle becomes more oval shaped with increased flexibility just as you did in the stationary circling exercise.

To start, step into a si liu bu stance with the ball cradled between your hands approximately at the dan tian level. Begin to inhale and initiate the movement from the forward foot up through your leg. As you start shifting your weight aft, twist the waist slightly to direct the ball on its horizontal circular path. From this initial movement aft, begin to close your chest and allow your arms to draw the ball back along the outside section of your circle (Figure 5-104).

Reaching your desired position aft, begin to twist your waist back while drawing the ball toward your body. From this position, you will transition back to rocking forward. Your chest will change from closing to opening and your breathing will change from inhaling to exhaling. Continue to twist your waist while initiating the shift forward. Allow the ball to continue on its forward path while exhaling and opening the chest (Figure 5-105). Once you have reached your desired position forward, transition back to rocking aft.

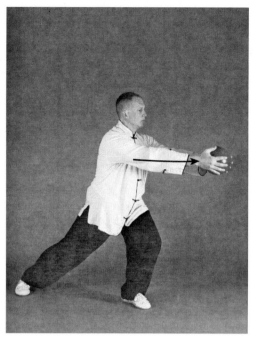

Figure 5-105

Each time you move forward and aft, increase the distance of rocking as well as the size of your circle. It is important to twist the waist as far as you can to increase your flexibility and strength. Reaching your maximum range of motion, you should repeat the pattern for 12 repetitions. Decrease the rocking pattern back to the original position and step back into a ma bu stance.

Now step into the si liu bu stance with the opposite foot forward and repeat the circling pattern. Once again, continue to horizontally circle for at least 12 repetitions. You should also change the height of the pattern just as you did in the stationary drill. Repeat this action for another 12 repetitions for each leg forward; then decrease the pattern back to its original starting point. Finally, step back up into a ma bu stance for closure.

3. Straight Line Stepping (*Zhi Xian Xing Bu,* 直線行步)

Now perform the horizontal circling pattern while stepping. In addition to the two methods of stepping previously discussed, there are two stages of momentum stepping that we will describe in this section. One involves allowing the center of the ball to travel laterally no more than the distance of the shoulders. The other method is more elaborate and involves the visualization of two horizontal yin-yang circles.

Begin by placing the ball between your palms while standing in a ma bu stance. Step into the si liu stance with either leg forward. Start your clockwise horizontal pattern while rocking as previously explained. Continue this rocking until you have reached your maximum range of motion.

To move forward using the first method of stepping, begin from your most aft position in rocking. The horizontal path of the ball will be no farther laterally than the width of your shoulders. You should be transitioning from inhaling to exhaling and your chest movement will be from closing to opening.

Pushing off the aft foot, allow the energy to be transferred from your foot through the leg into the waist (Figure 5-106).

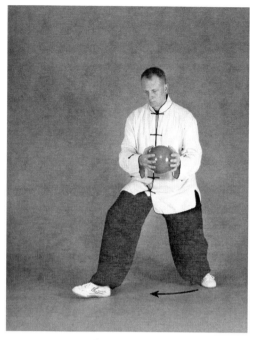

Figure 5-106

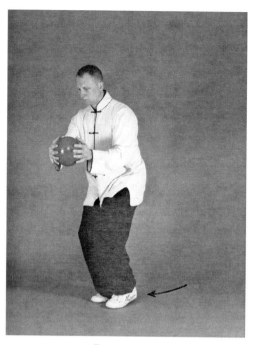

Figure 5-107

As the body shifts forward, the energy is now displaced from your waist though the body, out your arms, and into the ball (Figure 5-107).

This area of energy displacement is known as the transitional stage or wuji point of the body. It is where you are able to change the path of energy, without interruption. If you wish to remain in the rocking position, simply keep the waist and forward foot in their fixed position, allowing the energy to transfer back down into the forward foot. In our situation, this energy, transferred to the ball, is pulling your body forward with its accelerated momentum. Place the opposite foot down in front of your body and continue to circle the ball on a horizontal path (Figure 5-108).

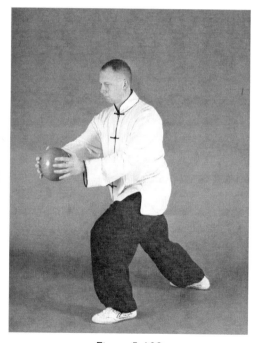

Figure 5-108

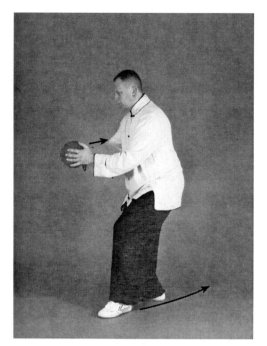

Figure 5-109

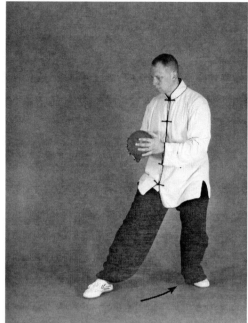

Figure 5-110

Continue to step forward until you've traveled to the end of your practice area.

From this position, practice the same technique while stepping backward. This will be done from the most forward position of circling while in transition from exhaling to inhaling with the chest changing from opening to closing. Push off the forward foot and draw the ball back toward you. Once again, in this stage the ball should move no more than the width of your shoulders. Slide your foot aft and continue to circle the ball horizontally (Figures 5-109 and 5-110).Continue to practice this stepping until you have reached your original position in the practice area.

The second method of momentum stepping allows you to circle your ball beyond shoulder width while stepping. In this situation, the ball will travel through the center of your existing circle, exit out the side, and then enter the center of the new circle through its side (Diagram 3). The stepping, breathing, and chest movements remain the same as before.

When moving forward, push off the aft foot, transfer the weight forward, and slide the aft foot forward shifting into your si liu bu stance. Once the ball reaches the center of your new circle, you will either continue with the yang circle, or if necessary, you will complete a smaller yang circle before expanding back out to your original size. The difference in your motion is dependent upon which foot is forward. Continue to step forward using this method while horizontally circling in the yang pattern until you have reached the end of your practice area. It is also a good idea to pause occasionally to practice rocking.

Next, practice stepping backward while using the same method. To step backward, initiate the movement from your most forward position in the rocking pattern. Begin

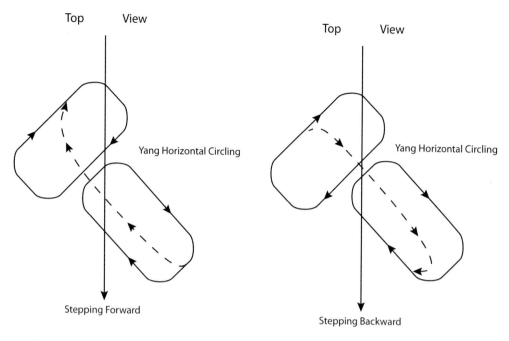

Diagram 3. Horizontal circling—
stepping forward.

Diagram 4. Horizontal circling—
stepping backward.

to inhale, push off your forward foot, and start to close your chest. Allow the ball to initiate its transition to the next circle by passing through the center of the original circle and exit out the side. Your body should continue to pull the ball as you shift your weight back on to the rear foot. Place the forward foot aft and continue to move the ball into the side of the new horizontal circle. While you shift your weight aft, turn the forward foot inward to realign the foot with the body. Once the ball reaches the center of the new circle, you will either continue on your original yang pattern, or, if necessary, you will complete a smaller circle before expanding back out to your original size. Continue to step backward until you are back to your original position in your practice area. Be sure to pause in between steps occasionally to practice rocking as well.

The following diagram will illustrate the action of the ball while stepping (Diagram 4). Your breathing techniques and chest movements will follow the same procedure as in the rocking pattern.

The final stage of this exercise is to practice the stepping using the balance method. This movement is the same as in the vertical circling exercise. You will slide the aft foot next to the other one when the ball moves back; then slide either leg backward when the ball moves forward. This can be done either linearly or on angles. Continue to practice this exercise until you are able to perform the action smoothly. When you have finished, gradually decrease the size of horizontal circling until you are back to your original starting position. Finally, step back into your ma bu stance for closure.

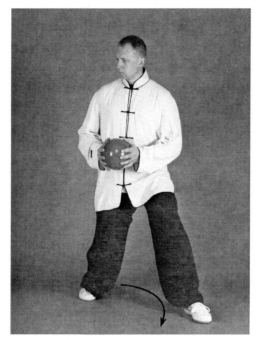

Figure 5-111

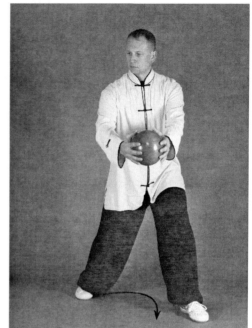

Figure 5-112

4. Bagua Stepping (*Bagua Xing Bu,* 八卦行步)

The final stage of horizontal circling is practicing it while bagua stepping. This movement will prove to be more difficult than the vertical circling bagua stepping. When you circle to the right and step forward with the right foot, you will have to turn into the right hip joint, or kua, for part of the circle. Depending on your flexibility, this may not be easy to do. Be aware of your body. Do not twist beyond the point where you can maintain the correct body alignment. With continued practice, you will be able to twist your waist farther and farther. To begin this pattern, cradle the ball lightly between your hands in front of your dan tian while standing in your ma bu stance. Step into a left si liu bu stance, twist your waist to the right and begin the horizontal yang circling pattern while rocking (Figure 5-111). Now, using the bagua stepping pattern, begin moving forward in a circular path to the right.

With the correct timing, you should feel the movement initiate from the foot, move up the legs, and continue through the waist. The waist will start twisting to the left, redirecting the energy. The chest will be opening up from the closed position, and the ball will be pulled along from the outside right section of the existing circle to the outside left section of the new circle (Figure 5-112).

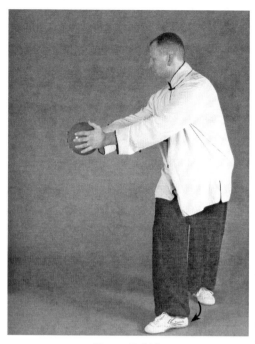

Figure 5-113

As the ball transfers from one circle to the next, the momentum will carry your body on to the next step. The breathing pattern will remain the same as before, inhaling while rocking aft, and exhaling while rocking forward. Continue to step forward until you have walked around in a complete circle and returned to your original position. Repeat this pattern until you have completed walking in twelve complete circles.

You must also practice this pattern while stepping backward. Start from a left si liu bu stance. To step backward, push off your left foot and shift your weight back over the right one. Simultaneously draw the chest inward while pulling the ball from the far outside section of your existing circle, back to the right outside section of your new circle (Figure 5-113).

Placing the left foot behind you, the ball will travel around the backside of the new circle while the chest is now opening. Complete the circle with the ball traveling from the left side of the circle to the forward section. Remember to inhale while rocking backward, and exhale while moving forward. Continue stepping backward until you have walked around 12 complete circles. When finished, decrease your horizontal circling back to the center and step back to your ma bu stance for closure.

After you practice for a while, you do not have to practice your stepping moving only in one direction. You should be able to move in either direction comfortably throughout the stepping process. In addition, you can also change the bagua circle stepping from the right side to the left side.

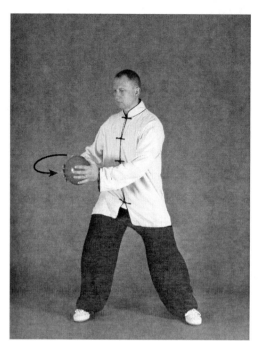

Figure 5-114

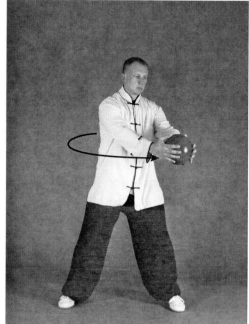

Figure 5-115

Yin Circling (*Yin Rao,* 陰繞)

FOLLOW ALONG
HORIZONTAL CIRCLING— COUNTER- CLOCKWISE (YIN)

1. Stationary (*Ding Bu,* 定步)

The next step of circling is the yin horizontal stationary movement. As before, the movement is begun in ma bu. Start the motion by twisting the body slightly to the right, closing the chest, inhaling, and moving the ball on its inward projected path of the circle. Reaching the desired point, twist back toward the left allowing the chest to open up. The ball should be on its way out and to the left while you are exhaling (Figures 5-114 and 5-115).

Continue these movements back and forth until you have increased the circle as much as you can. Use caution when the ball is extended out in front of you because there is a tendency to allow the upper body to lean over.

The next stage of this exercise is to circle the ball horizontally at different heights. Simply circle the ball at different intervals from shoulder height to waist height while practicing the pattern (Figures 5-116 and 5-117).

Repeat each stage of the pattern for 12 complete circles, and then slowly and gradually reduce the circle until you reach the originating point.

2. Rocking (*Qian Hou Dong,* 前後動)

The next step is to practice the yin horizontal circle while rocking. Begin in ma bu with the ball between your hands. Step into si liu bu with your right leg forward. Now start rocking into the aft position, close the chest, pull the ball toward you, and inhale. In the aft position, twist the waist to the right while leading the ball out and around the back side of the circle. Start exhaling, relax the chest, and rock forward while pulling the ball forward around the far side of your circle. Continue this movement back

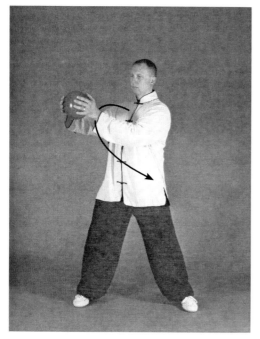

Figure 5-116

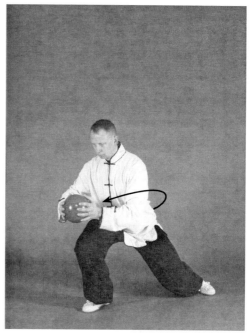

Figure 5-117

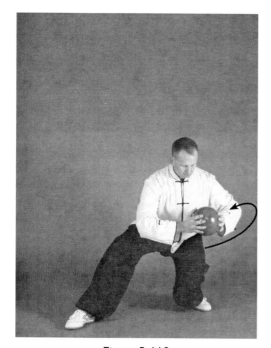

Figure 5-118

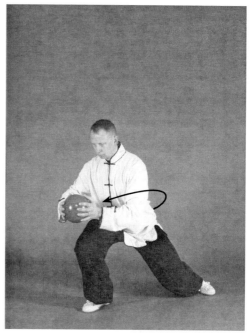

Figure 5-119

and forth, increasing the size of your circle to your maximum range of motion (Figures 5-118 and 5-119).

Remember to keep your shoulders and hips aligned throughout the movements. Once you are comfortable with this stage of circling, move on to the next stage and circle the ball at different heights. Continue each section for 12 repetitions, decrease your circle back to the original position, and step back into ma bu.

Now repeat the yin pattern with your left foot placed forward. You will notice this pattern will actually feel the same as your yang pattern with the right foot forward. When moving forward, you should be exhaling, your chest should be opening, and the ball will be on the left side of your circle. When moving aft, you will be inhaling, the chest will be closing, and the ball will be traveling on the right side of your circle. Repeat these patterns, including circling at different levels, for at least 12 repetitions, and then decrease your pattern back to the original position. Finally, step back into ma bu.

3. Straight Line Stepping (*Zhi Xian Xing Bu,* 直線行步)

Next, practice the same stepping technique while circling the taiji ball horizontally using a yin pattern. Essentially this stepping pattern remains the same as in previous exercises. The only difference is the direction of the horizontal pattern. Once again, be mindful of the timing of the ball with stepping forward or backward. The momentum must be initiated from the feet, travel up the legs to the waist, and finally out through the ball. Due to the similarity of this exercise to the previous one, we will not explain it in detail here. Be sure to practice both methods of stepping forward and backward previously explained as well as the balance method of stepping.

4. Bagua Stepping (*Bagua Xing Bu,* 八卦行步)

To complete this stage, you should now practice the same movement while practicing the horizontal circling in a yin pattern. Due to the similarity of this pattern to the previous one, we will not explain it in detail. The stepping, breathing, and chest movements all remain the same as previously explained; only the direction of the horizontal circle is different. Be sure to practice this pattern while stepping forward and backward to both the left and right sides. Also include different heights of horizontal circling as well.

Yin-Yang Exchange Circling (*Yin-Yang Hu Huan,* 陰陽互換)

1. Stationary (*Ding Bu,* 定步)

Moving on to the next exercise, we will describe the method of exchanging the horizontal pattern between yin and yang without interrupting the pattern. To begin this exercise, stand in ma bu and start the stationary horizontal circling pattern using a yang pattern. Once you have increased the size of the circle to your maximum range of motion, repeat the pattern for a few repetitions. Now to exchange from yang to yin, allow the ball to move out to the far left-hand side of your circle. As the ball continues on its path, start to draw it into your body. This time the ball will follow a horizontal 'S' shape while it passes through the center of the circle. Once it has reached the center of the circle, or wuji point, you will redirect the ball to its yin path (Figures 5-120, 5-121, and 5-122).

Allow the ball to continue its yin pattern for a few repetitions before you redirect it back to the yang pattern. Using the same method as before, allow the ball to reach the far right-hand side of its circle, and then redirect its path through the center of

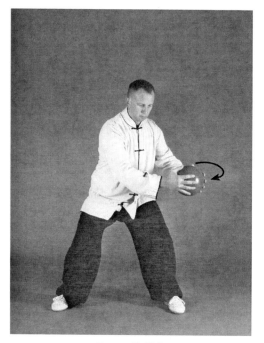

Figure 5-120

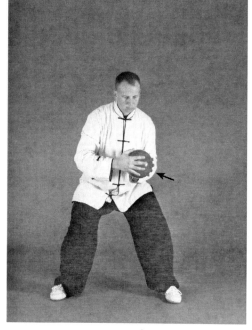

Figure 5-121

the circle and back into the yang pattern. Continue to practice this exercise, changing your movements from yin to yang and back again until you are comfortable exchanging smoothly, without interruption, and then reduce your circling pattern back to your original starting point.

2. Rocking (*Qian Hou Dong*, 前後動)

The next stage we will describe is to combine the yin-yang exchange with rocking. The exchange while rocking to one side is the same as you have done while stationary. Simply pass through the center of your circle. We will only describe the yin-yang exchange, which combines your rocking action with changing the direction you are facing while executing the horizontal circling pattern. As you will see from the description, this will follow the same rules you employed in the vertical yin-yang exchanging pattern. Once again, you will

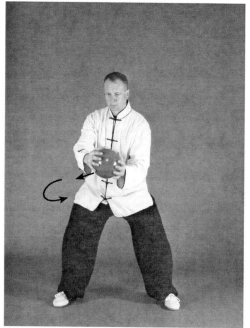

Figure 5-122

become the wuji point as you turn your body from one side to the other.

Begin with the horizontal clockwise circling pattern with the rocking motion.

Increase the diameter of the circling pattern until you have reached your maximum range of motion. To change your direction, begin with your body and the ball in the most forward position. Pushing off the forward foot, pull the ball toward your body just as you did in the horizontal circling pattern previously described. With the ball moving toward you, shift your weight back while simultaneously turning your forward foot in toward you. Twist your waist in the opposite direction while turning the opposite foot out (Figure 5-123).

The ball should maintain its path across your dan tian. Continuing with this movement, you will end up in a si liu bu stance, facing the opposite direction, and the ball will be moving on its outbound path. From this position, begin to rock forward and continue with your new horizontal circling counterclockwise pattern. Repeat this circling pattern for a few repetitions; then practice changing the direction of the pattern back to the original side.

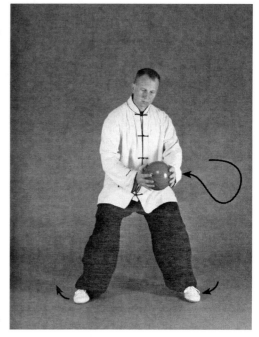

Figure 5-123

When you are comfortable switching back and forth, practice the exchange of directions along with an occasional exchange back and forth between yin and yang while on the same side. Repeat this exercise back and forth until you are comfortable and can perform it smoothly without interrupting the pattern.

3. Straight Line Stepping (*Zhi Xian Xing Bu,* 直線行步)

The next step is to practice the yin-yang exchange while stepping back and forth in a linear direction. Begin in si liu bu and begin your normal horizontal circling pattern in a clockwise direction. Continue until you have reached your maximum range of motion. Now begin to step forward and backward, and practice the exchange while using the two methods of stepping we have described in the stepping section of horizontal circling.

The first method involves keeping the path of the ball within the distance between the shoulders. The center of the ball will remain out in front and will not pass beyond shoulder width. In this case, you will simply pass through the center of the pattern as you step forward and backward. The second method allows the ball to extend laterally beyond the shoulders thus utilizing your maximum twisting ability. To execute

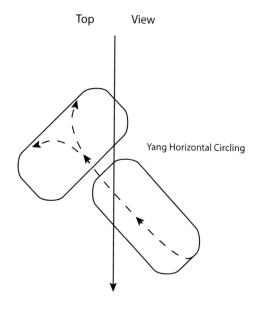

Diagram 5. Horizontal circling yin-yang exchange stepping forward and backward.

this exchange, you will pass through the center of the existing pattern, and then pass through the center of the new pattern as you step forward or backward (Diagram 5). This will become your wuji point and is where you will change to the opposite direction of horizontal circling.

Continue to step forward and backward using both methods of stepping until you are able to execute the exchanges smoothly. The next stage of this exercise is to perform the exchange while using the balance method of stepping. This exchange is done the same as the vertical one, only on a horizontal path. You may choose to exchange either while the ball is traveling aft or while it is traveling forward. Practice this method until the exchanges are smooth. When you are finished, reduce your circling pattern back to your dan tian and step into ma bu for closure.

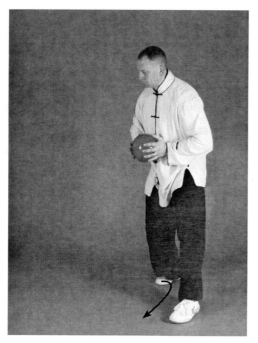

Figure 5-124

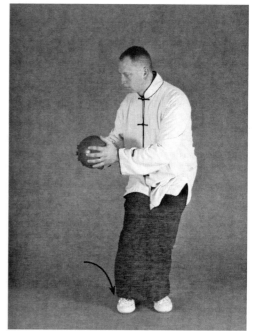

Figure 5-125

4. Bagua Stepping (*Bagua Xing Bu,* 八卦行步**)**

The final stage of horizontal exchanging is to perform it while stepping in a bagua pattern. Step into si liu bu, left leg forward. Twist your body to the right until you are facing the center of the circle you are about to walk. Initiate your normal horizontal circling in a clockwise direction while rocking until you have reached your maximum range of motion. To exchange from yang to yin while you are stepping bagua, start from your most aft position with the ball circling close to your body (Figure 5-124).

While pushing off your aft foot, begin to exhale and open your chest. As the ball begins to move forward, redirect its path toward the center of the circle you are walking (Figure 5-125).

Stepping forward, allow the ball to continue on its path forward and into a yin pattern. With the proper timing, you will simultaneously end with the ball on the far outside section of your yin circle and the opposite foot forward (Figure 5-126).

To change back to a yang direction while stepping, start from your most aft position with the ball circling on your right aft section of the pattern. Push off the aft foot while exhaling and opening the chest. As the ball moves forward, redirect its path to the center of the circular pattern. Step forward with the opposite foot, and allow the ball to follow through to the opposite side the circle moving in a yang pattern.

Practice this exchange while moving aft as well. Each time you exchange in this direction you will begin to do so from your most forward position in the pattern. The ball should also be in its forward section of the pattern and shall pass through the center of the existing pattern on each exchange. Continue to practice this pattern with the exchange occurring on both your forward movement and backward movement until it can be executed smoothly. In addition, the exchange should be done while bagua stepping both to the right and left.

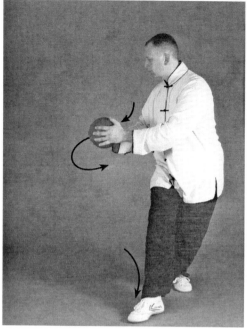

Figure 5-126

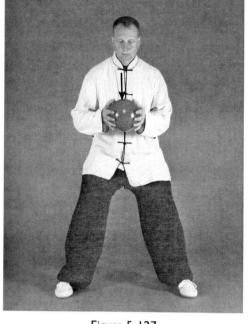

Figure 5-127

5.6.2.3 Vertical-Horizontal Yin-Yang Exchange Circling (Chui Zhi Shui Ping Yin Yang Hu Huan Rao Quan, 垂直水平陰陽互換繞圈)

The next stage of yin-yang circling exchange will be a complete freestyle movement where you are exchanging not only between yin and yang, but also between vertical and horizontal. Practice this exchange while stationary, rocking, straight line stepping, and bagua stepping.

Up to this point we have described two locations where you are able to exchange between yin and yang. One is located in the center of the pattern while the other is located in front of your dan tian. Now that you are going to add exchanges between vertical and horizontal patterns, you may discover additional areas to execute your exchanges. For example, while stationary you may exchange from vertical to horizontal by

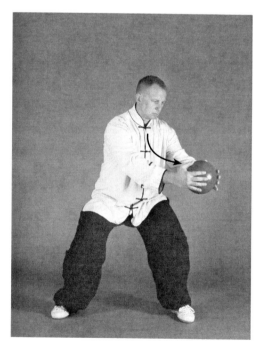

Figure 5-128

moving through the center of the pattern or by simply turning your waist as the ball is descending in the pattern (Figures 5-127 and 5-128).

There can be many different locations for this to occur. The wuji point is not an absolute location or point. The prevailing rule for exchanging is that the ball may not stop within the pattern to reverse its direction. For each of these patterns, we will begin with a yang vertical circling pattern. You may, however, elect to start with either the vertical or horizontal pattern in either the yin or yang direction.

1. Stationary (Ding Bu, 定步)

The first exchange will be performed while stationary. Standing in ma bu, begin to vertically circle the ball in a yang direction. Increase the size of the pattern to your maximum range of motion. The vertical yin-yang exchange will remain the same as previously described. To exchange from vertical to horizontal, simply pick a spot within the circle. Next, move the ball into the center of the pattern. Once it has reached this position, redirect the ball onto its horizontal circling path. You may also select whether you will continue on a yang direction or change to a yin direction. Continue with the horizontal pattern and exchange between yin and yang a few times. Now switch back to vertical. Once again, allow the ball to pass through the center of the pattern. From this wuji point, you may choose to remain on the existing direction or change to the other side. Once you are comfortable using this method of exchanging, practice the exchange by turning your waist and redirecting the ball from vertical to horizontal, or horizontal to vertical. Continue this exercise until you are able to exchange between both horizontal and vertical circling patterns as well as yin and yang from any position in the circling pattern without interrupting the pattern.

2. Rocking (Qian Hou Dong, 前後動)

The next exercise combines the use of rocking with a directional change while executing your vertical and horizontal exchanges. The exchanges while rocking are similar to those in stationary. As a result, we will only describe the directional exchanges here.

Step into si liu bu and begin your normal vertical circling pattern in a yang direction while rocking. Continue to increase the size of the pattern until reaching your maximum range of motion. To exchange from vertical to horizontal while changing the direction you are facing, begin from the forward position of rocking. Shifting aft, draw the ball toward you as it descends in its pattern (Figure 5-129).

Simultaneously turn the forward foot toward you and turn your body in the opposite direction. The ball will now be passing in front of your dan tian and from this point you will change its pattern to a horizontal circling pattern. You may choose whether to continue with a yang pattern or yin pattern.

To complete the exchange, turn your opposite foot out ending in a si liu bu stance 180 degrees from your original position. Shift forward into your deng san bu stance and continue with the horizontal pattern in either the yin or yang direction. Practice a few exchanges between yin and yang while rocking in one direction before going back to the opposite direction. Continue to practice this exchange back and forth. You may create any combination of exchanges you wish. Continue this exercise until you are able to comfortably exchange between yin and yang while rocking as well as when changing directions.

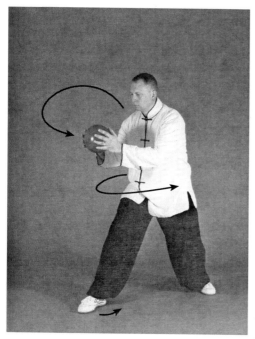

Figure 5-129

3. Straight Line Stepping (*Zhi Xian Xing Bu*, 直線行步)

The next stage of vertical-horizontal exchanging is to practice it while stepping in a linear direction using both the momentum and balance methods of stepping. To begin, step into your si liu bu stance and initiate your vertical circling pattern in a yang direction until you have reached your maximum range of motion. In order to exchange to horizontal, move the ball through the center of your vertical pattern; then twist the waist accordingly to redirect the ball as you are stepping forward. You may continue with the horizontal pattern in either a yin or yang direction.

To change back to vertical circling, use the first method of horizontal stepping by allowing the ball to move no further than shoulder width. Step forward while moving the ball into the center of the pattern. From this position, lead the ball out of the center into the vertical circling pattern in either the yin or yang direction.

To step backward simply perform the same movements in reverse order. From vertical to horizontal, draw the ball through the center of the existing pattern while stepping backward. Then lead the ball into the horizontal pattern in either direction. From horizontal to vertical once again draw the ball into the center of the pattern while stepping backward. Finally, lead the ball into the vertical circling pattern to finish the exchange.

Practice this stage of exchanging back and forth between vertical and horizontal while stepping forward and backward until you are comfortable with this exercise. In the next stage, practice the exchanges while allowing the ball to travel beyond the shoulder width, allowing an increase in your twisting range.

You may notice that there are other areas where the ball may seem to flow into the next pattern without passing through the center of the existing pattern. While stepping forward and backward, you should practice exchanging between vertical and horizontal, yin and yang, using these combinations as well.

Finally, practice your exchanging while using the balance technique of stepping. This will be no different than before. Each time you step, one leg will slide aft while the ball moves forward. The only difference is that the ball will now change from vertical to horizontal or vice versa.

Each stage of straight line stepping should be practiced until you can execute each exchange smoothly and without interrupting the pattern.

4. Bagua Stepping (*Bagua Xing Bu,*** 八卦行步)**

The final stage of the vertical-horizontal exchange is to perform it while bagua stepping in a circle. The rules remain the same for the exchange, whether vertical or horizontal, yin or yang. Each exchange may occur either by passing through the center of the existing pattern or by twisting the waist and redirecting the ball accordingly. At this stage, you should be comfortable with both the vertical and horizontal yin-yang exchanging. Therefore, we will not describe this exercise in full detail. Be sure to practice your exchanging between vertical and horizontal, yin and yang, while circling both forward and backward as well as to the right and left.

5.6.3 Rotating (Zhan Zhuan, 輾轉)

The next pattern we will describe is known as rotation. It is a good drill for training the kua (胯), i.e., the hip joint area, knees, and ankles and contains two elements. The first element is the circling motion you have been practicing in the previous section. This action is produced from the dan tian, travels up the spine, and exits through the arms into the ball. The second element involves the actual rotation of the ball within the circular path.

The rotation is produced by the continuous twisting action of the waist. This movement will cause one hand to be drawn backward as the other moves forward, resulting in the rotation of the ball. It is important to use your waist to lead the rotation as well as to keep it aligned with your shoulders; otherwise, your wrist will become tense causing the hand to rise off the ball when it travels close to your body. This creates a disruption in the flow of your qi. Practice this pattern slowly while focusing on keeping your hips and shoulders vertically aligned while twisting back and forth. In addition, your hands should not slide around on the ball but remain attached in the same position throughout your rotation.

The rotation pattern contains four separate directions: two are related to vertical, and two are related to horizontal. Similar to our circular pattern, rotating vertically forward is known as yang vertical rotation, while rotating vertically backward is known as yin vertical rotation. Rotating in a horizontal clockwise direction is known as yang horizontal rotation, and rotating in a counterclockwise direction is known as yin horizontal.

The vertical rotation is accomplished by placing your hands on the sides of the ball and then utilizing the twisting of your waist back and forth to initiate the rotation. As you increase the size of pattern, the hands will appear to move from the sides of the ball to the top and bottom. Horizontal rotation will begin with the hands on the top and bottom of the ball. As you increase the size of this pattern, the hands will appear to move out toward the sides of the ball. As you continue to practice this pattern, you may elect to rotate the Taiji ball more than once throughout the circular portion of rotation. The number of rotations per circle is up to you. This will also hold true while practicing horizontal rotations.

Once again, we have selected 12 repetitions as a sufficient number to condition the body, breath, mind, qi, and spirit. Although these patterns are more difficult than the previous ones, the preceding drills should provide you with the foundation to understand this pattern. By starting with basic drills, your body is gradually and safely conditioned.

These exercises should be practiced first without a ball, then with the ball. Again if you are not comfortable with 12 repetitions, simply choose a lower number and work your way up to this number. As your body becomes more comfortable, you may elect to increase the number of repetitions.

5.6.3.1 Vertical Rotation (Chui Zhi Zhan Zhuan, 垂直輾轉)

Yang Rotating (Yang Zhuan, 陽轉)

I. Stationary (Ding Bu, 定步)

The first direction we will describe will be the yang vertical rotation while standing in a stationary position. The direction of the rotation will follow the same direction of your circling. For this pattern, the hands will move forward when on top the ball and backward when under the ball.

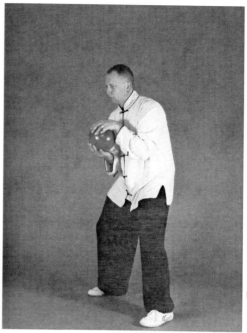

Figure 5-130

FOLLOW ALONG
VERTICAL ROTATION— FORWARD (YANG)

To begin, stand in ma bu with the ball held in front of your dan tian. Take a moment to lead your qi to your dan tian with a few deep breaths. Inhale and start moving the ball toward you using the same technique you used in the stationary circling exercise. As this occurs, simultaneously begin to twist your waist back and forth (Figure 5-130). Try to keep the sliding action of the hands on the ball to a minimum. As you increase the twisting action of the waist, your hands will eventually remain on the top and bottom of the ball.

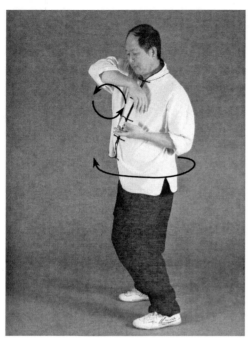

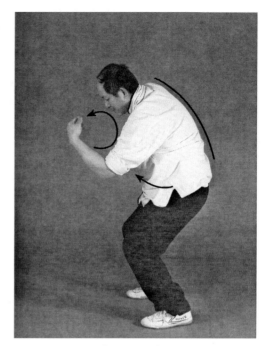

Figure 5-131   Figure 5-132

The breathing method and chest movement will follow the same flow as previously practiced in the yang circular pattern. Inhalation should be accomplished while the path of the ball is coming toward you while exhalation should be done as the ball moves away from you. The chest opens while the ball is moving toward the body and closes with the ball moving away from your body (Figures 5-131 and 5-132).

Once you have completed 12 repetitions of yang rotations, continue with the pattern and move the ball diagonally from one shoulder to the opposite hip. Repeat for an additional 12 repetitions; then twist your waist so your upper body faces both the left and right side. Repeat the pattern for each side for 12 repetitions. When you have completed this stage of rotations, return to your center and slowly decrease the pattern back to your original starting position.

2. Rocking (*Qian Hou Dong,* 前後動)

Next, practice the yang vertical rotation while rocking. Just as in the previous exercise, we are building upon your circling skills.

Begin in ma bu, taiji ball in front of your dan tian cradled between your hands. Turn your left foot out, and step into si liu bu, right leg forward. Breathe deeply and lead the qi into your dan tian. Begin with small movements. Inhale, push off the right foot, close the chest, and twist the waist back and forth while drawing the ball toward you. Allow the ball to follow through the bottom half of its circular path and begin its ascent (Figure 5-133).

Next, begin your forward rocking motion. Push off the back foot, exhale, close the chest, and allow the ball to continue on its circular path away from the body (Figure 5-134).

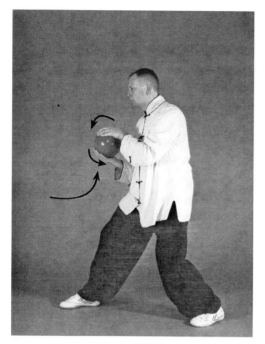

Figure 5-133

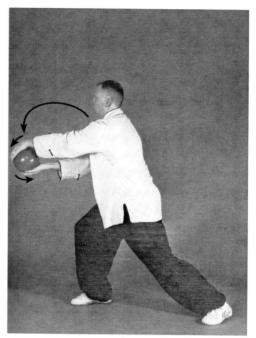

Figure 5-134

All of this is occurring simultaneously with your continuous twisting of the waist and rotation of the ball. Continue this pattern until you have expanded the size of the pattern to your maximum range of motion. Repeat this exercise for 12 repetitions, and then practice moving the ball diagonally from one shoulder to the opposite waist.

Once you have completed each stage for 12 repetitions, return to your center and decrease the pattern back to your original starting point. Step back into ma bu, turn the right foot out, and step into si liu bu, left leg forward. Repeat each stage of the pattern as previously described for 12 repetitions, decrease it back to your original starting position, and then step back into ma bu for closure.

3. Straight Line Stepping (*Zhi Xian Xing Bu,* 直線行步)

Now that you have practiced your rotation while rocking, it is time to continue on to the different methods of stepping. The same rules apply to rotation and to circling. It is crucial to find the correct timing to transition from one stance to the next. It is equally as important to begin with a constant slow speed throughout the stepping process, and to keep your hips and shoulders aligned vertically throughout the maneuver. Increasing the speed of rotation too rapidly often results in a disconnection between the two and you will end up rotating the ball using your hands and not your body. Remember the waist is the driver, as well as the connection between the legs and the torso.

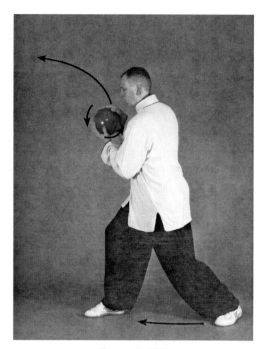

Figure 5-135

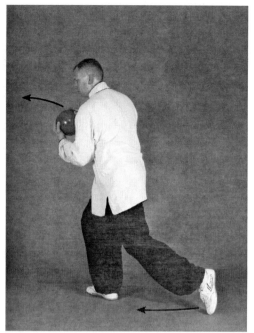

Figure 5-136

To begin the momentum stage of linear stepping, start in ma bu, and then step into si liu bu. Breathe deeply while leading the qi to your dan tian. Next, vertically rotate the ball in a yang direction while rocking as previously described. Increase the rotation pattern until you reach your maximum range of motion. To step forward and backward, use the same stepping methods as you did in circling. While in si liu bu, turn the forward foot out and allow the ball's momentum to pull you forward (Figures 5-135, 5-136, and 5-137).

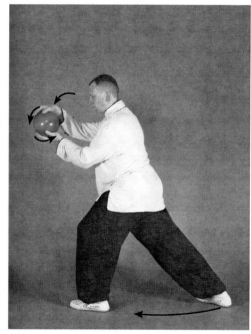

Figure 5-137

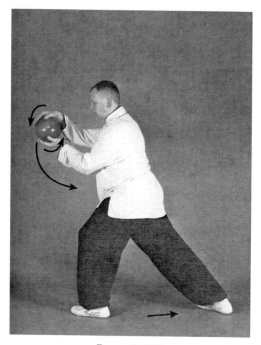

Figure 5-138

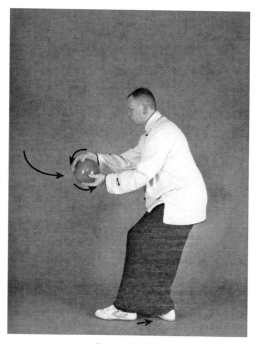

Figure 5-139

To step backward, begin from deng san bu and draw the ball toward you while stepping back (Figures 5-138, 5-139, and 5-140).

Continue to step back and forth in your practice area until you are able to do so comfortably while rotating the ball.

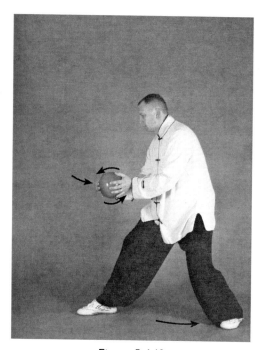

Figure 5-140

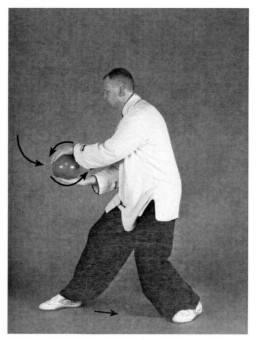

Figure 5-141

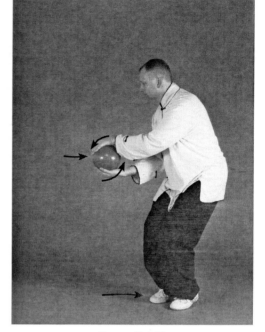

Figure 5-142

The next stage of stepping involves the balance method. In this situation you will be moving the ball forward while one leg moves aft. Just as you have practiced in your circling exercises, this may be done linearly or on angles (Figures 5-141, 5-142, and 5-143). You should continue to practice this stage of stepping until you are able to do so smoothly and without interrupting the pattern.

In the final stage of this exercise, you should combine both methods of stepping. In addition, you should include taking more than one step when moving forward and/or backward. Once you have completed all the stages of stepping, decrease the rotations back to your original starting point and step back into ma bu for closure.

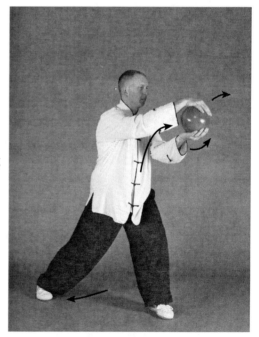

Figure 5-143

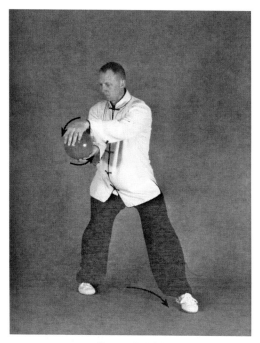

Figure 5-144

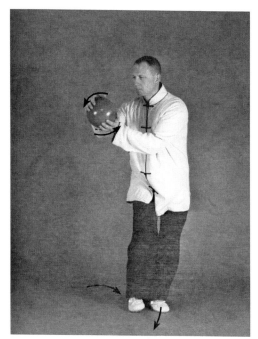

Figure 5-145

4. Bagua Stepping (*Bagua Xing Bu,* 八卦行步)

The final stage of vertical rotation is practicing it while moving in bagua stepping. This will take some time to master due to the twisting of the waist for rotating the ball.

With your taiji ball in front of you, step from ma bu to si liu bu, left leg forward. Now twist your waist so that your upper body is facing to the right and begin the rotation pattern as previously described in the rocking section (Figure 5-144). Continue to rock forward and aft a few times until you are comfortable rotating in that direction.

From this position, start your bagua stepping to the right. Depending on the flexibility of your waist, you will find a certain degree of difficulty with the right leg forward. Overall, the actions involved in rotational bagua stepping are fundamentally the same as circling. Moving forward, you are pushing off the rear leg, your chest is closing, you are exhaling, and the ball is traveling over the top of its circular rotation as well as moving away from you (Figure 5-145).

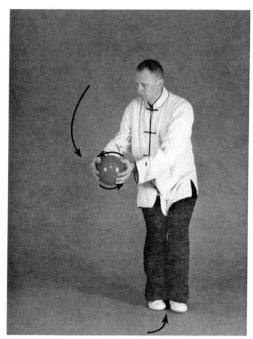

Figure 5-146

Moving aft, push off the forward foot; your chest begins to open, and you inhale while you draw the ball toward you in its descent (Figure 5-146).

Continue to step forward and backward in your bagua circle until you have reached your original starting point.

Practice this stepping until you are able to perform the pattern effortlessly while moving forward and backward in bagua circles. To finish stepping in this direction, twist the body back facing forward, slowly decrease your rotations back to the center, and step back into ma bu.

Next, make your circle to the left by stepping into si liu bu with your right leg forward. Twist your upper body to the left and begin your rotation while rocking. From this point continue your rotating and start your normal bagua stepping to the left. Continue to step in bagua circles to the left until you are able to perform the pattern effortlessly while stepping forward and backward.

To end, twist your body back to facing forward, slowly decrease the rotation of the ball back to the center while rocking, and finally step back into ma bu. Once again, if you are comfortable with bagua stepping, you may simply change from the right circling to the left and back without stopping the rotations.

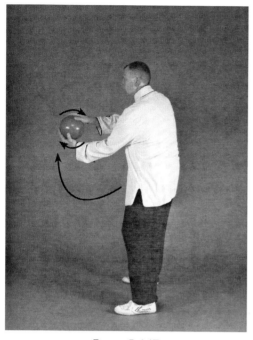

Figure 5-147

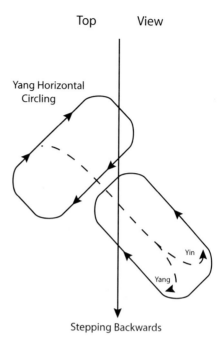

Diagram 6. Breathing and chest movements-
yin rotating.

Yin Rotating (*Yin Zhuan,* 陰轉)

I. Stationary (*Ding Bu,* 定步)

Next, practice the yin vertical rotation. This exercise is the same as the previous one with the exception that the movement is in the reverse direction. The rotation section of this pattern is now done by twisting the waist and moving the hands backward while over the top of the ball and forward while moving under the ball.

Position yourself in ma bu with the taiji ball in front of your dan tian. Breathe deeply while leading the qi into your dan tian. To begin the yin pattern, slowly twist the waist back and forth in small increments while allowing the body to initiate the movement of the ball up and away from the body on its circular path (Figure 5-147).

The breathing method and chest movement follow the same principles of the yin circular pattern. Inhale with the chest closing when the ball is traveling toward the body. Then exhale with the chest opening as the ball travels away from the body (Diagram 6). Continue to increase the size of this pattern until you have reached your maximum range of motion; then complete 12 repetitions of the yin vertical rotations.

FOLLOW ALONG
VERTICAL ROTATION—
BACKWARD (YIN)

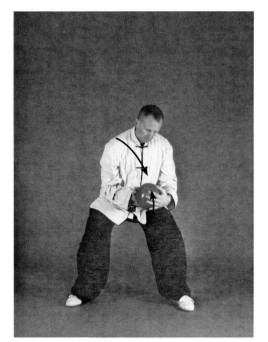

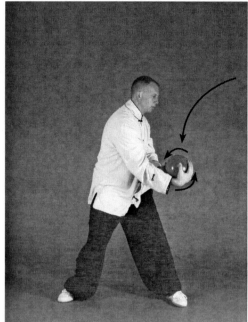

Figure 5-148   Figure 5-149

Next, move the ball diagonally from one shoulder to the opposite hip while rotating the ball (Figure 5-148).

Finally, twist your waist both to the left and right while in ma bu and complete 12 repetitions of vertical rotations in the yin direction (Figure 5-149). You may also include a diagonal motion for each side as well. Once you have completed this, return to the center and decrease the size of the pattern to your original starting point for closure.

2. Rocking (*Qian Hou Dong,* 前後動)

The next exercise is the vertical rotation in a yin direction while you are rocking. To start this exercise, step into si liu bu with your taiji ball in front of your dan tian. Using small slow movements, twist your waist back and forth to initiate the rotation of your ball. Push off your forward foot to rock aft while the ball ascends and is then drawn down toward your body on its circular path. You should be inhaling and your chest should be closing (Figures 5-150 and 5-151).

Pushing off your aft foot to rock forward, begin your exhaling and open the chest allowing the ball to follow through the bottom of the rotational pattern and return to the starting point (Figures 5-152 and 5-153).

Continue to increase the size of the pattern in small increments until you have reached your maximum range of motion; then repeat the patterns for 12 repetitions.

The next step is to move the ball diagonally while rocking, just as you have done while stationary. Repeat this section for an additional 12 repetitions. Finally, return to the center; decrease the size of rotations until you have arrived back at your original starting position, and step back into ma bu. Now step into si liu bu with the opposite foot forward, and repeat each section of the pattern for an additional 12 repetitions.

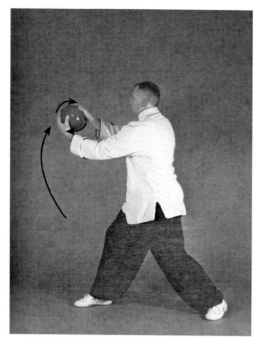

Figure 5-150

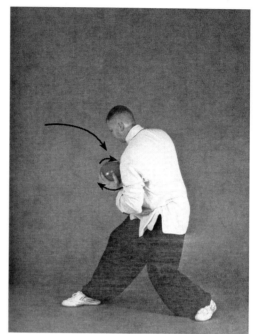

Figure 5-151

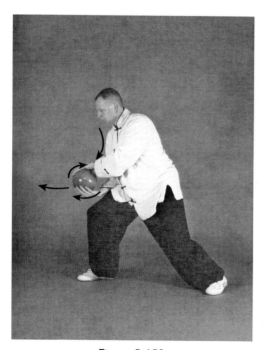

Figure 5-152

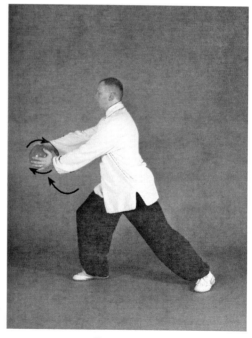

Figure 5-153

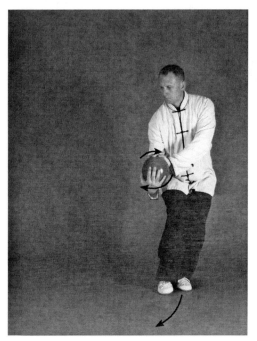

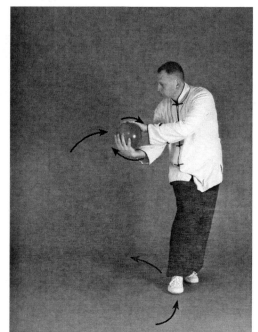

Figure 5-154   Figure 5-155

3. Straight Line Stepping (*Zhi Xian Xing Bu,* 直線行步)

Next, you should practice the yin vertical rotation using both the momentum and balance methods of stepping. Due to the similarity of this exercise to the previous one, we will not go into a detailed description. At this stage, you should be able to step forward and backward very easily while circling and rotating both in a yin and yang direction. Practice this exercise moving forward and backward until you are able to do so smoothly and without interrupting the pattern. This should include the balance method as well.

4. Bagua Stepping (*Bagua Xing Bu,* 八卦行步)

To complete the vertical portion of rotating, the next step is to practice the vertical rotations in a yin direction while bagua stepping. Due to the similarities of this movement to the yang side of bagua stepping, we will not describe this pattern in full detail. Remember that now your forward movement will entail exhaling, chest opening, and the ball traveling through the bottom of its circular rotation (Figure 5-154).

The aft movement will consist of inhaling, chest closing, and the ball traveling over the top of its circular rotation while being drawn toward you (Figure 5-155).

Continue to practice this exercise until you have completed 12 full bagua circles both to the right and left.

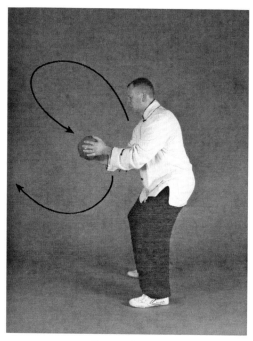

Figure 5-156

Yin-Yang Exchange Vertical Rotating (*Yin Yang Hu Huan Chui Zhi Zhan Zhuan,* 陰陽互換垂直輾轉)

The next set of exercises will involve practicing the yin-yang exchange while rotating the ball vertically. These exercises will be described using a stationary position, followed by rocking, straight line stepping, and bagua stepping. Each exchange will begin with a yang vertical rotation. You may choose to begin with the yin pattern if so desired.

I. Stationary (*Ding Bu,* 定步)

The first exercise is the stationary vertical yin-yang exchange while rotating the ball. Standing in ma bu, begin your normal vertical rotations in a yang direction. Reaching your maximum range of motion, continue with a few rotations until you have reached the top far end of your vertical rotation.

To exchange to a yin pattern, begin to lower the ball and draw it toward the body just as you have done in the circling yin-yang exchange. As you reach the center of this pattern, the next rotation of the ball should move the hands horizontally around the ball instead of over the top, or vertically (Figure 5-156).

This will be the way to change back and forth between yin and yang when executing the vertical rotations. Once the hands reach their opposite sides, you may now change the direction of the pattern to a vertical yin pattern. Allow the ball to continue its path down toward the body and resume the yin side of vertical rotations. Your breathing pattern and chest movement will follow the pattern as described previously in the circling yin-yang exchange.

To switch back to the yang side, perform a few repetitions of the yin rotation. Once the ball has reached the bottom far end of your vertical circular rotation, begin to raise

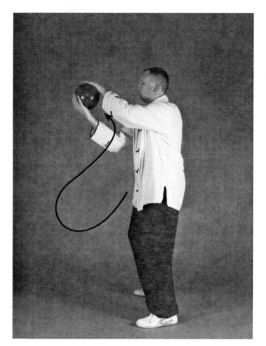

Figure 5-157

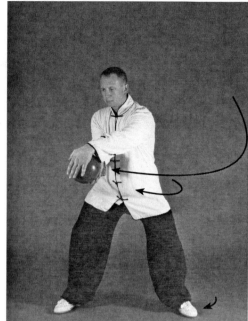

Figure 5-158

the ball while drawing it toward the body. As the ball reaches the central wuji point, change the rotation from a vertical one to a horizontal one. As the hands reach their opposite sides, change back to a vertical rotation in the yang direction (Figure 5-157). Continue to raise the ball toward you and resume the yang side of vertical rotations.

Practice exchanging back and forth between yang and yin rotations until you are comfortable executing the exchange smoothly, without interruption. As you become more comfortable with the exchange, you may attempt to exchange back and forth at different positions of the pattern.

2. Rocking (Qian Hou Dong, 前後動)

The next exercise to practice is the yin-yang exchange while rocking and changing the direction you are facing. To exchange while rocking, simply pass the ball through the center of the pattern, allow the hands to move horizontally around the ball, and then continue on with the vertical rotations in the opposite direction.

In order to perform the yin-yang exchanges while changing the direction you are facing, start from si liu bu, and begin to vertically rotate your ball in a yang direction. Increase the size of the pattern until you have reached your maximum range of motion. To execute your exchange, begin from the most forward position of rocking. Push off your forward foot and draw the ball through the center of the pattern toward your dan tian. While your weight is shifting aft, simultaneously turn your forward foot in toward you and twist your waist toward the opposite direction. Reaching the midpoint with the ball in front of your dan tian, you will change the rotation by allowing the hands to rotate the ball horizontally (Figure 5-158).

This will be followed by the vertical yin rotation. Turn the opposite foot out while continuing to turn the body to the other direction. You should now be in a si liu bu stance facing 180 degrees in the opposite direction.

From this position, you may now continue with vertical yin rotations while rocking. Practice a few exchanges while rocking; then perform the exchange while changing the direction you are facing. Once again, the exchange will occur as the ball passes your dan tian while turning to the opposite side. At this stage the hands will rotate the ball horizontally. This will be followed by vertical rotations in the opposite direction, and you will continue this pattern while facing the opposite direction. Continue to practice your exchanging back and forth until you are able to execute the exchange effortlessly.

3. Straight Line Stepping (*Zhi Xian Xing Bu,* 直線行步)

The next stage of yin-yang rotational exchanging is to practice it while using the momentum method of linear stepping as well as the balance method of stepping. The exchange is executed the same as you have done in your vertical circling exchange. The only difference is the addition of the rotational element. When stepping forward or backward and exchanging between yin and yang, it is best to initially practice it with the ball descending through the center of your pattern (Figure 5-159). This will assist you in remaining rooted throughout your stepping.

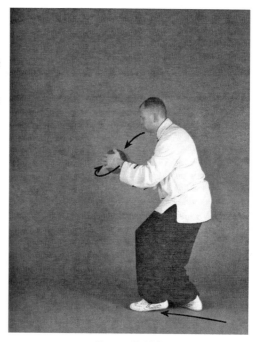

Figure 5-159

Once the ball has reached the center, horizontally rotate the ball once; then follow through with a vertical rotation in the opposite direction from which you were previously performing.

To execute the exchange while balance-stepping, start with the ball at the far end of the pattern. Draw the ball into the center of the pattern and perform the exchange while simultaneously sliding the aft foot up next to the forward one. Shift the weight onto your other foot; then slide the opposite foot aft while moving the ball away from the body in the opposite direction. Practice this exercise until you are able to exchange between yin and yang smoothly while using both methods of stepping.

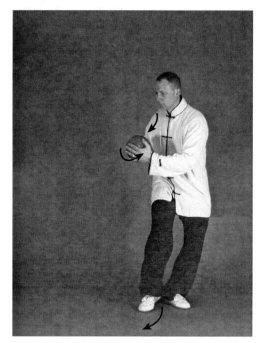

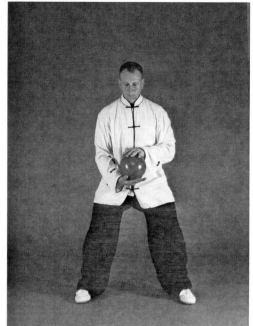

Figure 5-160   Figure 5-161

4. Bagua Stepping (*Bagua Xing Bu,* 八卦行步)

The final stage of this exercise is to practice the yin-yang exchange while bagua step-ping. This exercise is practiced the same as your vertical circling exchange. Begin a ver-tical rotational pattern in a yang direction while facing your bagua circle. Increase your pattern size until you have reached your maximum range of motion.

To switch, perform the exchange to the opposite direction, allowing the ball to de-scend through the center of the pattern while stepping in the circle. As the ball reaches the center, change to one horizontal rotation (Figure 5-160). Follow this rotation with a vertical rotation in the yin direction. You may now continue with the vertical rotation in a yin direction until you decide to switch back to your pattern in a yang direction.

Continue to practice this exchange until you are able to do so without interrupting the flow of the pattern. In addition, you should be able to perform this exchange while moving forward and backward in the bagua circle for both the left and right side.

5.6.3.2 Horizontal Rotation (Shui Ping Zhan Zhuan, 水平輾轉)

Now that you have practiced vertical rotating, it is time to move on to the next direction known as horizontal rotation. This rotation also contains the two elements of circling and rotation of the ball. The first element is the circular motion of the ball similar to the horizontal circling pattern. The second element is the rotation of the ball on a horizontal plane. You will remember from vertical rotating that your hands started on the sides of the ball. As the size of the pattern increased, the hands moved to the top and bottom of the ball. In order to practice the horizontal pattern correctly, your hands will begin on the top and the bottom of the ball slightly crisscrossed (Figure 5-161). As the size of your pattern increases, the hands will move to the sides of the ball.

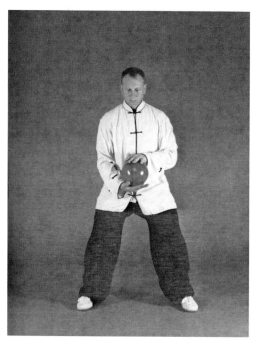

Figure 5-162

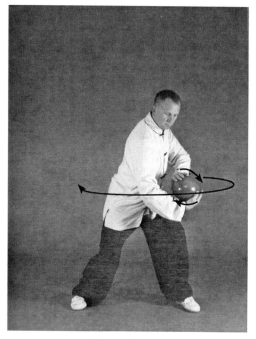

Figure 5-163

At first, you will find it is slightly more difficult to perform than the previous exercise. In most cases you will find your wrists are not flexible enough to make a completely horizontal path around the ball. Simply go as far as you can. It is more important not to tense the wrist and stop the free flow of qi. Also keep in mind, as you get more comfortable with this feeling of rotation, you may elect to increase the number of rotations within each circular motion. You are not restricted to only one rotation per circle.

The direction of rotations is considered the same as circling. Rotating the ball in a clockwise movement is considered a yang pattern, while rotating in a counterclockwise movement is considered a yin pattern when viewed as a right-handed movement.

Yang Rotating (*Yin Zhuan*, 陰轉)

1. Stationary (*Ding Bu*, 定步)

The first pattern to practice is the horizontal rotation while stationary. This will be described with only one rotation per circle for simplicity sake. You may increase the rotations per circle as you get more comfortable.

Stand in ma bu with your taiji ball placed between your hands in front of your dan tian. Take a moment to lead your qi to the dan tian. To begin the horizontal rotation, rotate your hands on the ball so that the left one is on the top and the right one is on the bottom. This will be the starting position (Figure 5-162).

Begin to inhale, close your chest, and slowly twist the waist to the left while drawing the ball toward you. This will start the ball on its horizontal circular path just as you did in the circular pattern. For the rotation element, your right hand will move to the left and aft while the left hand will move to the right and forward. Continue to twist to the left while inhaling and closing the chest until you reach the desired position (Figure 5-163).

FOLLOW ALONG
HORIZONTAL ROTATION— CLOCKWISE (YANG)

From this point, you will start to twist back to the right, and begin to exhale. The right hand will be moving forward and to the right while the left hand will be moving left and aft. Continue to twist your waist to the right while moving the ball out to the right, then back toward you (Figure 5-164). Reaching your original position, repeat the pattern and gradually increase the size of your circles and rotations.

The largest size of horizontal rotating should be where your arms are extended, far out in front of the body without locking the elbows on the outside section of the circle. Be careful not to lean over when you are rotating the ball away from your body. Complete this pattern for 12 repetitions.

Next, continue the exercise by changing the level or height of the horizontal rotations. The highest point of the pattern should be level with your shoulder. After you have completed at least 12 repetitions

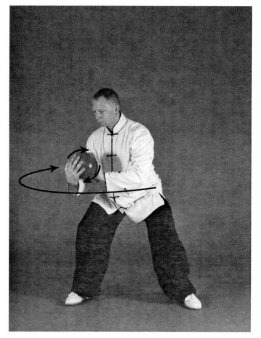

Figure 5-164

at different levels, you will need to twist your waist both to the left and right so you may repeat these exercises for both sides. Upon completion, return to your center and decrease the size of the pattern back to your original starting point for closure.

2. Rocking (*Qian Hou Dong,* 前後動)

The next exercise is the horizontal rotation pattern while rocking. Step into si liu bu, right leg forward, with the taiji ball held in front of your dan tian. Next, rotate the ball so your right hand is under the ball and the left hand is on top. Breathe deeply while leading the qi to the dan tian.

To begin the pattern, start to inhale, close the chest, and twist the body slightly to the left while pushing off the forward foot to rock aft. The ball will be drawn back and to the left on its circular path. The right hand will move aft and to the left while the right hand moves to the right and forward for the horizontal rotation of the ball. Next, push off the aft foot to rock forward while exhaling and opening the chest. Twist the body to the right while moving the ball forward. The right hand will now move forward and to the right while the left hand moves to the left and aft thus continuing with the rotation of the ball. Continue to increase the rotations with rocking until you have reached the maximum range of motion desired (Figures 5-165 and 5-166). Repeat this exercise until you have completed 12 repetitions.

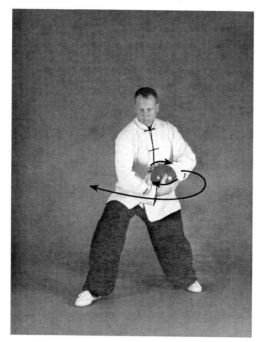

Figure 5-165

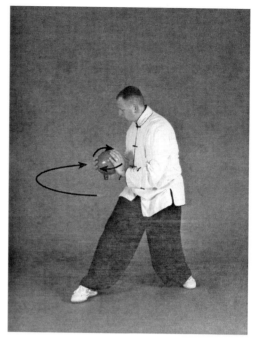

Figure 5-166

Next, practice rotating the ball horizontally, at different heights, while rocking. Then decrease the size of the pattern to the original size. Step back into ma bu, and then step forward into si liu bu with the left leg forward. Once again, rotate the ball so your right hand is on the bottom and the left hand is on the top. Start the clockwise rotation with rocking and continue to increase the pattern each time until reaching your maximum desired range of motion. Repeat the pattern for 12 repetitions. Include practicing at different heights.

Finally, decrease the size of rotations back to the original starting position and step back into ma bu for closure.

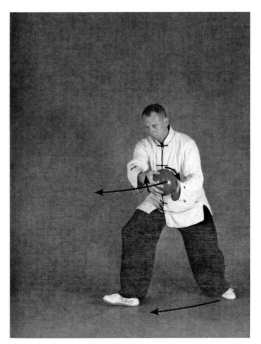

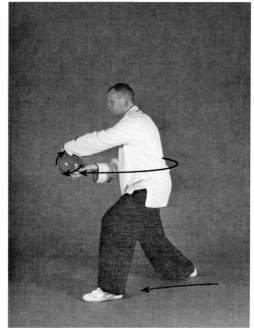

Figure 5-167   Figure 5-168

3. Straight Line Stepping (*Zhi Xian Xing Bu,* 直線行步)

Now that you have practiced the horizontal pattern while rocking, practice horizontal rotating while stepping. Practice using both the momentum and balance methods of stepping. Also practice linear momentum stepping using both techniques described in the horizontal circling section.

The first technique restricts the horizontal path of the ball to shoulder width when stepping. The second technique increases your range of motion and uses the visualization of yin-yang symbols for transitioning from one pattern to the next. If necessary, you may return to the horizontal circling section to review the correct movements for both patterns.

To begin the first stage of momentum stepping, step into si liu bu with the ball in front of your dan tian. Rotate the ball so that your left hand is on top of the ball and the right hand is on its bottom. Begin to horizontally rotate the ball while rocking. Increase the size of rotations to your maximum range of motion.

In order to step forward or backward while using the first technique, keep the path of the ball between the widths of your shoulders (Figures 5-167 and 5-168).

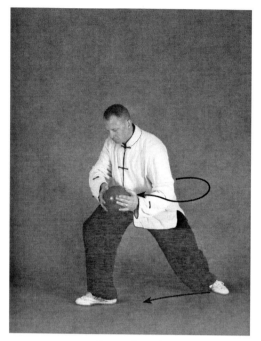

Figure 5-169

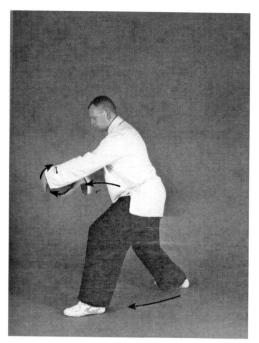

Figure 5-170

To step forward or backward using the second technique, your horizontal circle will be larger. This will allow you to move the ball through the center of the existing pattern; then enter the new circle through the side as you step forward (Figures 5-169 and 5-170).

Depending on which foot is forward, you will either allow the ball to continue on its yang path or make a smaller yang circle before expanding back to your original size. Continue to practice both techniques of stepping until you are able to comfortably move back and forth across your practice area.

Next, practice the balance method of stepping. Once again, this is no different than the horizontal circling exercise. Simply move the ball forward in the pattern while simultaneously sliding one leg aft.

Continue to practice each stage of stepping as well as combinations of each method until you are able to perform this exercise smoothly. Be sure to include rotating the ball at different heights throughout this exercise as well.

4. Bagua Stepping (*Bagua Xing Bu,* 八卦行步)

The final stage of horizontal rotating is to practice it while stepping in a bagua pattern. From ma bu, step into si liu bu with the right foot forward. Twist your body to the right and begin your horizontal rotations clockwise. This should be done the same as if you were facing forward and rocking. Increase the size of rotations while rocking until you have reached your maximum range of motion.

Next, step forward using the methods we initially described in horizontal circling. Stepping forward, your ball will be traveling forward, your chest is opening, and you are exhaling. Stepping aft, draw the ball toward the body, your chest is closing, and you are inhaling. Continue to step until you have completely walked around in a circle and reached your original starting position. Repeat this pattern until you have completed 12 full bagua circles. Change the bagua stepping to the other direction and complete 12 circles in that direction as well. Finally decrease your rotations, and step back into ma bu.

Yin Rotating (*Yin Zhuan,* 陰轉)

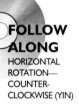

FOLLOW ALONG
HORIZONTAL ROTATION—COUNTER-CLOCKWISE (YIN)

1. Stationary (*Ding Bu,* 定步)

The next exercise is the horizontal rotation in a counterclockwise, or yin direction, while stationary. Once again we will describe this exercise with one rotation per circle. As you become more comfortable, you may increase the number of rotations per circle.

To begin this exercise, stand in ma bu with your hands placed on the ball in front of your dan tian. Rotate the ball so that your left hand is on the bottom and your right hand is on the top. Begin to inhale and close your chest while twisting the waist slightly to the right. The left hand should be moving slightly aft and to the right while the right hand moves slightly forward and to the left (Figure 5-171).

Next begin to twist the waist back to the left while opening the chest and exhaling. The left hand should now move forward and slightly to the left while the right hand moves aft slightly and to the right (Figure 5-172).

Continue this action back and forth while increasing the size of the horizontal circular element of the pattern. Once you have reached your maximum range of motion, continue to practice this exercise for 12 repetitions.

The next stage is to practice this pattern at different heights or levels. Once this has been completed, return to your center. Finally, reduce the size of your pattern until you have reached your original starting position with your taiji ball for closure.

2. Rocking (*Qian Hou Dong,* 前後動)

Next, practice the horizontal rotations in the counterclockwise, or yin pattern, while rocking. Begin in ma bu, step into si liu bu with the right leg forward. With the ball in front of your dan tian, rotate it so your left hand is now on the bottom of the ball and right hand is on the top. Take a moment to lead your qi into the dan tian. Start your counterclockwise rotation of the ball while simultaneously rocking backward. Inhale and close the chest while rocking aft, and then exhale and open the chest while rocking forward (Figure 5-173).

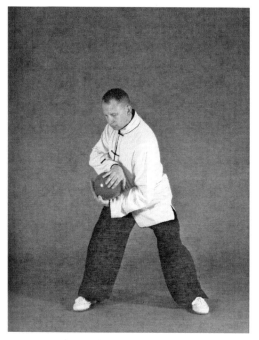

Figure 5-171

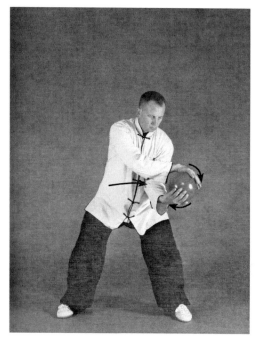

Figure 5-172

Continue to increase the size of the rotations until you have reached your maximum range of motion and repeat the pattern for 12 repetitions. After you have completed the 12 repetitions, practice this horizontal rotation at different heights. Repeat for 12 repetitions; then reduce the size of the rotations to the original starting point. Transition to si liu bu with the opposite foot forward and repeat each stage of the exercise for 12 repetitions. Finally, reduce the size of the pattern and step back into ma bu for closure.

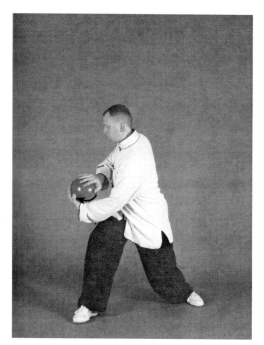

Figure 5-173

3. Straight Line Stepping (*Zhi Xian Xing Bu*, 直線行步)

The next exercise is the horizontal rotation while stepping in a linear direction using both the momentum and balance methods. The process is the same as it is in the yang rotation, except now your left hand will start on the bottom and the right hand will start on the top. Please refer to the exercise using yang rotation for a detailed description of the exercise. Repeat each stage of this exercise for 12 repetitions moving both forward and backward. Be sure to include the balance method of stepping. Upon completion, reduce the size of your pattern and step back into your ma bu stance for closure.

As you become more comfortable with this pattern, you may elect to step forward or backward more than once, or you may decide to combine your stepping forward and backward. You may also step on an angle when using the balance method of stepping. Any combination is possible.

4. Bagua Stepping (*Bagua Xing Bu*, 八卦行步)

The final stage of horizontal rotations is to practice the pattern while bagua stepping. This pattern is similar to the yang rotations and so will not be described again in full detail. Remember to initially rotate the ball to allow the left hand to be on the bottom of the ball and the right hand on top.

The same rules apply in your bagua stepping as in the linear stepping. You may elect to move forward, then backward, or choose to step forward or backward more than once. Finally, you may also decide to step to the right and change to the left, half way through the circle. The choice is yours. Complete at least 12 full bagua circles in both the clockwise and counterclockwise directions.

Yin-Yang Exchange Horizontal Rotating (*Yin Yang Hu Huan Shui Ping Zhan Zhuan*, 陰陽互換水平輾轉)

1. Stationary (*Ding Bu*, 定步)

The next stage is to practice the yin-yang exchange while rotating the ball horizontally. Stand in ma bu, and begin to horizontally rotate your ball in a yang direction until you reach your maximum range of motion. Allow the ball to continue on its path until it reaches the far left side of the circular rotation. Start drawing the ball toward your body, rotating it into the centerwhile inhaling and closing the chest. When the ball has reached the center of your body, change the horizontal rotation to a vertical rotation (Figure 5-174).

Once the hands have completed one vertical rotation, change back to the horizontal rotations. You should be moving in a yin pattern with your right hand on top of the ball and the left hand on the bottom. Continue to move the ball to the right while inhaling.

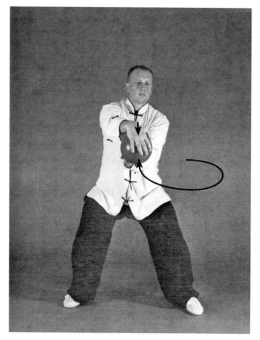

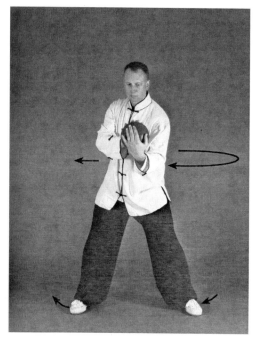

Figure 5-174   Figure 5-175

Reaching the original size of your horizontal pattern, proceed to move the ball around in the yin pattern. Complete a few horizontal yin rotations; then practice your exchange back to your yang pattern. To begin the transition, allow the ball to move to the far right- hand side of your horizontal circular rotation. Draw the ball in to the center toward you. Change the horizontal rotation to a vertical rotation once the ball has reached the center of your body. Once the hands have reached the opposite sides of the vertical rotation, change back to horizontal rotations this time using the yang pattern. Continue to change back and forth between yin and yang patterns until you can execute each exchange smoothly.

2. Rocking (*Qian Hou Dong,* 前後動)

Now practice the yin-yang exchange while rocking and changing the direction you are facing. The rocking section of this exercise is completed the same as in stationary. Simply pass through the center of the pattern while executing a vertical rotation; then continue the pattern in the opposite direction. In order to exchange the pattern while changing the direction you are facing, you will follow the same movements as the horizontal circling. The obvious difference is the rotation of the ball.

Each exchange from one side to the other must pass through the center of your body. This is the wuji point of exchange. As you may have guessed, the transition from yin to yang or yang to yin will occur when the ball is in front of your body and you are transitioning from si liu bu in one direction to si liu bu in the opposite direction. This is where you will execute one vertical rotation followed by a horizontal rotation in the opposite pattern (Figure 5-175).

Continue to move back and forth until you are comfortable with exchanging between yin and yang while rocking, as well as changing from your left and right directions.

3. Straight Line Stepping (*Zhi Xian Xing Bu,* 直線行步)

The next stage of yin-yang exchange is to practice it while horizontally rotating the ball and stepping in a linear direction utilizing the different stages of momentum and balance exercises. Start in si liu bu. Begin to horizontally rotate the ball in a yang direction while rocking. Continue to increase the size of the pattern until you have reached your maximum range of motion.

Next step forward and exchange the pattern to the yin direction using the first stage of momentum stepping. The ball will travel laterally no more than the width of your shoulders and the exchange will occur while the ball passes through the center of the pattern. Upon reaching the center, change the direction of the pattern by performing one vertical rotation. This will be followed by the horizontal rotations in the opposite direction. Continue to step forward and backward a few times while executing the exchange until you are comfortable doing so.

Next, practice stepping forward and backward using the second method of momentum stepping. In this situation, the ball will pass through the center of the existing pattern and into the center of the new pattern. From this position, you will change to a vertical rotation; then continue with your horizontal pattern in the opposite direction. To change back, simply perform the same movement as described above. Continue to practice this stage until you are able to exchange back and forth between yin and yang without interrupting the flow of the pattern.

Next, practice the exchange while using the balance method of stepping. This is done in the same manner as horizontal circling exchanges. While the aft foot slides forward to be next to your other foot, the ball moves aft and into the center of the pattern for the exchange. Perform the vertical rotation; then change to horizontal rotations in the opposite direction. Shift the weight onto the foot that was slid forward, and then slide the other one back all while the ball now moves forward along the horizontal pattern. Practice this stage of exchanging until you are able to do so smoothly.

The final stage of this section is to combine all the stages of stepping. This will include stepping on angles as well.

4. Bagua Stepping (*Bagua Xing Bu,* 八卦行步)

The final stage of horizontal yin-yang exchanging is to practice it while stepping in a bagua circle. To begin this exercise, step into the si liu bu stance, twist the body to the right, and initiate your horizontal rotational pattern in a yang direction. Once you have increased the size of the pattern to your maximum range of motion, you may begin the exchange between yin and yang.

To exchange while stepping forward, start from your most aft position in the pattern. Push off the aft foot and begin moving the ball into the center of the pattern. As the ball passes through the center of the pattern, change the rotation to one vertical rotation; then change to a horizontal rotation in the yin direction. Continue to slide the foot forward while moving the ball out into the new horizontal pattern. You should now be in si liu bu, left foot forward, with the upper body twisted to the right and the ball now moving in the yin direction.

Rock back and forth for a few repetitions, and then switch back to the yang direction, while stepping backward in the circle. To perform this action, simply start from your forward position, push off the forward foot, draw the ball back through the center of the pattern, and once again execute one vertical exchange before moving into the horizontal rotations in the opposite direction. Practice exchanging until you are comfortable enough to do so effortlessly. This should include moving forward and backward while stepping both clockwise and counterclockwise in the bagua circles.

5.6.3.3 *Vertical-Horizontal, Yin-Yang Exchange Rotating (Chui Zhi Shui Ping Yin Yang Hu Zhuan, 垂直水平陰陽互轉)*

Once you have become adept in the previous exercises, it is time to combine the vertical and horizontal patterns. This should be done while stationary, rocking, straight line stepping, and bagua stepping. These exercises will all be introduced with the vertical rotation in a yang direction. You may choose to begin with any pattern. You may be beginning to discover more locations in the pattern to execute the exchanges. There will be more areas for this to occur as you add more patterns and directions. We cannot explain all the different locations. There are an infinite number of locations for pivoting the exchange. You are encouraged to explore these possibilities on your own. The rule is that the ball should not come to a complete stop before moving on to the next direction or pattern. There should be a continuous flow of action throughout.

1. Stationary (*Ding Bu*, 定步)

The first set of exercises shall be done while stationary. Stand in ma bu, and begin your vertical rotation in a yang direction. Rotate until you reach your maximum range of motion. To exchange to horizontal rotations, simply move the ball into the center of your pattern, change to the horizontal rotation, and lead the ball out of the pattern on the horizontal plane. You may choose either the yang or yin direction. To exchange back to vertical, once again move the ball into the center of the pattern, change it to a vertical rotation, and lead the ball out on the vertical plane. Continue to practice this exchange back and forth between vertical and horizontal until you are able to do so without interruption.

2. Rocking (*Qian Hou Dong*, 前後動)

The next exercise is to practice your vertical/horizontal exchange while rocking and changing directions. Step into your si liu bu stance and begin your normal vertical rotations in a yang direction while rocking. In order to exchange back and forth from vertical to horizontal while rocking, you will use the same technique as you did in the stationary exercise. Allow the ball to be drawn into the center of the pattern while rocking aft, perform the exchange, and then continue onto the new pattern or direction while rocking.

To change from vertical to horizontal while changing directions, rock aft and draw the ball toward your body. While transitioning from one side to the other, allow the ball to pass the wuji point in front of your waist; change the rotations to horizontal and continue with this pattern while turning to the opposite direction. You may choose either yin or yang for the direction. Practice this vertical/horizontal exchange while rocking and changing directions until you are able to do so smoothly without interruption.

3. Straight Line Stepping (*Zhi Xian Xing Bu,* 直線行步)

The next stage of vertical/horizontal yin-yang exchanging is to practice it while stepping. Step into your si liu bu stance and begin your vertical rotations in a yang direction while rocking. Increase the size of your pattern until you reach your maximum range of motion. To change to horizontal, step forward while moving the ball down into the center of the pattern. Once the ball has reached the center of your pattern, change to horizontal rotations and lead the ball out on its horizontal path in either the yin or yang direction.

To change back to vertical rotations, move the ball through the center of the existing horizontal pattern while stepping forward. As the ball reaches the center of the pattern, change the rotations to vertical, either in the yin or yang direction. Allow the ball to continue on its path forward while stepping into si liu bu. From this position, you will rock forward while simultaneously moving the ball to the far end of your pattern.

Next, practice exchanging while using the balance technique of stepping. Simply draw the ball toward the body while one foot slides forward. Make the exchange as the ball moves through the center of the pattern; then simultaneously move the ball out on the new pattern while sliding the opposite foot back.

You should practice exchanging between vertical and horizontal rotations until you are able to perform each exchange without interrupting the flow of the pattern, using each method of stepping. The balance stepping, of course, may be done on angles as well.

4. Bagua Stepping (*Bagua Xing Bu,* 八卦行步)

The final stage of vertical/horizontal yin-yang exchanging is to perform the exercise while stepping in a bagua circle. Step into si liu bu with the ball held in front of your dan tian. Twist your upper body to the right and begin your normal vertical rotations in a yang direction while stepping around a bagua circle.

To change the pattern to horizontal, apply the same technique that you used in the vertical/horizontal circle exchange while bagua stepping. Moving forward or backward, allow the ball to pass through the center of your pattern before changing to the horizontal pattern. This can be done in either the yin or yang direction. The same applies to exchanging back to the vertical rotations.

Continue to practice this exercise until you are able to execute the exchange smoothly, while moving both forward and backward around the bagua circle, moving clockwise and counterclockwise.

5.6.3.4 Vertical-Horizontal, Yin-Yang, Circling-Rotating Mixed Training (Chui Zhi Shui Ping Yin Yang Rao Quan Zhan Zhuan Hun He Lian Xi, 垂直水平陰陽繞圈輾轉混合練習*)*

The next stage of vertical/horizontal yin-yang exchanging is to add the element of exchanges between your rotating and circling pattern. (As you can see, each stage is building upon the last.) These exercises should be practiced while stationary, rocking, straight line stepping, and bagua stepping. As mentioned earlier, you may discover more possibilities to exchange your patterns than we are going to describe. Each time you add another element, you will increase the number of places to exchange from one

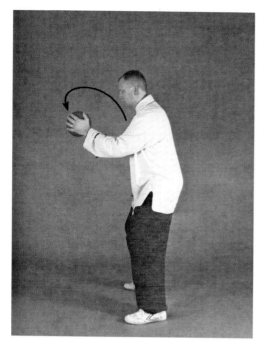

Figure 5-176

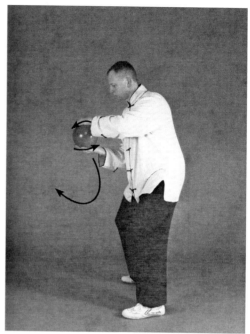

Figure 5-177

pattern to another. You are free to explore these possibilities. Keep in mind that the ball should not stop in its progression to reverse the direction. When you step, the ball should not be on the far outside section of a horizontal pattern. This will create a misalignment, which will become more apparent as you continue to practice and increase the size of the ball.

The following exercises will be introduced with the vertical circling pattern in a yang direction. You may choose to begin the exercise with the yin direction or the rotating pattern in either the yang or yin direction.

I. Stationary (*Ding Bu,* 定步)

The first set of exercises will be done stationary. Stand in ma bu, begin your vertical circling pattern in a yang direction, and increase the size of the pattern until you have reached your maximum range of motion. To exchange the rotations, simply lead the ball to the center of your pattern. Once the ball reaches the center, change the pattern to rotating and lead the ball out of the center on a vertical or horizontal plane in the direction you wish to perform (Figures 5-176 and 5-177).

To return back to the circling pattern, lead the ball back into the center or wuji point and perform the exchange as previously explained. The one minor difference will be when the ball reaches the center. The ball will rotate halfway to allow the hands to return to the side of the ball for the circling pattern.

Continue to practice this exchanging back and forth until you are able to do this exercise smoothly. It should be done using various combinations of rotating and circling as well moving in different directions.

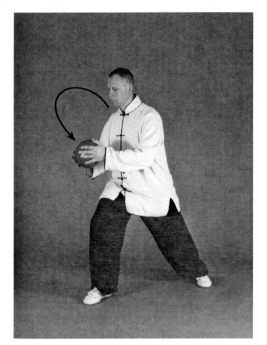

Figure 5-178

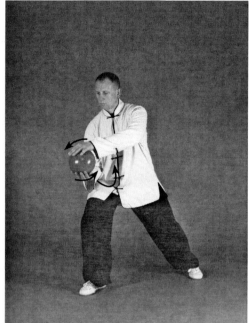

Figure 5-179

2. Rocking (*Qian Hou Dong*, 前後動)

The next stage of this exercise is to perform it while rocking and changing directions. Overall, the exchanging is performed the same as the previous exercise; therefore, we will not explain it in full detail. The exchange can occur either in front of your body, while in transition from facing one direction to the next or at the center of the pattern when rocking (Figures 5-178 and 5-179).

Once again, you should not restrict yourself to moving back and forth solely between circling and rotations. You should also combine directions of the pattern as well. Continue to practice this exercise until you are able to perform each exchange smoothly.

3. **Straight Line Stepping (***Zhi Xian Xing Bu,*** 直線行步)**

The next stage of vertical/horizontal yin-yang exchanging is to practice it while using the different stages of momentum stepping as well as using the balance method of stepping. Begin in si liu bu with your vertical circling pattern in a yang pattern while rocking. Increase the size of the pattern to your maximum range of motion; then start to exchange patterns and directions while stepping forward and backward. Each time you change from a horizontal pattern, initially keep the pattern of the ball the width of the shoulders. This will simplify the exchanges.

Once you are comfortable, increase the size of the horizontal pattern and practice the exchanges using the second stage of stepping. This will involve the use of passing through the center of the existing horizontal pattern then moving into the center of your new pattern. Continue to practice this until you are able to perform each exchange smoothly and without interrupting the flow of the pattern.

Next, practice the balance method of stepping. This is no different than the previous exercises. Simply draw the ball toward the body and exchange your pattern as you normally would while simultaneously sliding the aft foot next to the other foot. Now move the ball outbound on its new path while sliding one foot aft. This can also be done on angles. Continue to practice this until you are able to execute your exchanges smoothly.

Finally, you should combine your methods of stepping with the exchanging of patterns and directions. Practice this exercise until you are able to execute the exchanges using all combinations of stepping previously described.

4. **Bagua Stepping (***Bagua Xing Bu,*** 八卦行步)**

The final stage of this exercise is to practice it while stepping in a bagua circle. This exchange, regardless of change in patterns or directions, will follow the same principles that were described in the previous sections of yin-yang vertical/horizontal exchanging; therefore, we will not describe this action in full detail here. By this stage, you should be very familiar with exchanging and be able to do so comfortably. Be sure to practice this exchanging both forward and backward as well as to the left and right.

FOLLOW ALONG
WRAP COILING

5.6.4 Wrap-Coiling (Chan Zhuan, 纏轉)

Now that you are familiar with the circling and rotating exercises, the next pattern you will explore is known as wrap-coiling. This pattern will build upon the last section of exercises. This additional element will be the coiling action of your wrist and will occur throughout the rotational section of the pattern. Vertically wrap coiling the ball so that it moves forward while at the top of the pattern is considered the yang direction. The yin direction is the when the ball is moving in the opposite direction. Horizontally, the yin and yang directions are the same as circling and rotating.

In order to assist you with the wrap-coiling action, the following exercises may be practiced before continuing on to other exercises in the pattern. It is recommended you perform the following standing over a soft surface such as your bed or over a soft mat. This will provide a soft area for the ball to land if it is dropped.

Place one hand on the far side of the ball with the palm facing it. Place your other hand on the side of the ball closest to you. This hand should be facing you. Next, slide it up slightly so your wrist is now touching the ball. Now roll your hand over the ball and twist, or coil, your hand over so that it faces the ball as it reaches the opposite side (Figures 5-180 and 5-181). The other hand will simply hold the ball.

Once the hand reaches the other side, continue to move the hand around the ball until your hand returns to its original position on the ball, facing you. Repeat this exercise for 12 repetitions. Switch hands and repeat the exercise for an additional 12 repetitions using your other hand.

As you continue with this exercise, try to wrap-coil the ball using any part of your hand, wrist, or, arm. Wrap-coiling the ball, using the finger tips, will build strength and increase qi flow in the fingers. This exercise focuses on using the hand closest to you as the one to initiate the wrap-coiling action. You may also use this wrap-coiling exercise as a tool to train the opposite hand as well. Simply swap the wrap-coiling action to the hand on the far side of the ball.

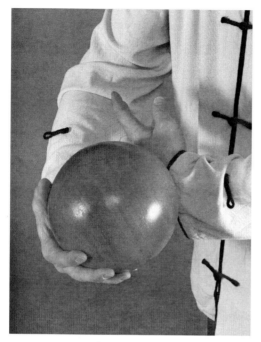

Figure 5-180

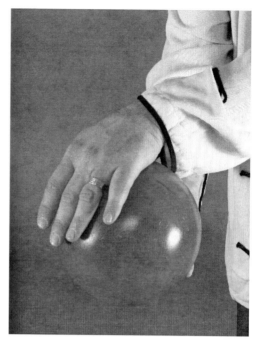

Figure 5-181

Another exercise you may attempt is to wrap-coil on a table. It is shown later in Chapter 6 that describes applications. Place the ball in front of you and practice moving it forward and backward on the table with one hand. As you continue this movement, you should start with your palm facing away from the ball; then roll the ball forward and coil your palm over to face the ball. Continue to practice this movement until you are comfortable; then, switch hands. Remember to turn your waist as you move the ball across the table. Further details on this will be explained in a later section.

Once again we have elected to choose 12 repetitions as a minimum training number. As previously explained, you may elect a lower number and increase these numbers accordingly as the body is conditioned and becomes more comfortable with the movements. The method of training remains the same. Begin each exercise without a ball; then change to using a ball when the body is comfortable.

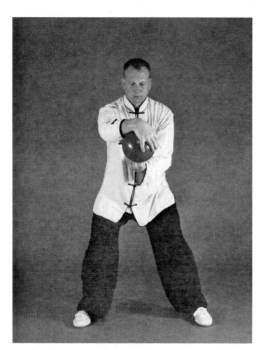

Figure 5-182

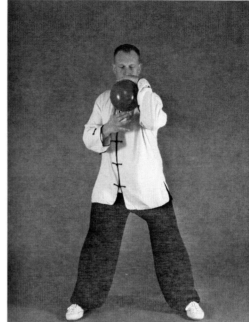

Figure 5-183

5.6.4.1 Vertical Wrap-Coiling (*Chui Zhi Chan Zhuan,* 垂直纏轉)

Yang Wrap-Coiling (*Yang Chan Zhuan,* 陽纏轉)

1. Stationary (*Ding Bu,* 定步)

To begin this exercise, stand in ma bu with your taiji ball held in front of your dan tian. Breathe deeply while taking a moment to lead your qi to the dan tian. Start to wrap-coil the ball in a yang direction by inhaling and moving the dan tian to initiate the circular element of the pattern. Twist the body slightly to the left to commence the rotational element of the pattern. Move your left hand aft and under the ball. Coil the wrist so that your palm is now facing you. Move the right hand forward and over the ball while the hand remains palm touching the ball (Figure 5-182).

Now begin twisting to the right side and continue the rotation of the ball. As the right hand moves under the ball, coil the hand so it now faces you. Simultaneously coil the left hand so the palm faces the ball (Figure 5-183).

Each time the ball makes a rotation, one hand will be facing it and the other will be facing you. Continue to slowly and gradually increase the circular element of wrap-coiling until the pattern increases to your maximum range of motion.

In order to practice this exercise correctly, perform the following action. With the ball on the far end of the pattern, you will perform the wrap-coiling by dropping the elbow of the hand which is coiling on the ball. This will give the arm more of a vertical wrap to the ball (Figure 5-184).

When the ball moves closer to the body, allow the arm to stay in a horizontal position (Figure 5-185). This will cause you to lead the action with the shoulder followed

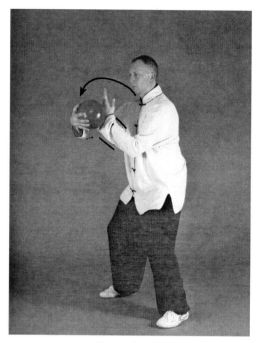

Figure 5-184

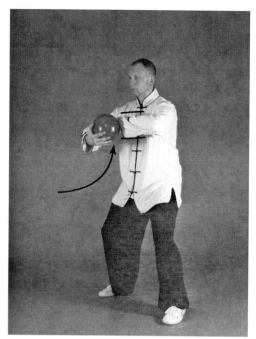

Figure 5-185

by the elbow, arm and hand while coiling vertically over the ball.

The breathing and chest movements are similar to those of vertical rotation. While the ball is ascending toward you, inhale and begin to open your chest. While the ball is descending away from you, exhale and close your chest. Continue this pattern for 12 repetitions.

Next, you will vertically wrap-coil the ball in the yang direction by moving it from one shoulder diagonally to the opposite hip. This should be followed by twisting the waist both to the left and right and repeating the procedures for both sides. Complete 12 repetitions for each stage of the exercise; then return to your center. Finally, decrease the pattern until you have reached your original starting position.

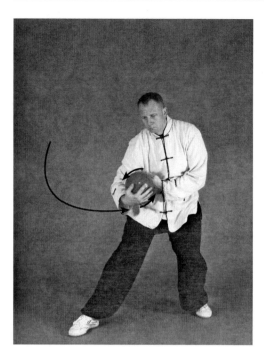

Figure 5-186

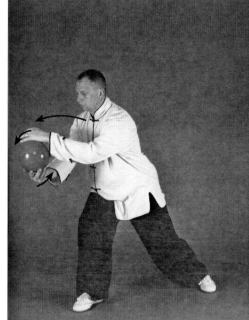

Figure 5-187

2. Rocking (*Qian Hou Dong,* 前後動)

The next stage of vertical wrap-coiling is to practice it while rocking. Essentially it is performed the same as vertical rotation. Stand in ma bu with the taiji ball in front of your dan tian. Step into si liu bu with the right leg forward. Starting with small movements, begin to twist your waist while slowly wrap-coiling the ball as you did in the stationary exercise. Push off the forward foot to rock aft and draw the ball toward you as it descends. At this point, your chest should be opening slightly and you should begin to inhale. Continue with the circular element of the pattern by raising the ball up in front of your body. Moving forward in the rocking position, close your chest and exhale while the ball continues on its path away from the body (Figures 5-186, 5-187).

Continue to increase the size of the wrap-coiling until you have reached your maximum range of motion and repeat this exercise for 12 repetitions.

Next, move the ball diagonally from one shoulder to the opposite hip for 12 repetitions. Return to the center of the rocking pattern and decrease the wrap-coiling motion until you have arrived back to the original starting point. Step into ma bu, and then step back into si liu bu with your left leg forward. Repeat each stage of the exercise for an additional 12 repetitions. Finally, step into ma bu for closure.

3. Straight Line Stepping (*Zhi Xian Xing Bu,* 直線行步)

The next exercise is yang side vertical wrap-coiling while using both momentum and balance methods of stepping. To practice this exercise, begin in si liu bu, right leg forward, with the ball in front of your dan tian. Begin to wrap-coil the ball while rocking, just as you did in the previous exercise. Increase the size of the pattern until you reach your maximum range of motion.

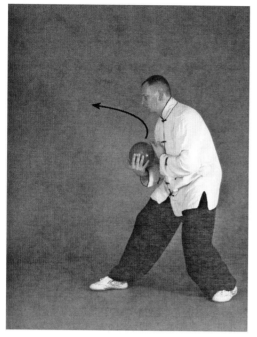
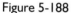

Figure 5-188

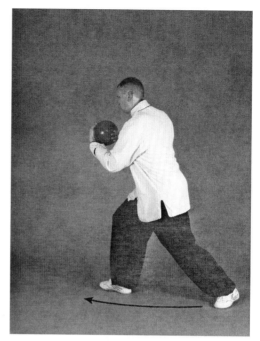

Figure 5-189

To step forward, initiate the movement from the most aft position of rocking. Pushing off the left foot, begin to shift forward. Continue the forward momentum, allowing your left foot to slide up alongside the right one; then place it out in front, ending in a si liu bu stance.

The ball will continue on its path forward while your body rocks forward into the deng san bu stance (Figures 5-188, 5-189, and 5-190).

The movement of the chest and breathing will follow the same action as the previous exercise. Continue to step forward, occasionally pausing between steps, until you have reached the limit of your practice area.

Next, practice stepping backward. Begin in the most forward position of rocking. Pushing off the forward foot, begin to draw the ball toward your body. Shifting your body weight backward, slide your forward foot back and place it behind you. Continue to step back, occasionally pausing in between, until you have reached your starting position.

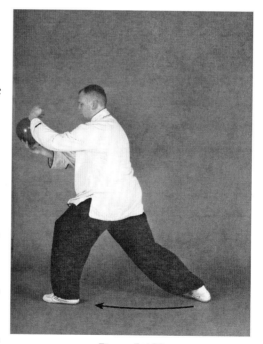

Figure 5-190

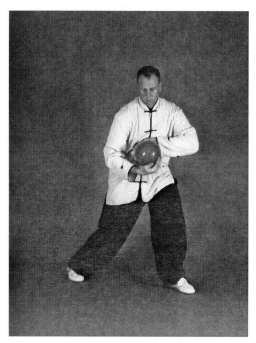

Figure 5-191

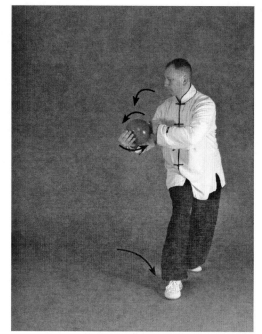

Figure 5-192

Next, practice this exercise while using the balance method of stepping. This is fundamentally done the same as the previous balance stepping exercises. Simply draw the ball toward the body as the aft leg slides forward, and then move the ball forward in the pattern while one leg slides aft. This may also be done on angles. Practice this until you are able to perform each movement smoothly and without interrupting the flow of the pattern.

4. Bagua Stepping (*Bagua Xing Bu,* 八卦行步)

The final set of exercises to practice is the yang vertical wrap-coiling as you step around a bagua circle. To begin, step into si liu bu, left leg forward, with the taiji ball held in front of your dan tian. Now twist your waist to the right so you are now facing the center of the circle around which you will be stepping (Figure 5-191).

Slowly begin to wrap-coil the ball while rocking back and forth, as you did in the previous rocking exercise. While the ball descends and is drawn toward your body, open your chest and inhale. As the ball is ascending and moving away from your body, close your chest and exhale. Increase the size of your wrap-coiling until you have reached your maximum range of motion.

Now it is time to step to the right and complete a circle using bagua stepping. From your aft position, push off the aft foot. Following the momentum of the ball, slide the right foot forward and set it down in front of you (Figure 5-192).

Complete a few wrap-coiling movements with the right leg forward; then step forward in the circular path once again. Continue to step around until you have reached the starting position. Complete 12 full stepping circles clockwise while occasionally pausing between the steps to rock back and forth a few times. You may also elect to

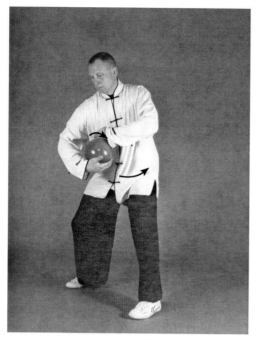

Figure 5-193

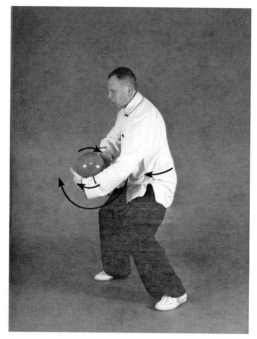

Figure 5-194

take more than one step at a time or take a step backward within the circling. At this stage of practice, you should be comfortable enough in bagua stepping to move back and forth accordingly.

Completing the stepping clockwise, reduce the size of the wrap-coiling to its original position. Twist your waist to the left so you will now face center of your circle. Complete 12 full stepping circles counterclockwise. Finally, decrease the size of wrap-coiling until you have returned to your original position. Twist your waist back to the center and step back into ma bu.

Yin Wrap-Coiling (*Yin Chan Zhuan,* 陰纏轉)

I. Stationary (*Ding Bu,* 定步)

Now practice the yin side of vertical wrap-coiling. Stand in ma bu, twist your waist to the left and rotate the ball using a yin rotation. As the left hand moves over the ball and aft, allow your hand to coil and face you. The right hand will move forward and under the ball. It will perform the opposite action and face the ball (Figures 5-193 and 5-194).

Start twisting to the opposite direction and continue the rotational element of the ball. As this occurs, the right hand will now coil so the palm faces you as it moves aft over the ball. The left hand simultaneously moves forward and under the ball with the palm to coiling to face the ball. Increase the size of your wrap-coiling until you have reached your maximum range of motion, and then repeat the movement for 12 repetitions.

Next, wrap-coil the ball in a yin direction diagonally from one shoulder to the

FOLLOW ALONG
VERTICAL WRAP COIING— BACKWARD (YIN)

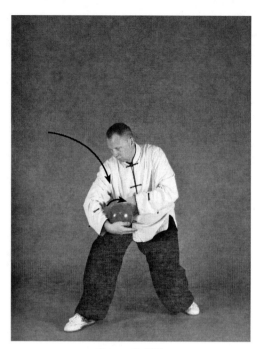

Figure 5-195

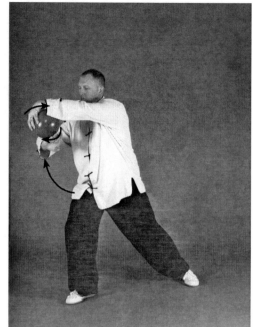

Figure 5-196

opposite hip. Perform 12 repetitions; then twist the upper body to the left and right in order to reach additional angles for strengthening the body.

Repeat for 12 repetitions for each side. To end, twist back to the center and simply decrease the wrap-coiling until you have returned to your original starting point.

2. Rocking (*Qian Hou Dong,* 前後動)

The next stage of yin wrap-coiling is to practice it while rocking. From ma bu, step into si liu bu, right leg forward. Begin your vertical wrap-coiling in a yin direction as you did in the stationary exercise. This time as you rock aft, the ball should be descending and traveling toward your body. Close the chest, and inhale (Figure 5-195).

Rocking forward, the ball will be ascending and traveling away from your body. This is the area within which you should be opening the chest and exhaling (Figure 5-196).

Gradually increase the size of the wrap-coiling exercise until you have reached the maximum range of motion. Repeat for 12 repetitions; then practice the same movement while twisting the upper body to the left and right in order to reach additional angles for strengthening the body.

Once you have completed this action for 12 repetitions, reduce the pattern to your original starting point. Step back to ma bu, and then place your left foot forward in si liu bu.

Repeat each stage of the exercise for 12 repetitions. Finish this section by decreasing the size of the pattern back to the original position and stepping back into ma bu.

3. Straight Line Stepping (*Zhi Xian Xing Bu,* 直線行步)

The next exercise is yin vertical wrap-coiling while stepping. Due to the similarity to the yang side of straight line stepping, we will not describe this exercise in detail. Remember to properly time the transition of stepping by leading it off the aft foot when moving forward, or the forward foot when moving aft. Continue to move across your practice area until you reach the end; then move backward until reaching your original point.

The next exercise should be done while using the balance method of stepping. Finally, practice combinations of stepping until you are able to move continuously throughout your practice area. Finish the exercise by decreasing the size of the pattern and stepping back into ma bu.

4. Bagua Stepping (*Bagua Xing Bu,* 八卦行步)

The final exercise of vertical wrap-coiling in a yin direction is to practice it while stepping around a bagua circle. Due to its similarity to the yang side, we will not describe this in full detail. The pattern should be repeated for 12 full stepping circles, clockwise and counterclockwise. It should also be completed with an occasional pause between steps, stepping more than once, as well as occasionally stepping backward within each bagua circle. Be sure to inhale and close the chest while the ball moves toward your body. Exhale and open the chest as the ball moves away from your body. Complete the exercise by decreasing the size of the pattern until you reach your original starting position. Finally, step back into ma bu for closure.

Yin-Yang Exchange Wrap-Coiling (*Yin Yang Hu Huan Chan Zhuan,* 陰陽互換纏轉)

The final stage of vertical wrap-coiling is to perform the yin-yang exchange. You should practice this in the same manner as you did when practicing the circling and rotating yin-yang exchange. Begin with vertical exchanging in the stationary position, followed by rocking, straight line stepping, and bagua stepping. Each exercise will start with the vertical wrap-coiling in a yang direction. You may start with the yin direction if you wish.

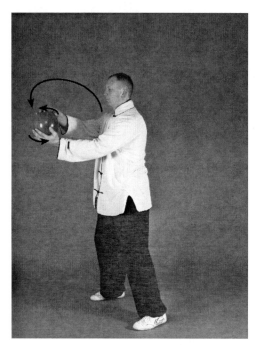

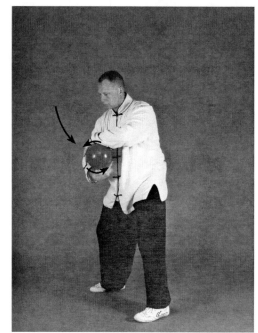

Figure 5-197   Figure 5-198

I. Stationary (*Ding Bu,* 定步)

First, we will practice the vertical wrap-coiling yin-yang exchange while stationary. Stand in ma bu and begin your normal vertical wrap-coiling pattern in a yang direction. Once you have reached your maximum range of motion, start your exchange. To do so, allow the ball to reach the top far end of its circular path. From this position, draw the ball into the center of the pattern, as in the previous exercises (Figures 5-197 and 5-198).

Once the ball has reached the center of the pattern, change the direction to the yin side. This is done by wrap-coiling the hands horizontally once. As the hands reach the opposite sides of the ball, change the movement back to the vertical wrap-coiling pattern in a yin direction (Figure 5-199).

Once again, the breathing pattern and chest movements will remain constant and flow with the existing circular movement of the pattern. Continue the yin side of the pattern for a few repetitions, and then change back to the yang side of the pattern.

To change back to yang, draw the ball back into the center of the pattern from the lower far end. When the ball has reached the center of the pattern, wrap-coil the hands horizontally. Once the hands have reached the opposite sides of the ball, change the pattern back to vertical wrap-coiling in a yang direction.

Continue to practice this vertical yin-yang exchange back and forth until you are comfortable with the exchange and can perform it anywhere in the pattern.

2. Rocking (*Qian Hou Dong,* 前後動)

The next stage of this exercise is to practice the exchange while rocking and changing the direction you are facing. Step into si liu bu, right leg forward. Begin your vertical

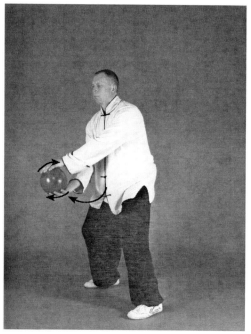

Figure 5-199

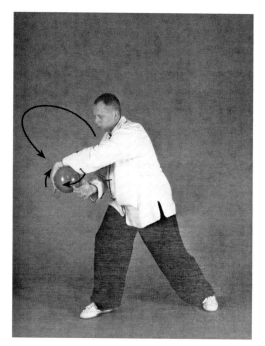

Figure 5-200

wrap-coiling pattern in a yang direction while rocking. Expand the size of your pattern until you reach your maximum range of motion. To vertically exchange between yin and yang while rocking, simply pass the ball through the center of the pattern and perform one horizontal wrap-coil movement before changing to the opposite direction (Figure 5-200).

To execute the exchange while changing your direction, repeat the movements from the vertical rotation yin-yang exchange exercise. This time you will perform one horizontal wrap-coil pattern as your ball passes in front of your dan tian; then continue with the vertical wrap coil pattern in the opposite direction (Figure 5-201).

Continue to practice exchanging, in both the rocking position and while changing the direction you are facing, until you are able to smoothly execute the yin-yang exchange without interruption.

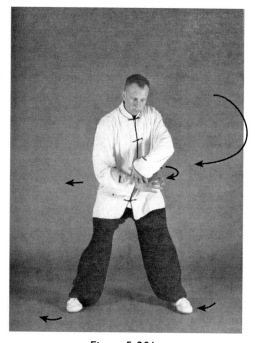

Figure 5-201

3. Straight Line Stepping (*Zhi Xian Xing Bu,* 直線行步)

The next stage of the vertical yin-yang exchange is to practice it while stepping. Practice both methods of stepping.

Step into si liu bu. Begin to vertically wrap-coil the ball in a yang direction while rocking, and increase the size of the pattern to your maximum range of motion. To change from yang to yin, step forward while leading the ball from the top end of the pattern closest to the body down through the center. Reaching the center, execute one horizontal wrap-coil before changing vertically to the yin direction (Figure 5-202).

Continue to step forward into si liu bu with the opposite leg forward while simultaneously wrap-coiling the ball in the yin direction.

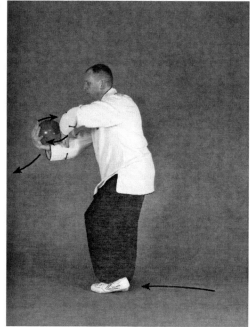

Figure 5-202

To step backward and exchange the direction of the pattern, once again draw the ball down into the center of the pattern. Change the wrap-coiling to a horizontal direction; then continue the vertical wrap-coiling pattern in the opposite direction. Continue to practice this vertical yin-yang exchange while stepping both forward and backward until you are able to execute each maneuver smoothly.

The next stage of this exercise is to practice the yin-yang exchange while using the balance method of stepping. This is similar to the previous exercises. Simply move the ball in to the center of the pattern and execute one horizontal wrap-coil while simultaneously sliding the aft leg up next to the opposite one. Continue with the vertical pattern in the opposite direction and slide one leg aft while the ball travels forward. Continue this exchange until you are able to execute each one smoothly.

The final stage is to practice combinations of stepping while exchanging the direction of the patterns.

4. Bagua Stepping (*Bagua Xing Bu,* 八卦行步)

The final stage of the yin-yang vertical wrap-coiling exchange is to practice it while stepping in a bagua circle. Begin your normal vertical wrap-coiling pattern in a yang direction while stepping around a bagua circle. Reaching your maximum range of motion, step forward and perform the yin-yang exchange. The exchange is performed in essentially the same way as the other exercises. Simply lead the ball to the center of the pattern and perform one horizontal wrap-coil movement before continuing on to the vertical wrap coil pattern in the opposite direction (Figure 5-203).

Continue this exercise until you are able to execute each exchange, forward and backward, smoothly throughout the bagua circle. This includes moving to the counter-clockwise and clockwise directions.

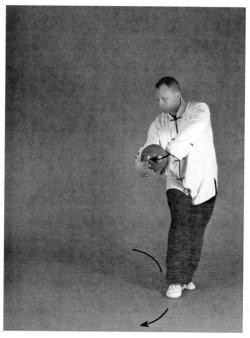

Figure 5-203

5.6.4.2 *Horizontal Wrap-Coiling (Shui Ping Chan Zhuan,* 水平纏轉)

The next set of exercises is the yin and yang horizontal wrap-coiling. This set may prove to be one of the most difficult to perform. One of your hands will be facing away from the ball periodically as it horizontally moves around the ball. It is noticeably more difficult as you reach your maximum range of motion. You should initially practice this over a mat, which can cushion your ball if and when you drop it. Overall, this pattern is the same as the horizontal rotation with the exception of the coiling of your hands on the ball.

FOLLOW ALONG
HORIZONTAL WRAP COILING—CLOCKWISE (YANG)

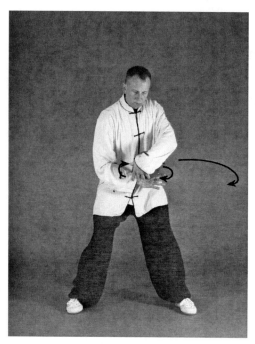
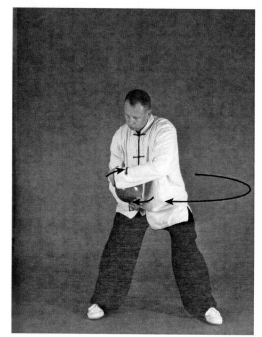

Figure 5-204   Figure 5-205

Yang Wrap-Coiling (*Yang Chan Zhuan,* 陽纏轉)

I. Stationary (*Ding Bu,* 定步)

The first set of exercises will be practiced stationary. Stand in ma bu with the ball held in front of your dan tian. Rotate the ball so your right hand is underneath the ball, palm facing up, and your left hand is over the ball, palm facing down. This will be your starting position.

Inhale, begin closing your chest, and start twisting your body to the left. Your right hand should be moving aft and left with the palm slightly lifting away from the ball. The left hand will subsequently be moving forward and to the right (Figure 5-204).

Now slowly change the direction by twisting your body back to the right. Begin to exhale, as well as open the chest. Move the left hand aft and to the left while the right hand moves forward and to the right. As this occurs, allow the right palm to settle back on the ball while the palm of the left hand coils away from the ball (Figure 5-205).

Continue this action, gradually increasing the size of the pattern. Each time you increase the size of wrap-coiling, allow your hands to make larger coiling movements on the ball. If you are flexible enough, you will eventually have one hand completely on the side of the ball, palm facing away, while the other one is on the opposite side, palm facing the ball.

Repeat the exercise for 12 repetitions. Practice this horizontal pattern at different heights as well. To finish this exercise, gradually decrease the wrap-coiling until you have returned to your original starting position.

2. Rocking (*Qian Hou Dong,* 前後動)

The next exercise is the horizontal wrap-coiling pattern in a yang direction while rocking. This will be done the same as the horizontal rotation while rocking. The exception is now you will have one hand facing away from the ball at some point throughout the pattern.

Step into si liu bu with your taiji ball in front of your dan tian. Rotate the ball so your right hand is on the bottom of the ball and your left hand is on top. Begin to inhale, close your chest, and start your horizontal wrap-coiling as previously described. Continue this motion while increasing each movement until you have reached your maximum range of motion.

Complete 12 repetitions, including at different heights, and then decrease the size of your wrap-coiling back to the original position. Change the forward leg by stepping back into ma bu and placing the opposite leg forward in si liu bu. Repeat the pattern once again for 12 repetitions; then decrease the size of your pattern back to the starting position. Finally, step back into ma bu.

3. Straight Line Stepping (*Zhi Xian Xing Bu,* 直線行步)

Now practice the yang horizontal wrap-coiling with stepping. By now you should be comfortable with the horizontal wrap-coiling pattern. You should also be comfortable with stepping while both horizontally circling and rotating the ball.

Step into si liu bu, right leg forward, and begin your horizontal wrap-coiling while rocking, as previously described. Next, practice stepping forward while horizontally wrap-coiling the ball. Continue this forward movement, occasionally pausing between steps, until you have reached the end of your practice area.

Next, practice the pattern while stepping backward until you have arrived back at your starting position. Be sure to practice this pattern using both methods of momentum stepping as described in the previous horizontal patterns.

Once you have completed this stage of the exercise, move on to the balance method of stepping. Finally, try combining all the different methods of stepping while practicing the pattern.

4. Bagua Stepping (*Bagua Xing Bu,* 八卦行步)

The final stage of this section is to practice horizontal wrap-coiling in a yang direction while stepping around a bagua circle. Step into si liu bu and twist your body toward the center of the circle. Rotate the ball so your right hand is on the bottom of the ball and the left hand is on top.

Begin your horizontal wrap-coiling pattern in a yang direction as described in the rocking section. Reaching your maximum range of motion, begin to step forward and backward in the circle as desired. Overall, this is performed no differently than in the exercises for horizontal circling or rotation patterns while bagua stepping. The only change is the element of wrap-coiling the ball.

Continue with this exercise until you have completed 12 bagua circles, counterclockwise and clockwise. Reduce the size of the pattern back to the original position and step back into ma bu.

Yin Wrap-Coiling (*Yin Chan Zhuan,* 陰纏轉)

1. Stationary (*Ding Bu,* 定步)

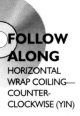

The next exercise is wrap-coil in the yin direction while stationary. This is done essentially the same as you did while practicing the yang side. One major difference will be the hands. When you begin this pattern, your left hand will be on the bottom of the ball while the right one is on the top (Figure 5-206).

Of course, the ball will also be moving in a counterclockwise path on the horizontal plane as well. Increase the size of your wrap-coiling until you reach your maximum range of motion. Practice each stage of this pattern for 12 repetitions, and then decrease the pattern back to the original position.

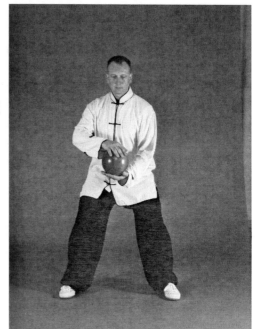
Figure 5-206

2. Rocking (*Qian Hou Dong,* 前後動)

The next exercise in this section is the horizontal wrap-coiling pattern in a yin direction while rocking. Aside from the direction, the yin side of this exercise is the same as the yang side. Due to this similarity, we will not describe it in full detail here.

In this pattern, your left hand will now be placed on the bottom of the ball during the initial rotation of the ball, and the direction of wrap-coiling will be counterclockwise. Once you have reached your maximum range of motion, continue to practice this pattern for 12 repetitions.

Be sure to practice this exercise at different heights as well. Once you have completed the exercise, reduce the size of your pattern to the original starting position and step back into ma bu.

Step into si liu bu with the opposite foot forward and repeat each stage of the exercise for 12 repetitions. Finally reduce the size of the pattern to your starting point and step back into ma bu for closure.

3. Straight Line Stepping (*Zhi Xian Xing Bu,* 直線行步)

The next stage of horizontal wrap-coiling is to practice it in the yin direction while stepping. This exercise is performed the same as it is with the yang side of wrap-coiling. The exceptions are the initial placements of the left and right hands on the ball and the direction of the pattern. For more detailed information refer back to the previous horizontal wrap-coil stepping section. Continue to practice this exercise using all combinations of stepping described.

4. Bagua Stepping (*Bagua Xing Bu,* 八卦行步)

The final stage of this pattern is horizontal wrap-coiling in a yin direction while stepping in a bagua circle. The pattern is essentially the same as the horizontal rotation exercise with the exception of the horizontal wrap-coiling. For this reason, we have decided to omit the full description of this exercise here.

Step into si liu bu and twist your body to the right. Begin your horizontal wrap-coiling in a yin direction while rocking. Next, step around in your bagua circle and complete 12 full circles. Upon completion of this, twist your body to the left and repeat the 12 full circles to the left. Reduce the size of the pattern to your original starting position and step back into your ma bu stance.

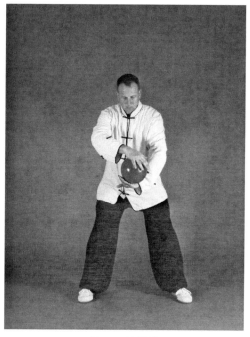

Figure 5-207

Yin-Yang Exchange Wrap-Coiling (*Yin Yang Hu Huan Chan Zhuan,* 陰陽互換纏轉)

The next set of exercises involves changing the direction of the horizontal wrap-coiling between yin and yang. This will be described while stationary, rocking, straight line stepping, and bagua stepping. Each exercise will begin with the horizontal wrap-coil pattern moving in a yang direction. You may choose to begin with the pattern in the yin direction. In addition, we will describe one or two places for exchanging. As you will discover there is more than one place to execute an exchange in a pattern.

I. Stationary (*Ding Bu,* 定步)

The next exercise is the yin-yang exchange of horizontal wrap-coiling. As you may already guess, the exchange will occur in the center of the circular element of the pattern, and you will change the direction by utilizing one vertical wrap-coil.

Stand in ma bu. Begin your horizontal wrap-coiling pattern in a yang direction as previously described. Reaching your maximum range of motion, prepare to change to the yin side. Allow the ball to reach the far left hand side of the pattern; then draw the ball toward the center of the pattern (Figure 5-207).

After reaching the center, change the horizontal pattern to one vertical wrap-coil. Once the hands have completed the one vertical movement, resume the horizontal pattern in a yin direction. Continue for a few repetitions; then change back to the yang side using the technique previously described. For this exchange, allow the ball to reach the far right end of the pattern before drawing the ball into the center.

Practice this exercise exchanging back and forth between yin and yang until you are comfortable exchanging anywhere in the pattern.

2. Rocking (*Qian Hou Dong,* 前後動)

The next exercise is the horizontal wrap-coiling yin-yang exchange while rocking and changing the direction you are facing. Step into si liu bu and begin to wrap-coil the ball horizontally in a yang direction while rocking. These exchanges will be performed the same as they have been in the horizontal circling and rotating exchanges. When rocking, simply draw the ball through the center of the pattern and perform the exchange to the opposite direction.

In order to execute the exchange while changing directions, draw the ball through the dan tian area and perform your exchange. Continue to practice the exchange while rocking and changing directions you are facing until you are able to execute each exchange smoothly and without interrupting the flow of the pattern.

3. Straight Line Stepping (*Zhi Xian Xing Bu,* 直線行步)

The next stage of yin-yang exchanging is to practice it while stepping. Due to the similarity in movements of this exercise to horizontal rotating yin-yang exchanging, we will omit the full description of this exercise. Repeat this exercise until you are able exchange between yin and yang smoothly while using any combination of stepping.

4. Bagua Stepping (*Bagua Xing Bu,* 八卦行步)

The final stage of horizontal wrap-coiling yin-yang exchanges is to practice them while stepping in a bagua circle. Once again the exchanges are performed the same as they are in the horizontal rotating yin-yang exchanging exercise. Practice this exchange until you are able to execute your exchanges smoothly, without interruption, while stepping forward and backward in the bagua circle. This should be done while circling both to the left and right as well.

5.6.4.3 Vertical-Horizontal, Yin-Yang Exchange Wrap-Coiling (Chui Zhi Shui Ping Yin Yang Hu Huan Chan Zhuan, 垂直水平陰陽互換纏轉*)*

The next stage of yin-yang exchanging is to practice combinations of exchanges between both vertical and horizontal wrap-coiling patterns as well as yin and yang directions. We will introduce each pattern beginning with a stationary position, then rocking, straight line stepping, and bagua stepping. Each exercise will start with the vertical wrap-coil in a yang direction. You may choose to start with any wrap-coil pattern in any direction. We will describe one position for each exchange to occur. As we have discussed previously, you are encouraged to explore other possibilities.

1. Stationary (*Ding Bu,* 定步)

The first exercise is the vertical/horizontal yin-yang exchange of wrap-coiling while stationary. You will find that this exercise, as well as the others listed in the following sections, will follow the same movements of the vertical/horizontal yin-yang exchange of rotating described earlier. Stand in ma bu and begin your vertical wrap-coiling pattern. Increase the size of the pattern to your maximum range of motion. Each time you decide to exchange between yin and yang, or vertical and horizontal, simply lead the ball through the center of the existing pattern. Practice this exercise until you are able to execute each exchange smoothly anywhere in the pattern

2. Rocking (Qian Hou Dong, 前後動)

The next exercise of vertical/horizontal yin-yang exchanging is to practice it while rocking and changing directions. Step into si liu bu and start your vertical wrap-coiling pattern in a yang direction while rocking. Increase the size of the pattern to your maximum range of motion.

To exchange from the vertical pattern to the horizontal pattern while rocking, simply lead the ball through the center of the pattern, then on to its horizontal path in either a yin or yang direction. This can be done anywhere in the pattern.

To change to horizontal while changing the direction you are facing, allow the ball to pass in front of your dan tian while transitioning from one side to the next. From this position when you make the exchange you may choose either the yin or yang direction.

Practice this exercise until you are able to execute your exchanges between vertical and horizontal, as well as yin and yang, smoothly and without interrupting the movement of the ball.

3. Straight Line Stepping (Zhi Xian Xing Bu, 直線行步)

The next stage of this exercise is to practice the vertical/horizontal yin-yang exchange while using each method of stepping. Step into si liu bu. Begin to vertically wrap-coil the ball while rocking, and increase the size of the pattern to your maximum range of motion.

To change to horizontal while stepping forward or backward using momentum, lead the ball down through the center of the vertical pattern while stepping. From this position, you may lead the ball out from the center in a yin or yang direction.

To change back into the vertical pattern, apply the same technique. Lead the ball into the center of your horizontal pattern, then out of the center in the vertical pattern while simultaneously stepping forward or backward. The ball may be redirected to the yin or yang direction in the vertical pattern.

Next, practice exchanging while using the balance method of stepping. Slide one leg forward or aft while the ball is drawn through the center of the pattern. Exchange your pattern; then move the ball forward, vertically, or horizontally, in the new direction as one leg slides aft. This can also be done on angles. Continue with this exercise until you are able to do so smoothly.

Finally, combine the stepping techniques with your exchanges and repeat the movements until each exchange is smooth.

4. Bagua Stepping (Bagua Xing Bu, 八卦行步)

The final stage of this exercise is to practice this vertical/horizontal yin-yang exchange while stepping in a bagua circle. To perform your exchanges, simply allow the ball to pass through the center of the pattern while stepping forward or backward. This is regardless of whether you are exchanging vertical to horizontal, or horizontal to vertical. Due to these similarities, we will omit a full description of the exercise. Be sure to practice this exercise until you are able to execute your exchanges smoothly and without interrupting the movement of the ball.

5.6.4.4 Vertical-Horizontal, Yin-Yang, Circling-Rotating-Wrap-Coiling Mixed Training (Chui Zhi Shui Ping Yin Yang Rao Quan Zhan Zhuan Chan Zhuan Hun He Lian Xi, 垂直水平陰陽繞圈輾轉纏轉混合練習)

The final stage of this chapter requires you to perform your exchanges from any pattern to any pattern in any direction desired. You should be able to perform this while stationary, rocking, straight line stepping, and bagua stepping. Eventually you should be able to combine your stepping techniques as well. Ultimately you will be able to use any combination you wish and in doing so the ball will endlessly flow throughout your patterns.

These exercises will be introduced with the vertically circling pattern in the yang direction. You may begin these exercises with any pattern in any direction you wish. Once again, we will only mention one exchange in the following exercises. You are encouraged to explore other possibilities not mentioned.

I. Stationary (*Ding Bu,* 定步)

The first exercise is to practice the exchanges while stationary. Standing in ma bu, begin the vertical circling pattern in the yang direction, and increase the size of your pattern to your maximum range of motion.

In order to exchange from circling to any other pattern, you will simply lead the ball to the center of the existing pattern; then continue with your desired pattern, in the direction you wish. There is one minor difference in exchanging from wrap-coiling or rotating to circling. The exchange may involve a half rotation of the ball in order to place the hands in the proper position for the circling pattern. This may also occur when exchanging from circling to rotating or wrap-coiling. Continue to practice this exercise until you are able to execute your exchanges smoothly. You should be able to do so anywhere in the patterns.

2. Rocking (*Qian Hou Dong,* 前後動)

Next, practice your exchanges while rocking and changing the direction you are facing. The theory remains the same. Each exchange while rocking will involve leading the ball to the center of the existing pattern. Each exchange while changing the direction you are facing will involve an exchange when you have led the ball to your dan tian area. Just as you have done in the previous exercise, you may have to perform a half rotation when exchanging between patterns in order to properly position the hands on the ball. Continue to practice this exercise until you are able to execute each exchange in pattern and direction smoothly.

3. Straight Line Stepping (*Zhi Xian Xing Bu,* 直線行步)

The next stage of this exercise is to practice the exchanges while using each method of stepping discussed thus far. Starting with your vertical circling pattern in a yang direction while rocking, increase the size of the pattern to your maximum range of motion, and then begin to step forward and backward while exchanging between patterns and directions.

To perform the exchange, regardless of pattern or direction, simply pass through the center of the existing pattern into the center of the next one. Continue to practice this exercise until you are able to execute each exchange smoothly. Be sure to use combinations of stepping, including angles.

4. Bagua Stepping (*Bagua Xing Bu,* 八卦行步)

The final exercise is to perform your exchanging between patterns and directions while stepping in a bagua circle. By now, it should be clear as to where you may exchange between patterns and directions.

Begin this exercise with your vertical circling pattern in a yang direction while stepping in a bagua circle. Reaching your maximum range of motion, begin to step forward and backward while exchanging patterns and directions. Continue to practice this exercise until you are able to execute the exchange, forward and backward as well as left and right, smoothly and without interrupting the flow of the ball's movement in the pattern.

Notes

1. *The Body Electric*, Robert O. Becker, M.D. and Gary Selden, Quill, William Morrow, New York, 1985.

2. *Qigong, the Secret of Youth–Da Mo's Muscle Tendon Changing & Marrow Brain Washing Classics*, Dr. Yang, Jwing-Ming, YMAA Publication Center, Boston, 2000.

CHAPTER 6

Applications of Taiji Ball Qigong
(太極球氣功之應用)

6.1 Introduction (介紹)

At this stage, you should be able to practice the circling, rotation, and wrap-coiling patterns smoothly. You should also be able to perform each of these patterns comfortably while stationary, rocking, stepping, and bagua stepping.

In this section, we will introduce you to the applications of taiji ball. This will include solo exercises of attaching to the ball, as well as listening and following exercises practiced with a partner. Each stage of practice in this section will allow you to focus on further developing your listening jin (*ting jin*, 聽勁), jin (*zhan jin*, 沾勁), adhering jin (*nian jin*, 粘勁), and following jin (*sui jin*, 隨勁). These are necessary skills. They will assist in the continuous flow of qi as well as refine the sensing skills necessary to become a proficient martial artist.

Finally, we will introduce a few advanced drills not shown on the *Tai Chi Ball Qigong* DVD series. We include rooting on bricks, taiji patterns, and jin patterns that involve two people. From these drills, endless patterns can be derived, and it is only up to you to decide how far and deep you wish to experience taiji ball qigong.

Before we continue, we will take a brief moment to remind you of a few concepts previously mentioned in this section. First, what is jin? This word is defined in a Chinese dictionary as li-qi (氣力) or qi-li (力氣). We know from our definition in earlier sections that qi is representative of our bio-electricity. Li is known as physically manifested muscular power. Jin therefore is defined as the focused manifestation of muscular power.

Definition can also be derived from the structure of the word jin. This word can be broken down into two words meaning path (巠) and muscular force (力). When interpreted in this manner, jin is defined as directing the muscular power into a precise path. In order to execute this action, the mind must be focused.

The first type we will address is listening jin (*ting jin*, 聽勁). This jin involves the ability of a person to recognize his opponent's intention both before and after contact has been made. Attaching jin (*zhan jin*, 沾勁) is defined as one who attaches to the incoming force as it is initiated. Next, we will address adhering jin (*nian jin*, 粘勁), which refers to the individual's ability to remain in contact with his opponent. Finally, following jin (*sui jin*, 隨勁) is the ability of the person to follow his opponent's actions regardless of direction.

Each of these jins complements each other and for the most part, cannot be separated. For instance, in order to utilize following jin, you must be able to use your listening jin. Following jin also requires you to be able to use your skills in adhering jin, which in turn will occur as you exercise your attaching jin, by using your listening jin. To learn more about jin and the different types of jin, please refer to *Taiji Theory*, by Master Yang, Jwing-Ming, available from YMAA Publication Center.

6.2 Self-Practice (自我練習)

FOLLOW ALONG
SELF PRACTICE

The first section of applications will explore advanced solo maneuvering of the ball. You will learn to focus on attaching and adhering to the ball while it is on a table, your forearm, and various surfaces such as bricks, discs, and walls. Each exercise continuously builds upon the last. Eventually you will be able to practice all the patterns collectively in a freestyle manner.

6.2.1 Adhering to the Ball (Zhan Qiu, 粘球)

I. On the Table (Zhuo Shang Zhan Qiu, 桌上粘球)

The first exercise is known as returning the ball. You will need a table approximately waist height. The purpose of this exercise is to improve your ability to control the rotation of the ball using your body, and heighten your sensitivity/feeling. Just as you practiced in the previous exercises, begin your practice of this exercise using small movements and gradually increase the motion.

To start, stand in ma bu and place the ball in front of you on the table under your wrist, palm down. Take a moment to lead the qi to the dan tian with a few deep breaths. Using the twisting action of your waist, move the ball backward and forward along the table in front of you while keeping your palm facing down. Each time the ball is drawn back toward you, the chest will close and you will inhale. As you move the ball forward, exhale and open the chest (Figures 6-1 and 6-2).

Increase the movement until the ball moves from your fingertips to your elbow.

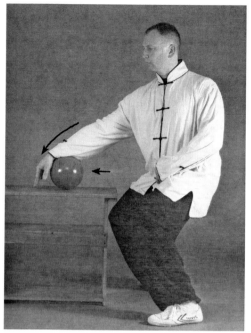

Figure 6-1

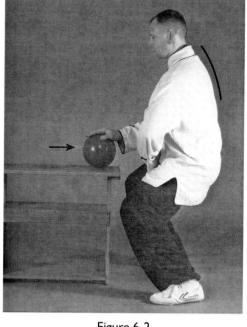

Figure 6-2

When you are comfortable, rotate your hand so that the palm faces up each time you move the ball forward. Rotating the palm up may also be practiced when moving the ball backward (Figure 6-3).

When you are able to comfortably control the movement of the ball, practice with your eyes closed. Remember the main point of this training is to develop your feeling, or sensing jin.

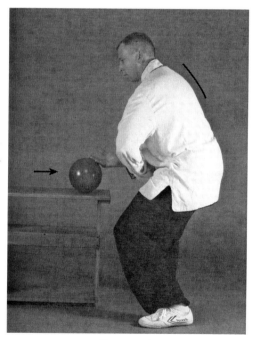

Figure 6-3

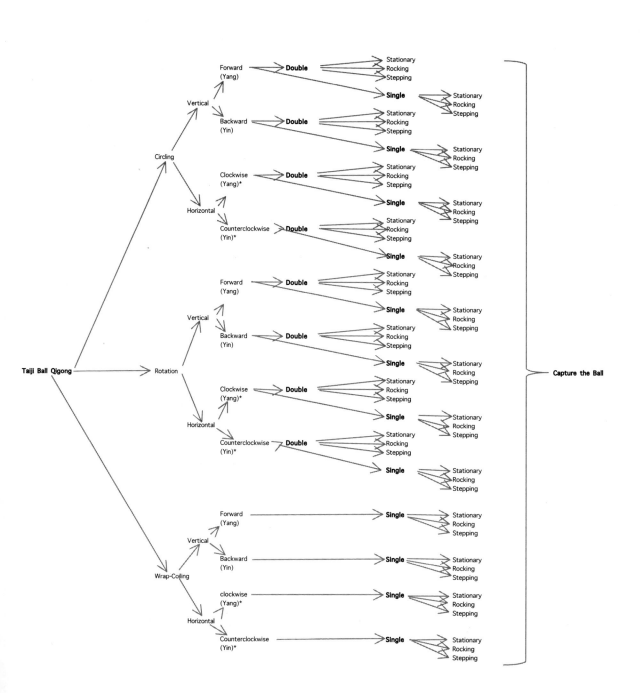

Tai Chi Ball Qigong Yin-Yang Training–Double

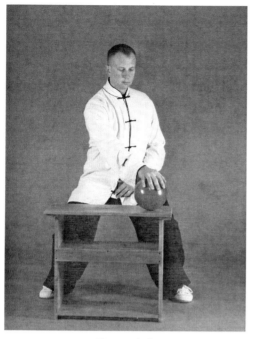

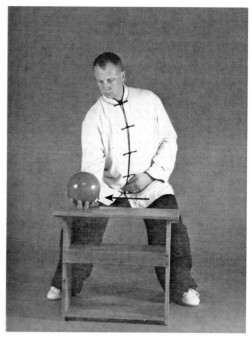

Figure 6-4   Figure 6-5

2. Attaching to the Ball (*Nian Qiu,* 黏球)

The next exercise is known as attaching to the ball. Simply put, you are allowing the rotational momentum of the ball to move it across the table into your palm to raise it into the air. To begin this exercise, place the ball on the table in front of the opposite shoulder of the hand you are using to control the ball (Figure 6-4).

With palm facing down on top of the ball, begin to inhale and twist the body to draw the ball across the table. Close the chest while the ball continues across the table. As you reach the shoulder of the hand you are using, rotate your palm face up and permit the ball to roll up into the palm of your hand. Finally, raise the ball up off the table while opening the chest and exhaling (Figures 6-5 and 6-6).

Continue practicing this exercise for each hand until the movements become effortless.

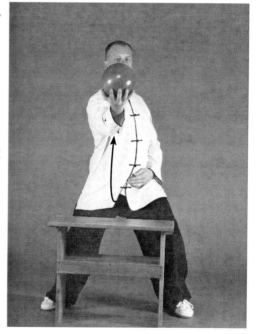

Figure 6-6

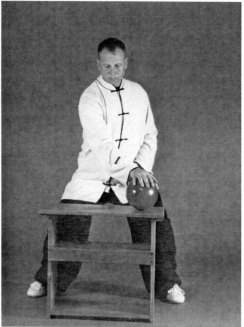

Figure 6-7

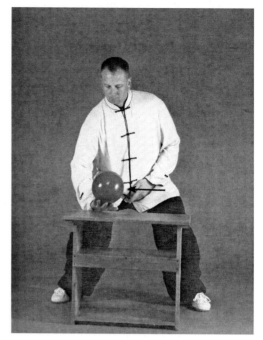

Figure 6-8

3. Sideways Attaching (*Zuo You Nian Qiu,* 左右黏球)

The next exercise you will practice is sideways attaching. To begin this exercise, place the ball on the table in front of the opposite shoulder of the hand moving the ball. Place your hand on top of the ball, inhale, and begin to move the ball across the table. As the ball is moved from one side of the table to the other, keep the palm facing down and allow the ball to roll up over the top of your hand. Next, begin to exhale, twist your body, and move the arm forward while raising the ball off the table. Rotate your palm face up and allow the ball to roll into the palm of your hand (Figures 6-7, 6-8, and 6-9).

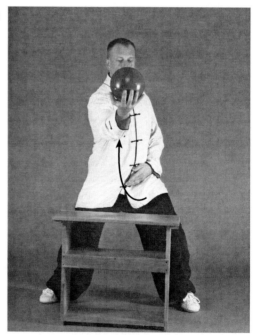

Figure 6-9

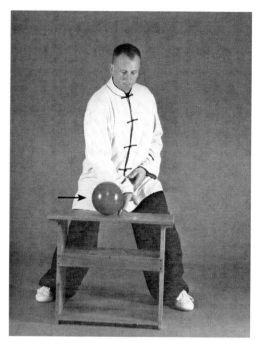

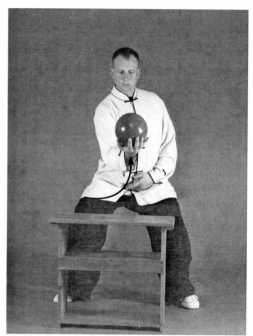

Figure 6-10   Figure 6-11

This can also be practiced by rolling the ball in the opposite direction. In this case, you will start with the ball in front of the same shoulder of the hand you are using. Roll the ball in the opposite direction while keeping the palm face down. Reaching the opposite shoulder, allow the ball to travel up over the top of your hand. Raise the ball off the table and rotate the palm up allowing the ball to travel once again into the palm of your hand (Figures 6-10 and 6-11). Continue to practice these exercises until the movements can be performed smoothly.

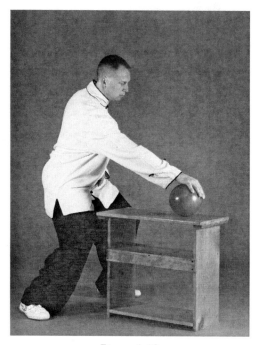

Figure 6-12

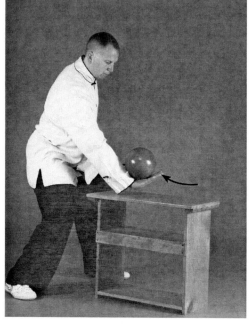

Figure 6-13

4. Forward-backward Attaching (*Qian Hou Nian Qiu,* 前後黏球)

The next exercise is known as forward-backward attaching. In this situation, you will move the ball from front to back, and then raise it off the table. It can be practiced while standing either in ma bu or while rocking. To practice this while standing in ma bu, you will start with the ball out in front of you on the table. With your palm facing down on the ball, begin to inhale, twist the waist, and draw the ball toward you. Allow the ball to roll over the backside of your hand, and then simultaneously twist your waist, and rotate your hand, palm up, allowing the ball to rest in your palm above the table (Figures 6-12, 6-13, and 6-14).

The breathing and chest movement should be as follows: inhale, chest closed while moving the ball backward, and exhale, chest open while raising the ball up

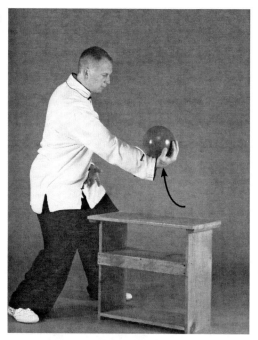

Figure 6-14

off the table. When you practice this exercise while rocking, begin in the most forward

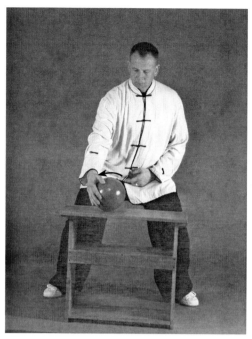 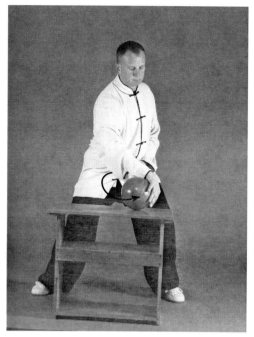

Figure 6-15 Figure 6-16

position; then rock aft as you draw the ball toward you. Finally, twist the waist while lifting the ball off the table. The breathing and chest movements remain the same. Continue with this exercise until you are able to move the ball across the table and lift it up smoothly.

6.2.2 Rotating the Ball (Zhan Zhuan, 輾轉)
1. On the Table (Zhuo Shang Zhan Zhuan, 桌上輾轉)

In this exercise, you will practice rotating the ball in a clockwise and counterclockwise direction both on a table and on your forearm. To practice this exercise on the table, stand in ma bu with the ball in front of you. Place your hand on the ball and begin to move it around the table in a clockwise direction by twisting the waist back and forth. Your palm should stay in contact with the ball at all times. As the ball moves away from you, expand your chest and exhale. While moving the ball toward you, close your chest and inhale (Figures 6-15 and 6-16).

In order to change directions from clockwise to counterclockwise, you must manipulate the ball through the center of the circular path. Remember, you do not want the ball to come to an abrupt stop to change to a new direction. This movement follows the same principles of the yin-yang exchange you performed in the previous chapter. In addition, you may also change hands while performing this exercise.

2. On the Forearm (*Bi Shang Zhan Zhuan,* 臂上輾轉)

Practice this technique using your forearms as the base for rotating the ball. Start with the ball in one hand, palm facing up. Raise the arm slightly to allow the ball to roll down the forearm toward the body. Once the ball reaches your shoulder, twist the waist resulting in the shoulder moving forward on the same side as the ball. This should assist in moving the ball across the front of the body to the other shoulder. Finally, twist your waist back and allow the ball to roll onto the opposite forearm ending in your other hand. With continued practice, you should be able to keep the ball moving from one hand to the next in an uninterrupted circle.

6.2.3 *Wrap-coiling the Ball (Gun Qiu,* 滾球)

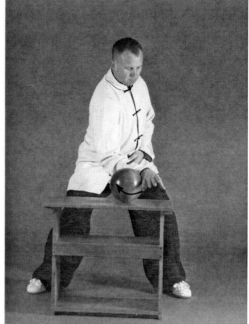

Figure 6-17

This exercise was described briefly in the wrap-coiling section and is very similar to rotating the ball on the table. Use the wrap-coiling technique as the ball moves in the clockwise and counterclockwise path on the table.

Place the ball on the table in front of you and begin to move the ball around in the clockwise path while wrap-coiling the hand on the ball. With each rotation, increase the size of this pattern until your hand moves around the sides of the ball (Figure 6-17). This is where it will be harder to control the direction of the ball.

It is most important to use the waist to control the direction of the ball. Just as in the last exercise, you may switch from one hand to the next as well as change the directions of the pattern by moving the ball through the center of the pattern.

Train this exercise on the forearm as well. Start with the ball in one hand, palm up. Simultaneously twist your wrist and raise your hand causing the ball to roll over your palm and down your forearm. If you are able, raise the arm slightly and allow the ball to travel down your arm, behind the neck, and onward to the other side. As the ball reaches the other side, lower that arm slightly; then twist the wrist from palm down to palm up allowing the ball to come to a rest in your hand.

1. Adhere-Connecting to the Ball (*Nian Lian Qiu,* 黏連球)

This section involves utilizing all the previous skills as necessary to free your mind into a free-style movement of the ball. Practice this using the table first. The main idea is to be able to move the ball in any direction, including lifting it off the table (sideways attachment and forward-backward attachment), without causing a bump. It builds upon your connecting, adhering, and most importantly, listening jin. When you are comfortable doing this exercise, try closing your eyes and see if you can continue the movements.

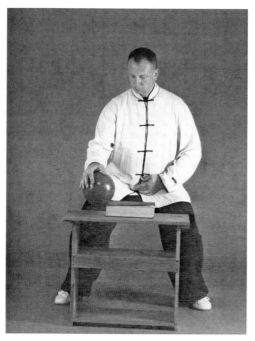

Figure 6-18

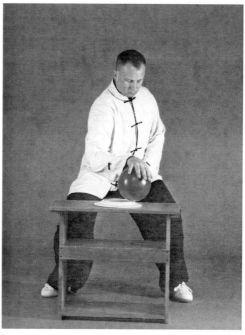

Figure 6-19

2. Flying Dragon Plays with the Ball (*Fei Long Xi Qiu,* 飛龍戲球)

This exercise builds upon the previous exercise by practicing the free-style motion while away from the table. You should be able to move freely across the floor while practicing all the patterns previously described. At this stage you will notice a basic mutual understanding developing between you and the ball. You will control the direction of the ball and yet it feels as though the ball is actually controlling your direction. In addition, practice with your eyes closed and focus more on the internal flow of qi through the ball. Keep your breathing steady, slow, and full.

6.2.4 *Walking Along the Edge Practice (Zou Yuan Lian Xi,* 走緣練習*)*

The following exercises will assist you in focusing your mind to a point beyond the ball. This type of training is considered crucial to taiji pushing hands skills. Your main focus is to find your opponent's center for uprooting. In our situation, we are focusing on the center of the object to which we are adhering.

I. Along the Right Angle (*Zhi Jiao Zou Yuan,* 直角走緣)

In the first exercise, place any object such as a book, plate, or cinder block on a table approximately the height of your dan tian. Now place the taiji ball along the top edge of the object. From this position, roll the ball around the edge of the object (Figures 6-18 and 6-19).

Do not allow the ball to slide up on top of the object or down the side. It should be rolled completely along the edge. You may have to change hands at one point in order to move the ball completely around the far edge of the object. Once you are comfortable with this feeling, the next step is to practice it with your eyes closed. Remember to twist the body in order to move the ball around correctly.

FOLLOW ALONG
FLYING DRAGON PLAYS WITH THE BALL

FOLLOW ALONG
ALONG THE EDGE PRACTICE

2. Circle on a Point (*Dan Dian Rao Quan,* 單點繞圈)

The next exercise is circling on a point. This exercise should be done in stages. For the first stage, use an object such as a chair for the point. Follow this by using the corner of a cinder block. The final stage requires the use of a knife or nail. We cannot emphasize enough how dangerous this can be if you are using such an object.

As you can see, each exercise trains the mind to focus on a central point. This will assist you with focusing on your opponent's center when you are engaged in your push hands training. Practice this exercise using both circling methods and wrap-coiling methods.

Place the object on the table in front of you approximately dan tian height. With one hand on the ball, begin to twist your waist back and forth while circling the ball on the point (Figure 6-20).

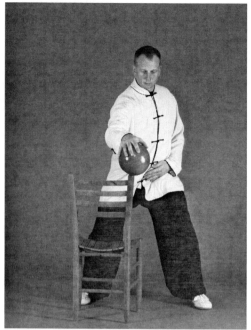

Figure 6-20

The ball should be moved on the point and not around it. Inhale when you are moving the ball toward you and exhale when moving the ball away from your body. Close your chest as the ball is moving toward you and open the chest while it moves away.

Once you are comfortable with this movement, try to wrap-coil the ball while continuing with the same movements as before. As you will notice, it is very important to move your body in order to keep the ball moving continuously on the point.

Finally, try this exercise with your eyes closed. This will increase your sensing jin and allow you to focus through the ball to the point.

The final stage is to practice this on the end of a knife or the head of a nail. In order to do this you will need to have the knife *secured* in place, approximately dan tian height. You may also hammer a long nail through a block of wood and secure it on top of the table with the nail facing up. *Be very careful* when practicing this exercise.

Practice circling first, then wrap-coiling. Finally, practice with your eyes closed. Of course it is strongly advised that you not do this until you have practiced the first stage of this exercise and have reached a sufficient skill level where you are confident enough to move on.

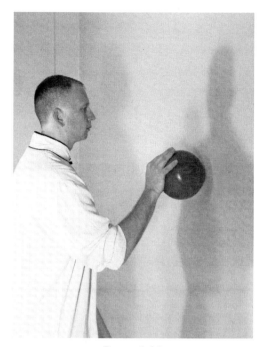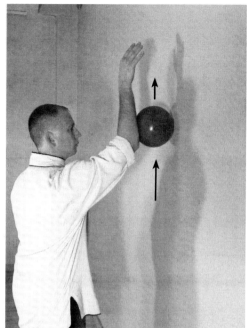

| Figure 6-21 | Figure 6-22 |

6.2.5 *Along the Wall Horizontal (Bi Shang Ping Mian Zou Yuan,* 壁上平面走緣*)*
I. Up and Down *(Shang Xia Zou Yuan,* 上下走緣**)**

The next set of exercises will be practiced while facing a wall. The purpose is to train your connecting jin (*lian jin,* 連 勁) and adhering jin (*nian jin,* 黏 勁). You will be focusing on the amount of pressure applied to the ball in order to keep it on the wall as well as the pressure necessary to allow the ball to roll as opposed to slide.

We will first practice the vertical section of the pattern, then move on to the horizontal section. To practice, face the wall with your ball in hand against it approximately chest height (Figure 6-21).

While standing in ma bu, twist your waist, roll the ball up the wall, and allow the ball to move up your arm to approximately elbow height (Figure 6-22).

Twist the waist back and roll the ball back down to the starting point. As the ball ascends, exhale and open the chest. As the ball descends, inhale and close the chest. Practice this movement for 12 repetitions; then switch hands and continue for another 12 repetitions.

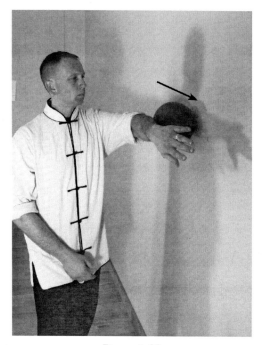

Figure 6-23

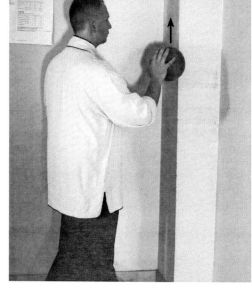

Figure 6-24

Next, practice moving the ball horizontally along the wall. Standing in ma bu, place the ball in front of you against the wall. The height of the ball should be approximately the same as your shoulder. With your palm facing the ball, twist at the waist and roll the ball along the wall until it has moved across your arm to your elbow (Figure 6-23).

Return to the original position allowing the ball to arrive back in your hand. Exhale and open the chest as you move the ball away from you, and inhale with the chest closing as you move back to your original position. Repeat for 12 repetitions as before; then switch hands and continue for another 12 repetitions.

The next stage of this exercise is to practice rolling the ball vertically along the edge of a wall.

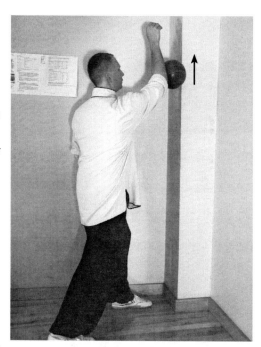

Figure 6-25

Placing the ball along the edge of the wall with your hand, roll the ball back and forth vertically allowing it to move from your hand to elbow (Figures 6-24 and 6-25).

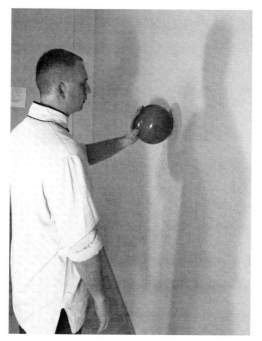

Figure 6-26

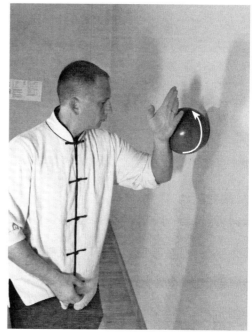

Figure 6-27

Close the chest and inhale as the ball is moved down the wall toward you, and open the chest while exhaling as the ball rolls vertically up the wall away from you. Continue to practice this for 12 repetitions, and then switch hands for 12 more repetitions.

The final stage of this exercise is to practice the wrap-coiling motion against the wall. Place the ball against the wall with your palm facing the ball. Begin to wrap-coil the ball in a clockwise and counterclockwise direction (Figures 6-26 and 6-27).

Repeat for 12 repetitions, switch hands and continue for an additional 12 repetitions.

The next two exercises are not found on the *Tai Chi Ball Qigong* DVD series. They are additional methods of training the body to reach deeper levels of conditioning for health and martial arts. Both of these exercises involve moving the ball across the wall horizontally while maintaining contact using your hands, arms, and back. This training will enhance your listening, attaching, adhering, and following skills beyond the hands.

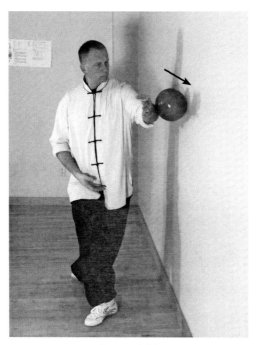

Figure 6-28

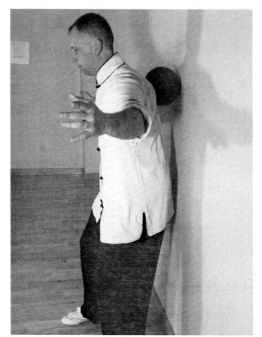

Figure 6-29

There are two ways to practice this exercise. Each is begun the same way. Stand facing the wall in ma bu and place the ball in front of you at approximately shoulder height. With your palm facing away from the ball, twist your body into zou pan bu and roll the ball across your arm (Figure 6-28).

As the ball continues to roll across your shoulder, turn your body away from the ball and step into ma bu. The ball will now be moving across your back (Figure 6-29).

Next, turn your body so you are in a si liu bu stance while allowing the ball to roll across your arm ending at the opposite hand, palm facing away from the ball (Figure 6-30).

From this position, simply roll the ball from one hand across your back to the other hand while shifting from si liu bu to ma bu, then back to si liu bu. Continue this exercise until you have completed 12 repetitions.

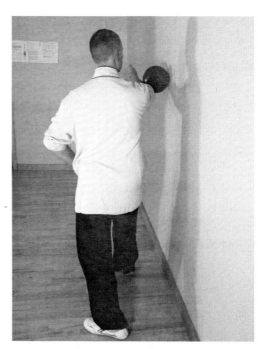

Figure 6-30

To finish, allow the ball to roll across your back while stepping backward into zou pan bu. From this position, simply twist the body back to face the wall while the ball rolls back to your original hand.

The second way to do this exercise involves practicing your wrap-coiling technique. Start by facing the wall in a ma bu stance with your ball against it at approximately shoulder height. With your palm on the ball, twist the body into a zou pan bu and wrap-coil your hand. Step across with your back foot into a ma bu facing away from the wall, and continue to roll the ball across your back toward the other hand.

As the ball reaches the other arm, step backward into a zou pan bu stance. To complete the movement, twist your body back to face the wall, and wrap-coil your hand ending in a ma bu stance with the ball in your opposite hand against the wall. From this position, step back to your original position using the same technique previously described. Repeat this exercise moving back and forth for at least 12 repetitions.

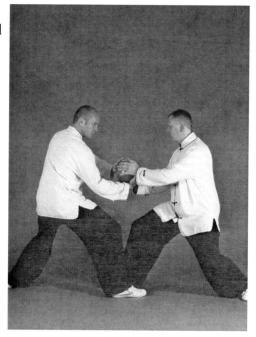

Figure 6-31

6.3 Train with Partners (*Yu Ban Tong Lian,* 與伴同練)

In the previous exercises, you have focused on practicing with the taiji ball or an inanimate object associated with the ball. In the next set of exercises, you will be practicing with a partner. This will allow you to focus on your sense of distancing as well as enhancing your connecting, adhering, and sticking jin skills. Whether you are practicing pushing hands or engaged with your enemy, these skills are necessary for positioning an opponent into a disadvantage and defeating them. In the following exercises, when it is recommended that one person at a time initiate a movement, the training for the passive partner is to stick to the ball and yield to the direction of the initiating partner. This is also an important element in training.

6.3.1 *Straight Line Listening and Following (Zhi Xian Ting Sui,* 直線聽隨*)*

The first set of exercises focuses on maintaining an equal distance between you and your partner while moving on a linear path. The whole concept of this training is to be able to read your opponent's body language by sensing or feeling his energy through the taiji ball. For this training, three separate stages have been established.

The first stage is to move linearly in one direction at a time with your partner while holding the ball in a fixed position between you. Stand in si liu bu, right leg forward. Your partner will also stand in si liu bu, right leg forward, facing you. The taiji ball will be held by you and your partner with both sets of hands on the ball level to the lower dan tian area (Figure 6-31).

FOLLOW ALONG
PRACTICE WITH A PARTNER

Start to rock back and forth. Both the ball and your partner should remain equally apart from you throughout the rocking movement.

Next, step forward slowly and attempt to close the distance between you and your partner. This is also known as attempting to occupy the central door (*zhong men*, 中 門). (If you wish to explore more information on this subject, you will find this subject further described in *Taijiquan Theory of Dr. Yang, Jwing-Ming: The Root of Taijiquan* by *Dr. Yang, Jwing-Ming*, available at YMAA Publication Center.)

As you step forward, your opponent should step back and maintain the same distance between you, the ball, and himself. In addition to maintaining this distance, your opponent should also be focusing on maintaining an equal amount of tension, or pressure, on the taiji ball. Allowing an increase of pressure is known as being double weighted. The increase of pressure will lead to tension in the muscles and disrupt the continuous flow of movement as well as disrupt the flow of qi.

The overall object is to be able to sense the incoming force, yield to it and lead it away from you, or neutralize the force. This is commonly known as using four ounces to deflect one thousand pounds. Continue to step forward until you have reached the end of your practicing area. Once you have reached the end of the practice area, switch roles with your partner.

Keep the eyes focused at approximately the heart level on your opponent. Your partner should do the same. Focusing the eyes on this area gives you an acceptable peripheral view of your opponent and surrounding area. It is a tool that will prove to be beneficial when engaging an opponent for self-defense.

Continue back and forth throughout the practice area until you and your partner, taking turns leading, are able to maintain equal distancing throughout the exercise. In addition, you both should break up the pattern by varying the number of successive steps or pausing between steps to simply rock back and forth.

The next stage of this exercise is similar to the last. The main difference is the person controlling the stepping is also allowed to step backward. The opponent will be responsible to sense the forward movement of attack as well as the retreating movement. Once they reach the end of the training area, the individuals will switch roles. The ball will remain in a fixed position between you and your partner throughout the stepping exercise.

When you both are comfortable with this exercise, mix the patterns using a free-style method. Start from the center of your practicing area. Either partner may take the lead. This exercise is more difficult and allows each of you to enhance your listening skills. Both you and your partner should continue to practice these exercises until each person can maintain an equal distance between each other while advancing and retreating.

The final stage of this exercise is to practice with your eyes closed. Closing off the visual will allow you to focus more on the tension between you and your partner and the taiji ball. As mentioned before, you want to avoid a double-weighted feeling. Practice each stage of this exercise until you and your partner are able to move back and forth smoothly.

6.3.1.1 Circling (Rao Quan, 繞圈)

The following exercises involve circling the ball with a partner. These are performed the same as the previous listening and following exercises; however, you will now add the element of circling the ball. In addition, you and your partner will practice the yin-yang circling exchange both vertically and horizontally. This will assist you in recognizing how to yield to an inbound force and redirect/neutralize the force. Ultimately, either person in this exercise may control this yin-yang exchange.

As you continue to practice this, you will realize that there are infinite numbers and sizes of circles that can be made. We will explain this in more detail later. To simplify your understanding of this exercise, practice the circling patterns vertically and then horizontally, using both hands, and then single hands. Practice these exercises while stationary, rocking, and stepping.

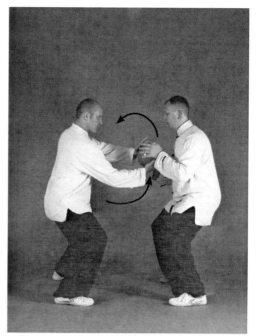

Figure 6-32

Yin-Yang Vertical Circling Training with a Partner (Chui Zhi Yin Yang Rao Quan Yu Ban Tong Lian, 垂直陰陽繞圈與伴同練)

The first set of exercises will be the vertical yin-yang circling patterns using both sets of hands on the ball, followed by each person using a single hand attached to the ball. When practicing the exercises using both sets of hands, the ball will be turned slightly along its horizontal axis allowing a crisscross pattern.

It is advisable to have one partner at a time lead the exchanges in the beginning. Follow this with the freestyle method of exchanging where either person may choose to change the direction of the pattern between yin and yang.

I. Stationary (Ding Bu, 定步)

The first exercise is the vertical yin-yang circling pattern while in a stationary position. The circling pattern as well as the exchanging between yin and yang are performed the same as you have done when practicing solo. One difference is that while you move in a yang direction, your partner will move in the yin direction. The opposite holds true when you move in the yin direction.

To start the exercise, stand in ma bu facing each other. With both your hands holding the ball in front of your dan tian, rotate it slightly and allow your partner to place both their hands on the ball. Begin to vertically circle the ball in a yang direction and expand the size of the pattern until you have reached a mutual maximum range of motion (Figure 6-32).

Double
Hands
(Shuang
Shou)
雙手

Continue to vertically circle the ball a few times, and then move on to your yin-yang exchanges. You may elect to execute the exchange anywhere in the pattern. Once you are able to execute the exchange smoothly, allow your partner to perform his exchanges until it can be done smoothly.

Follow this action by allowing either person to lead the exchange in a free-style manner. You may also elect to close your eyes to reach a deeper stage. Continue to practice this pattern until you are both able to perform the circling with exchanging, seamlessly, anywhere within the pattern.

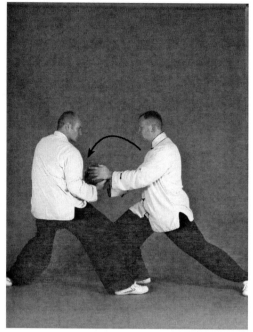

Figure 6-33

2. Rocking (*Qian Hou Dong,* 前後動)

The next partner exercise is the yin-yang vertical circling pattern while rocking. To start this exercise, face each other standing in si liu bu with the right foot forward. Your partner will place both hands on the ball while you hold it in front of your dan tian (Figure 6-33).

Initiate the vertical circling pattern in a yang direction, while rocking just as you have done while solo. Your partner will be rocking while circling the ball in the yin direction. Keep in mind that each time you and your partner rock backward you should be careful not to allow the ball to get too close to your body. This can cause unnecessary muscular tension resulting in restriction of the flow of qi. It also is not a good defensive position. Practice the vertical circling pattern until you and your partner are comfortable with the movement. It should be smooth and there should be no bumping throughout the rocking pattern.

Next, practice your yin-yang exchanges. Practice using a few different methods. First, practice the exchanging by allowing one person at a time to lead the exchange. Follow this exercise with a free-style exchange exercise, where either partner may initiate the exchange. The passive partner trains to follow the lead of the active partner. The active partner trains his awareness of how to initiate the exchange.

Finally, practice the exchanges in the following manner. Your partner will move the ball toward the center of the pattern, then directly toward the center of your body. You will yield to the incoming force and neutralize it by rocking aft and redirecting the ball in a different direction. Once you can perform this smoothly, allow your partner to perform the same task.

Follow this with free-style exchanging between partners. Continue to practice this until you both are able to perform the exchanges smoothly and without interrupting the pattern. Also practice with your eyes closed.

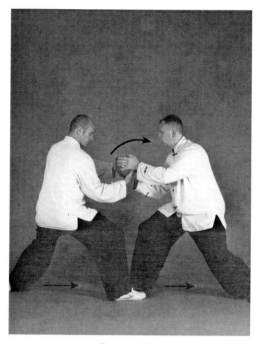

Figure 6-34

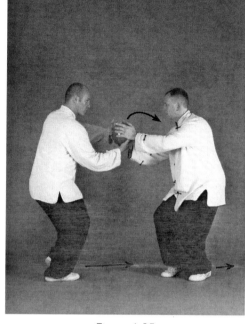

Figure 6-35

3. Stepping (*Dong Bu,* 動步)

The next stage is to practice this while stepping forward and backward. Begin this exercise facing your partner in si liu bu, either leg forward. With both sets of hands on the ball, start your yang vertical circling. Increase the size of the pattern to the maximum range, and then add stepping forward and backward across the practice area (Figures 6-34, 6-35, and 6-36).

Once you and your partner are able to move back and forth smoothly, move on to the yin-yang exchanging. First, have your partner continuously step forward while you execute the exchanges. Next, you step forward and allow your partner to execute the exchanges.

Once you and your partner are comfortable with this stage, begin to step forward and backward, and this time, both of you are allowed to initiate the exchange of the

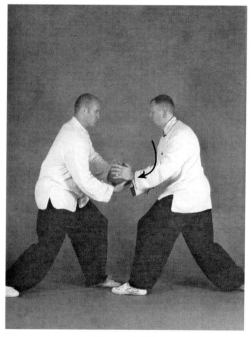

Figure 6-36

pattern back and forth. Pay particular attention to your following jin, connecting jin, as well as sticking jin while your partner steps backward. Continue this exercise until

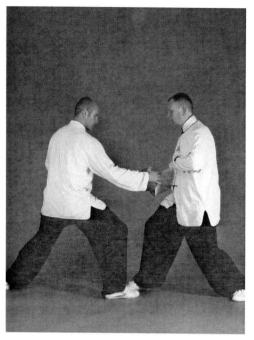

Figure 6-37

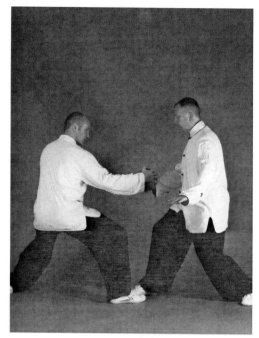

Figure 6-38

you have crossed the practice area several times. Remember to keep an equal distance between you and your partner.

The last stage is to practice this same exercise with your eyes closed. As before, this will enhance the sensing jin by taking away the element of sight.

In the next set of exercises, each partner places a single hand on the ball. The opposite hand should initially be placed on your dan tian. When you are comfortable with the exercise, you may place the second hand on your chest to assist with feeling the opening and closing of this area (Figure 6-37).

Next, practice the same exercise with one hand out to the side approximately level with your dan tian (Figure 6-38).

Finally, you may practice the exercise by placing the free hand near the elbow of the hand on the ball (Figure 6-39).

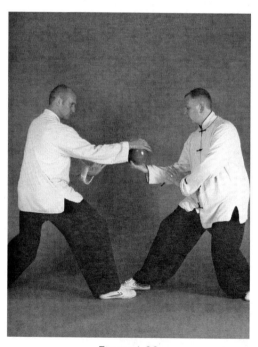

Figure 6-39

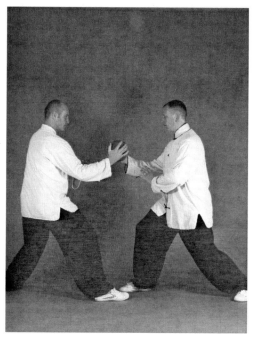

Figure 6-40

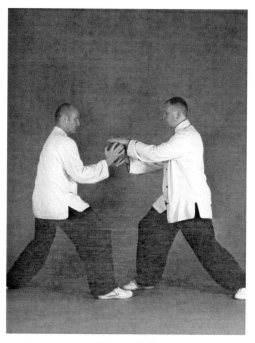

Figure 6-41

These patterns should be practiced while stationary, rocking, and stepping. In addition to the single hand exercises, practice switching hands. Do this by placing the non-active hand on the ball while performing the pattern. Once that hand is placed on the ball, rotate it on the horizontal axis while simultaneously lifting the other hand off the ball. Continue with the vertical circle exercise (Figures 6-40, 6-41, and 6-42).

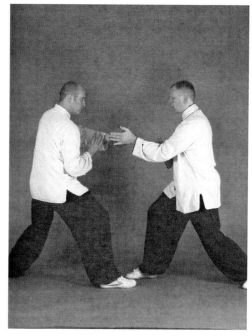

Figure 6-42

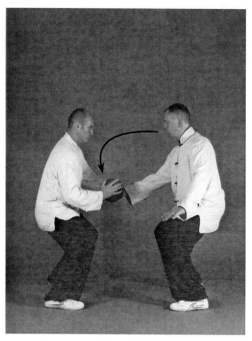

Figure 6-43

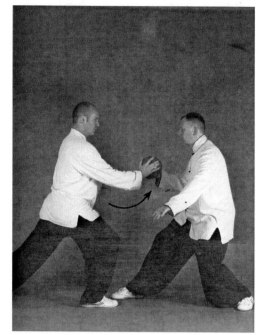

Figure 6-44

1. Stationary (*Ding Bu*, 定步)

To begin this exercise, stand in ma bu with your partner. Both of you should place one hand on either side of the ball and begin the vertical circling pattern (Figure 6-43).

Increase the size of the pattern until reaching the maximum range of motion mutually agreed upon. Continue to practice the circling until you and your partner are comfortable doing the exercise, and then practice the yin-yang exchanging.

Start by having one person initiate the exchange; then reverse roles. Next, either partner may initiate the yin-yang exchange in the pattern. Finally, the two of you should close your eyes and practice exchanging the direction of the ball between yin and yang. Continue this exercise until you and your partner are able to execute the exchange anywhere in the pattern smoothly.

2. Rocking (*Qian Hou Dong*, 前後動)

The next stage of this exercise is the single hand vertical circling pattern while rocking. Face each other in si liu bu, right leg forward. Each of you places one hand on the ball and circles the ball vertically, as previously described (Figure 6-44).

Reaching the desired maximum size of the pattern, begin to exchange the direction of the ball back and forth between yin and yang. Once again, practice this in stages by first allowing one person at a time to practice the exchange. This should be followed by allowing both partners to initiate the exchange at will. Next, you both close your eyes and practice the exchanging. Continue this exercise until you and your partner are able to execute the exchanges smoothly and without interruption in the pattern.

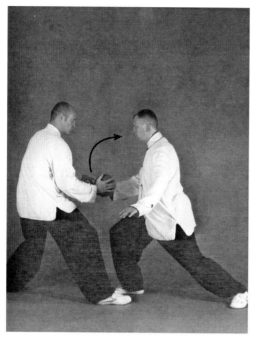

Figure 6-45

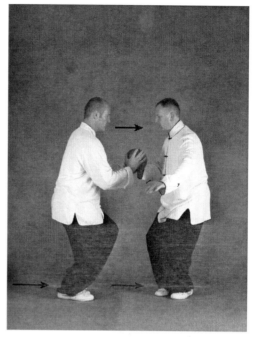

Figure 6-46

3. Stepping (*Dong Bu,* 動步)

The final stage of this exercise is stepping while using the single hand vertical circling pattern. Step into si liu bu with your partner and begin the vertical circling pattern as previously described in the rocking section. Increase the size of the pattern to the maximum range allowable, and then begin to practice stepping forward and backward (Figures 6-45, 6-46, and 6-47). This can also be done in stages if you wish.

Once you and your partner are comfortable doing so, add the element of the yin-yang exchange. Follow the same progression as you have in the past. One person at a time should execute the exchange followed by both people practicing the yin-yang exchange, back and forth. Finally, close the eyes and practice the same exercise. Continue this exercise until you and your partner are able to perform the exchanges smoothly.

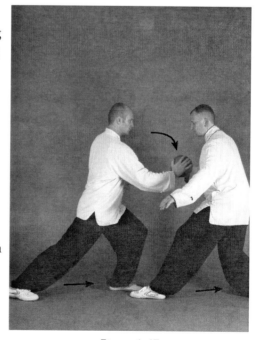

Figure 6-47

Yin-Yang Horizontal Circling Training with a Partner (*Shui Ping Yin Yang Rao Quan Yu Ban Tong Lian*, 水平陰陽繞圈與伴同練)

The next set of exercises will be practiced while horizontally circling the ball. They will be practiced with both sets of hands placed on the ball, then with a single hand placed on it. Each set of exercises will be practiced while stationary, rocking and stepping. Unlike the vertical two person exercises, you will notice that both you and your partner will be moving in the same direction whether yang or yin.

1. Stationary (*Ding Bu*, 定步)

Double Hands (*Shuang Shou*) 雙手

Stand in ma bu facing your partner; place both sets of hands on the ball. Begin to horizontally circle the ball and increase the size of your pattern until reaching a maximum range of motion for the two of you. Continue to practice the horizontal pattern until both of you are comfortable (Figure 6-48).

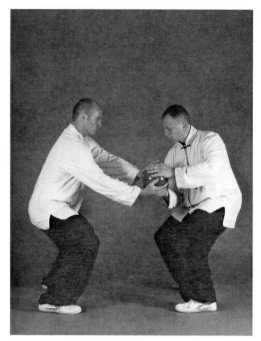

Figure 6-48

Next, practice while one person at a time initiates the exchange. When you are ready, either partner may initiate the exchange. One person has to initiate the exchange, but it does not mean the other cannot initiate his change right after. There is no limit to how, where, or when changes occur because the shape of the pattern will always change and the wuji point will always move. The pattern becomes a sphere.

These exercises are done in stages where one person does the exchanging while the other just follows, and then they switch roles. Finally, either partner may initiate the exchange.

Finally, close the eyes and practice exchanging the pattern between yin and yang. Continue this exercise until you are both comfortable exchanging between yin and yang anywhere in the pattern. It should be performed smoothly.

2. Rocking (*Qian Hou Dong*, 前後動)

The next stage is horizontal circling while rocking. Face your partner. Step into si liu bu, right leg forward, and place both sets of hands on the ball. Begin to circle the ball horizontally and increase the pattern to the size desired. Practice your horizontal circling pattern until you are both comfortable (Figure 6-49).

Next, start practicing the yin-yang exchange using the same stages of progression previously described. Continue to practice this exercise until you and your partner are able to execute the exchanges smoothly.

3. Stepping (*Dong Bu,* 動步)

The final stage of this exercise is to practice the yin-yang exchange while stepping. Standing in si liu bu with your partner, begin the horizontal circling pattern as described in the previous section. Reaching the maximum size desired, begin to step forward across the floor until you have reached the end of the practice area.

Next, allow your partner to step forward until you reach the other end of the practice area, or until you want to switch. You should then both move forward and backward until you are comfortable with this movement.

Next, practice the yin-yang exchanging while stepping. This exchange should be executed in stages similar to the horizontal exchange practiced solo. Once again, allow one person at a time to practice this yin-yang exchange; then move on to having either partner initiate the exchanges.

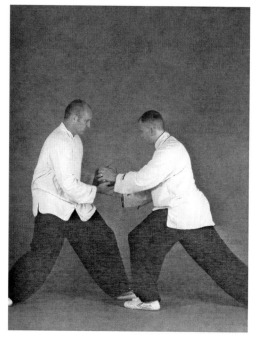

Figure 6-49

Finally, practice the yin-yang exchange while stepping with the eyes closed. Continue this exercise until you and your partner can perform the exchange smoothly.

For the next stage of horizontal circling, each partner will place one hand on the ball. You may elect to place the hands on the sides of the ball or on the top and bottom of the ball. By placing the hands on the top and bottom, you will prepare yourself for the rotational patterns that will be explained following the circling patterns. The other hand may be placed on the dan tian, or the chest, or out to the side approximately level to the dan tian. Finally, place the free hand by the elbow of the first hand while practicing the patterns. After you have completed the exercises, you may elect to go back and practice switching hands. This will be done the same as in your vertical circling exercises.

1. Stationary (Ding Bu, 定步)

Face your partner while standing in ma bu and place one hand on the ball (Figure 6-50). Begin to horizontally circle the ball and increase the size of the pattern until you have reached the desired range of motion. Continue to circle the ball until you both are comfortable.

Next, begin to practice your yin-yang exchange exercises. One person at a time should initiate the exchange. Once you have done this, both of you should practice exchanging throughout the pattern. The final stage is where you both close your eyes and practice exchanging throughout the pattern. Continue to practice the exercise until you and your partner are able to perform the exchanges smoothly.

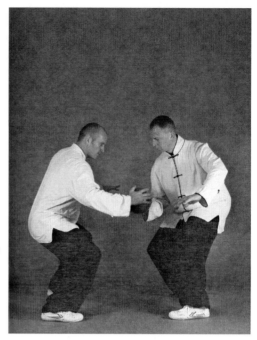

Figure 6-50

2. Rocking (Qian Hou Dong, 前後動)

The next exercise is the single hand horizontal circling pattern while rocking. Standing in si liu bu, face your partner, place one hand on the ball and begin the horizontal circling pattern while rocking. Reaching the maximum range of motion desired, complete a few circles; then begin to practice the yin-yang exchanges of the pattern. Be sure to follow the same progression of exchanging you have been using thus far. One person initiates the exchange followed by the other. Next, both partners practice the exchange followed by keeping the eyes closed throughout the exercise. Continue to practice this exercise until you and your partner can execute the exchange anywhere in the pattern. It should be done smoothly, without interruption.

3. Stepping (Dong Bu, 動步)

The final stage of this exercise is to practice the single hand horizontal circling pattern while stepping. Standing in si liu bu facing your partner, begin the horizontal pattern while rocking. Once you have reached the maximum range of motion desired, practice stepping forward until you have reached the end of your training area.

Next, allow your partner to practice the same stepping action forward until you have reached the original position in the practice area.

Now practice stepping forward and backward within the practice area until you and your partner can move back and forth comfortably while performing the horizontal circling pattern.

Next, step forward and simultaneously practice the yin-yang exchange. This should be done until you reach the end of your practice area. Now allow your partner to practice the same procedure until you arrive back at the desired position on the floor. Follow this by practicing the exchanges while moving forward and backward. Finally, both of you should close your eyes and practice the same exercise. Continue this until you and your partner are able to perform this exercise smoothly, without interruption.

Vertical-Horizontal, Yin-Yang Mixing Circling with a Partner (*Chui Zhi Shui Ping Yin Yang Rao Quan Yu Ban Hun He Lian Xi*, 垂直水平陰陽繞圈與伴混合練習)

Now that you have practiced the vertical and horizontal patterns with your partner, it is time to combine them. The following exercises may be done using both hands or with a single hand. You may also add combinations of moving from double hands to single hands or switching single hands. We will introduce each exercise with the vertical circling pattern; you may choose to begin with the horizontal pattern. Also keep in mind there will be more sections of the pattern to perform the exchanges than we will describe here.

1. Stationary (*Ding Bu*, 定步)

The first set of exercises will be done stationary. Standing in ma bu with your partner, begin to vertically circle the ball and increase the size of the pattern until you have reached the maximum range of motion desired. Practice the yin-yang exchange and include changing between vertical and horizontal patterns. Each exchange will follow the same technique you used in the solo practice. Once you are comfortable doing this, allow your partner to practice the same procedure.

In the next stage, you both may initiate the exchange at random. The training for the person who does not initiate the exchange is to yield and follow the pattern smoothly.

Finally, close the eyes and repeat the exercise. Continue to practice this exercise until you and your partner are able to execute each exchange smoothly and without interrupting the pattern.

2. Rocking (*Qian Hou Dong*, 前後動)

The next stage is to practice the exercise while rocking. Stand in si liu bu facing your partner. Begin the vertical circling pattern while rocking and increase the size of the pattern until you have reached an acceptable range of motion. Once again, you and your partner should progress through the different steps of exchanging the directions and patterns of the ball. The final stage, as always, will be practiced with your eyes closed. Continue this exercise until you and your partner are able to perform each exchange smoothly

3. Stepping (*Dong Bu*, 動步)

The final stage of this exercise is the yin-yang exchanges while stepping. The exercise essentially remains the same as previously described, only now you are going to step while you perform the exchange. The rules of exchanging will remain the same as it was for the solo exercises. Of course, you may notice a few instances where you are able to execute an exchange without maneuvering the ball through the center of the pattern. This is acceptable only if you have not disrupted the flow of the pattern. Continue this exercise until you and your partner are able to perform this exercise smoothly, without interruption. This includes performing the exercise with the eyes closed.

6.3.1.2 Rotating (Zhan Zhuan, 輾轉)

The next set of exercises is the vertical and horizontal rotation patterns while stationary, rocking, and stepping. Practice using single and double hands. You will notice the double hand exercise will prove to be more difficult due to the placement of sets of hands on the ball. To alleviate some of the difficulty, you and your partner will initiate the exercise by rotating the ball slightly on its horizontal axis creating a crisscrossed pattern on the ball. This will allow you and your partner better ability to rotate the ball. Of course, you will still need to twist the waist and keep the shoulders aligned with the hips to perform to rotations correctly.

Vertical Rotating (*Chui Zhi Zhan Zhuan,* 垂直輾轉)

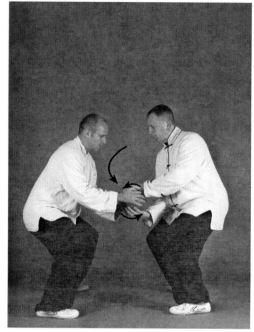

Figure 6-51

1. Stationary (*Ding Bu,* 定步)

Double Hands (*Shuang Shou)* 雙手

Stand in ma bu facing your partner, place both sets of hands on the ball, and rotate it slightly on its horizontal axis (Figure 6-51).

From this position, begin the vertical rotation pattern and slowly increase the size of the pattern. Although you will be able to increase the circular element of the pattern, you will notice you will not be able to increase the rotational element of the pattern as you have while practicing it solo. Simply increase the size of the pattern to the maximum size allowable for you and your partner. Continue to practice the vertical pattern until it becomes smooth, and then practice the yin-yang exchange using the same steps as you have done previously.

The exchange will be the same as in the solo exercise, through the center of the pattern with one horizontal rotation then continuing on with the vertical rotation in the opposite direction. Practice this exercise until you and your partner are able to execute the yin-yang exchange anywhere in the pattern smoothly.

2. Rocking (*Qian Hou Dong,* 前後動)

To begin the next stage, stand in si liu bu, right leg forward facing your partner. With both of you holding the ball, begin practicing the vertical rotation pattern while rocking. Increase the size of the pattern to the maximum range of motion that you and your partner are able. Continue to practice the pattern until both of you are comfortable. Next, execute the yin-yang exchanges using the same steps you have taken in the previous exercises. Continue this exercise until you and your partner are able to smoothly perform the yin-yang exchanges, without interruption. This includes performing the exercise with the eyes closed.

3. Stepping (*Dong Bu,* 動步)

The final stage of the double hand vertical rotation involves stepping while rotating. Due to the similarity of this exercise to the circling stepping exercise, we will not describe this in full detail. Some of the key points that should be noted are practice slowly so you can feel the connection between you and your ball as well as you and your partner, and try not to allow the ball to get too close to your body when moving aft. Always maintain an equal distance between you and your partner any time you are withdrawing. This exercise will also be practiced using the same progressive stages of the previous stepping exercises.

First, practice the stepping section; then add the yin-yang exchange. One person should initiate the exchanges followed by the other. Next, both partners may initiate the exchanges back and forth. The final stage is to practice the exercise with your eyes closed.

Once again, you focus internally on your listening skills. Continue to practice this exercise until you and your partner are able to comfortably step forward and backward while rotating the ball. In addition, you both should be able to smoothly exchange between the yin and yang directions.

The next set of exercises involves vertically rotating the ball with a single hand placed on the ball by you and your partner. For each of these exercises, the hand will initially be placed on the sides of the ball just as you have done when practicing the rotations solo. The hands will move toward the top and bottom of the ball when viewed from the side.

The second hand should be initially placed on the dan tian. If you are comfortable with this position, practice the patterns while placing the second hand over your chest. You may then practice the exercise by placing the free hand out to the side approximately level to the dan tian. Finally, place the free hand by the elbow of the first hand while practicing the patterns. You may also explore exchanging hands while practicing the pattern or during the exchanging section of the pattern.

1. Stationary (*Ding Bu,* 定步)

The first exercise is the stationary single hand rotation. Stand in ma bu facing your partner, place a single hand on the ball, and begin to vertically rotate the ball just

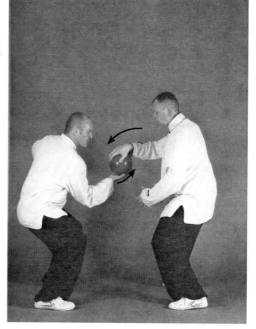

Figure 6-52

Single Hand (*Dan Shou*) 單手

as you have when solo. Increase the size of the pattern to the maximum range possible. Continue to practice this pattern until it is smooth (Figure 6-52).

Next, begin practicing the yin-yang exchanging exercise using the same steps you have previously. Continue to practice this exercise until you and your partner are able to perform the exchanges anywhere in the pattern smoothly.

2. Rocking (*Qian Hou Dong,* 前後動)

The next stage is single hand rotating while rocking. Stand in si liu bu, right leg forward facing your partner, place one hand on the ball and begin to vertically rotate the ball. Reaching the maximum range of motion possible, rotate the ball back and forth until you are both ready for the next stage.

Next, practice the yin-yang exchanges using the same sequence of steps you have taken in the previous exercises. Continue this exercise until you and your partner are able to execute the exchanges smoothly. This should also include practicing the exercise while keeping the eyes closed.

3. Stepping (*Dong Bu,* 動步)

The final stage of single hand vertical rotations is to practice them while stepping. To begin this exercise, simply step into si liu bu with your partner and start the vertical rotation pattern as you did when rocking. Once you have reached the maximum range of motion, it is time to practice the stepping section of the exercise. This will be followed by the yin-yang exchanging exercise. Finally, you will practice these exercises while the eyes are closed. Continue to practice this until you and your partner are able to perform each exchange smoothly.

Horizontal Rotating (*Shui Ping Zhan Zhuan,* 水平輾轉)

The next set of exercises will be done while horizontally rotating the ball. You and your training partner will practice this using double hand and single hand configurations while stationary, rocking, and stepping.

In order to horizontally rotate the ball using the double hand exercises, you and your partner will initially rotate it slightly on its horizontal axis. When using the single hand technique, one hand will be placed on the top of the ball while the other will be placed on the bottom.

To perform the yin-yang exchange, you will perform the same actions as you did when practicing it solo. In addition, you may also decide to practice switching hands while practicing the single hand patterns.

I. Stationary (*Ding Bu,* 定步)

The first exercise is the double hand horizontal rotation while stationary. Stand in ma bu with your partner and place both sets of hands on the ball. Rotate the ball slightly on its horizontal axis allowing the hands to form a crisscrossed pattern. Begin to horizontally rotate the ball and increase the size of the pattern to the maximum range of motion possible (Figure 6-53).

Next, practice exchanging between yin and yang using the same steps you have taken previously. Continue to practice this exercise until you and your partner are able to execute the yin-yang exchange from any position in the pattern smoothly. This should also be practiced with the eyes closed.

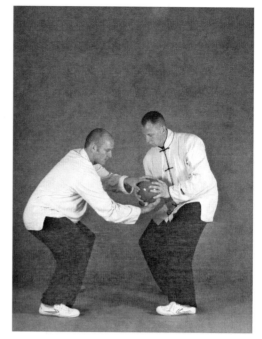

Double
Hands
(*Shuang
Shou*)
雙手

[Figure 6-53

2. Rocking (*Qian Hou Dong,* 前後動)

The next exercise is the double hand horizontal rotation. While standing in si liu bu with your partner, place both sets of hands on the ball and rotate it slightly on its horizontal axis. Begin the horizontal rotating pattern and increase the size of the pattern to the maximum range of motion possible. Continue with the pattern until both of you are comfortable.

Next, practice the yin-yang exchange using the same steps you have taken previously. Continue to practice this exercise until you and your partner are able to perform the yin-yang exchange smoothly. This includes practicing the exercise with the eyes closed.

3. Stepping (*Dong Bu,* 動步)

The final stage of horizontal rotations we will introduce in this section is rotating while stepping. Essentially, it is the same as the double hand vertical rotation exercise; therefore, we will not describe this exercise in detail. The exception is the ball is now traveling on the horizontal plane. You should progress through the same steps taken on the previous exercises. Continue to practice this exercise until you and your partner are able to both step and exchange smoothly, without interruption.

The next set of exercises will be practiced with a single hand placed on the ball by both you and your partner. For each of these exercises the hands will be initially placed on the top and bottom of the ball. As the size of horizontal rotations is increased, the hands will move toward the sides of the ball. The opposite hand may be placed over the dan tian, on the chest, out to your side, or next to the elbow of the first hand. You may also attempt to switch hands during each exercise by placing the opposite hand on the ball while it is rotating or during the exchange.

I. Stationary (*Ding Bu,* 定步)

The first exercise is the horizontal single hand rotation while stationary. Stand in ma bu with your partner, place one hand on the ball, and begin to horizontally rotate the ball in the yang direction. Increase the size of the pattern to the maximum range possible (Figure 6-54).

Next, practice the yin-yang exchanges following the same steps previously described. Continue with these exercises until you and your partner are able to perform the exchanges anywhere in the pattern smoothly.

2. Rocking (*Qian Hou Dong,* 前後動)

The next exercise is single hand horizontal rotations while rocking. Stand in si liu bu with your partner, place one hand on the ball, and begin the horizontal rotation pattern in a yang direction. Increase the size of the pattern to the maximum

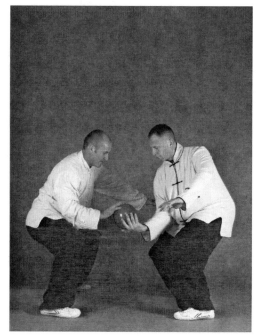

Figure 6-54

range of motion possible. Continue to practice the pattern until you and your partner are comfortable, and then start the yin-yang exchange exercise using the same method previously described in this section. Continue to practice this exercise until you and your partner are able to execute the exchanges smoothly. This should include doing the exercise with the eyes closed.

3. Stepping (*Dong Bu,* 動步)

The final stage is the single hand horizontal rotation while stepping. To begin this exercise, step into si liu bu with your partner and start the horizontal rotation pattern while rocking. Increase the size of the pattern to the maximum range of motion possible; then begin to practice the stepping exercises using the same steps you have taken previously.

Next, you and your partner should practice the yin-yang exchange exercises while stepping. Utilize the same method you have used thus far. Continue this exercise until you and your partner are able to perform the exchanges smoothly. Be sure to include closing your eyes while exchanging as well.

Vertical-Horizontal, Yin-Yang, Circling-Rotating Mixed Training with a Partner (*Chui Zhi Shui Ping Yin Yang Rao Quan Zhan Zhuan Yu Ban Hun He Lian Xi,* 垂直水平陰陽繞圈輾轉與伴混合練習)

The next set of exercises involves mixing the circling patterns with rotational patterns. You may mix any combination of vertical and horizontal patterns along with yin and yang directions. You may also combine this with double hands or single hands. This includes switching hands as well. As you continue to practice with your partner, you may find a few areas where you may perform an exchange without passing through the center of the circle. This is acceptable only if you do not interrupt the movement of the ball. Each exercise will be introduced with the vertical rotational pattern in a yang direction using both hands. You may choose any pattern and any direction when you start the exercise. In addition, you may choose to start with a single hand or double hand.

1. Stationary (*Ding Bu,* 定步)

To begin the exercise in the stationary position, you and your partner should stand facing each other in ma bu. Place both sets of hands on the ball and begin the vertical rotational pattern in a yang direction. Increase the size of the pattern to the maximum range of motion possible, and then begin to practice the yin-yang exchanging. Practice this exercise utilizing all the previous patterns and directions covered in this section. Continue this exercise until you and your partner are able to perform each exchange anywhere in the pattern smoothly. This should include performing the exchanges with the eyes closed.

2. Rocking (*Qian Hou Dong,* 前後動)

The next stage is to perform the exchanging exercises while rocking. Stand in si liu bu with your partner. Begin the vertical rotational pattern in a yang direction and increase the size of the pattern to the maximum size possible.

Next, you and your partner should practice exchanging all the patterns and directions you have practiced thus far. Continue practicing until you and your partner are able to execute the exchanges smoothly. This includes performing the exercises with the eyes closed.

3. Stepping (*Dong Bu,* 動步)

The final stage of this section is to practice your exchanging while stepping. It is similar to the previous stepping exercises. In this case, you are only adding the circling pattern to it. Be sure to practice all the patterns and directions in a free-style manner. Continue until you and your partner are able to execute the exchanges smoothly. This should include practicing with the eyes closed as well.

6.3.1.3 Wrap-Coiling (Chan Zhuan, 纏轉*)*

The next set of exercises will be done while wrap-coiling the ball both vertically and horizontally. One major difference here is that it will only be practiced utilizing a single hand placed on the ball by you and your partner. Using double hands creates an impossible pattern to practice due to the placement of the hands and arms. The double hands movement is more practical when attempting to capture the ball from your opponent.

Vertical Wrap-Coiling (*Chui Zhi Chan Zhuan,* 垂直纏轉)

The first set of exercises will be done while practicing the single hand vertical wrap-coiling pattern. Each of you will begin by placing a single hand on the ball. The hands should initially be placed on the sides of the ball and as the pattern increases in size they will move toward the top and bottom of the ball. The second hand will again initially be placed on your dan tian, by the chest, out to the side of the body, or next to the elbow of the hand on the ball. The exercises will be practiced while stationary, rocking, and stepping.

1. Stationary (*Ding Bu,* 定步)

Single Hand (*Dan Shou*) 單手

The first exercise is single hand vertical wrap-coiling while stationary. Standing in ma bu with your partner, place a single hand on the ball and begin wrap-coiling the ball in a yang direction (Figure 6-55).

Increase the size of the pattern to the maximum range possible, and then practice the exchanges using the same method as previously described. Continue this exercise until you and your partner are able to perform the exchanges anywhere in the pattern smoothly, without interruption. This should include closing the eyes as well.

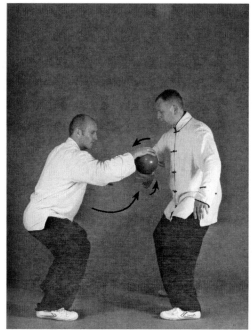

Figure 6-55

2. Rocking (*Qian Hou Dong,* 前後動)

The next stage is using the single hand vertical wrap-coiling pattern while rocking. This exercise is practiced the same as the previous vertical rocking patterns using the single hand technique. Continue this exchanging while rocking until you and your partner are able to execute the movements smoothly. Also practice with the eyes closed.

3. Stepping (*Dong Bu,* 動步)

The final stage of the vertical section is to practice the exercise while stepping. This exercise follows the same procedures as the previous single hand vertical circling and rotation stepping exercises. You now are simply adding the wrap-coiling patterns to the combinations. Continue this exercise until you and your partner are able to perform each exchange smoothly. Be sure to practice with your eyes closed as well.

Horizontal Wrap-Coiling (*Shui Ping Chan Zhuan,* 水平纏轉)

The next set of exercises will be done on the horizontal plane with a single hand placed on the ball by you and your partner. Initially, the hands will be placed on the top and bottom of the ball, then move to the sides of the ball as the size of the pattern is increased. Due to the complexity of the exercise, you may find that you and your partner may not be able to increase the size of the pattern such that the hands will end up on the sides of the ball. Simply increase the size of the pattern to the maximum size allowable for the two of you.

Remember that in order to perform the yin-yang exchange correctly, you will execute one vertical wrap-coil as the ball passes through the center of the pattern, and then follow this with the horizontal wrap-coil in the opposite direction. The second hand will follow the same positions previously described in the single hand sections.

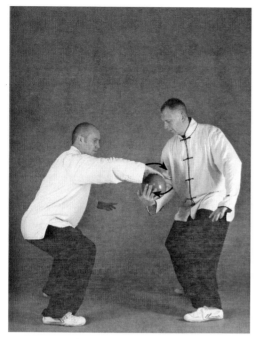

Figure 6-56

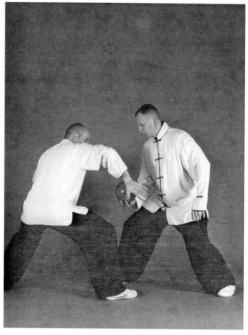

Figure 6-57

1. Stationary (*Ding Bu,* 定步)

The first exercise is single hand horizontal wrap-coiling while stationary. Stand in ma bu with your partner and place one hand on the ball. Begin the horizontal wrap-coiling pattern and increase the size of the pattern as large as possible (Figure 6-56).

Practice the pattern until you and your partner are comfortable, and then begin the yin-yang exchange exercise using the same method previously described. Continue to practice this exercise until you and your partner are able to execute the exchanges smoothly.

2. Rocking (*Qian Hou Dong,* 前後動)

The next stage of this exercise is single hand horizontal wrap-coiling while rocking. Standing in si liu bu with your partner, begin the single hand horizontal wrap-coiling pattern and increase the size of the pattern to the maximum size possible (Figure 6-57).

Continue with the pattern until you and your partner are comfortable practicing the yin-yang exchange exercise. Follow the steps in the same progression as described in the previous exercise. You and your partner should practice this until the exchanges are executed smoothly, without interruption.

3. Stepping (*Dong Bu,* 動步)

The final stage of this exercise is to practice stepping and exchanging while performing the single hand horizontal wrap-coiling pattern. Standing in si liu bu with your partner, begin the single hand horizontal wrap-coiling pattern and increase the size of the pattern to the maximum size possible.

Single
Hand
(*Dan Shou*)
單手

Next, you both should practice the stepping exercises followed by the yin-yang exercises using the same progression of steps previously described. Be sure to practice with your eyes closed, as well. Continue to practice this exercise until you and your partner are able to perform the exchanges smoothly while stepping.

Vertical-Horizontal, Yin-Yang, Circling-Rotating-Wrap-Coiling Mixed Training with a Partner (*Chui Zhi Shui Ping Yin Yang Rao Quan Zhan Zhuan Chan Zhuan Hun He Yu Ba Lian Xi,* 垂直水平陰陽繞圈輾轉纏轉混合與伴練習)

The next set of exercises will combine all the patterns previously discussed. This will include vertical, horizontal, yin and yang directions, and single or double hands. We have already mentioned that you cannot use double hands training for wrap-coiling. In this exercise, you may simply remove the second hand to transition to the wrap-coiling pattern.

By this stage, you and your partner should be very comfortable with exchanging, so we will not describe these exercises in full detail. Practice this exercise while stationary, rocking, and stepping. You should also practice with your eyes closed as part of the training. Continue to practice each exercise until you and your partner are able to execute each exchange smoothly.

6.3.2 *Capturing the Ball (Lu Qiu Lian Xi,* 擄球練習)

This exercise builds upon the last set of exercises. The main idea is to utilize the skills previously practiced to capture the ball from your partner. Through strategic stepping movements and proper angles, you should be able to capture the ball without using muscular force.

For many years, this exercise has been used in competitions held at parks. It was also not uncommon to see opponents utilize elbow strokes (*zhou,* 肘) and shoulder or knee bumping (*kao,* 靠), as part of their strategies. In today's society, we see attempts to capture the ball in the game of basketball. In most cases, basketball players exert a great deal of muscular force to steal the ball from an opponent.

To begin the exercise, face your partner standing in si liu bu, right leg forward. With both sets of hands on the ball, begin the exercise with any pattern in any direction and increase the size of the pattern to the maximum size desired. When you are both comfortable, you may start the capturing aspect of training. There is no set way to perform this task. You may decide to step forward and rotate the ball vertically, causing your opponent to release the ball (Figures 6-58 and 6-59).

You may also decide to step backward while performing a horizontal wrap coil action to capture the ball (Figures 6-60 and 6-61).

There are endless possibilities. Be careful, as your partner will also be attempting the same task. If you prefer, you may, in the beginning, take turns attempting to capture the ball for a set number of times. Remember to deemphasize muscular force and focus on stepping strategies as well as proper angles to capture the ball.

Practice this exercise until both you and your partner have successfully captured the ball for a total of 12 times each. If you want, you may also choose to practice this exercise with your eyes closed.

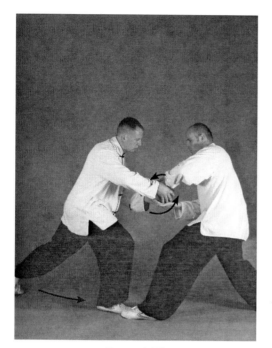

Figure 6-58

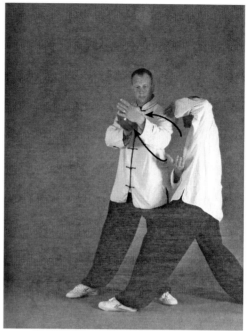

Figure 6-59

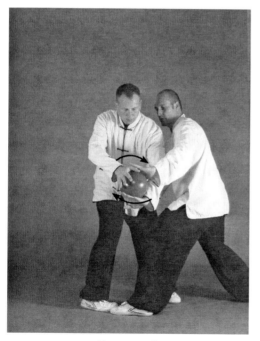

Figure 6-60

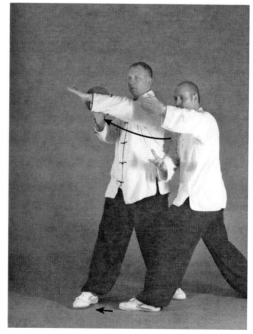

Figure 6-61

6.4 Advanced Taiji Ball Training (高級太極球之練習)

The following exercises are not found on the *Tai Chi Ball Qigong* DVD series. These exercises are a sample of how you may take your training even further. As you will see, there is no limit as to how much you can train. It is up to you to challenge yourself to reach deeper levels of understanding and excel at taiji ball training.

Now that you have a firm concept of solo exercise as well as practicing with a partner, it is time to challenge the body to reach greater strengths. This will include brick training, taiji patterns, and two-person jin patterns, or ball tossing.

6.4.1 Rooting Training (Zha Gen Lian Xi, 紮根練習)

The purpose of brick training is to develop a firmer and deeper sense of being rooted. What is meant by rooting? If you remember from our description in part one of regulation of the body, it involves feeling centered and balanced on both a physical and mental level.

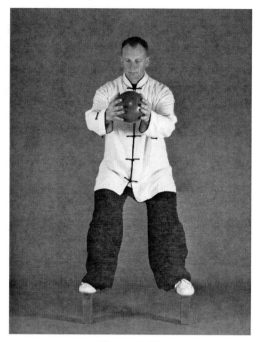

Figure 6-62

At each stage of brick training, keep your mind focused at least six inches below the ground. Begin with two bricks flat on the floor, approximately shoulder width apart and train the stationary circling, rotating, and coil-wrap sets (Figure 6-62).

Next, place a few bricks in a line. They will be used for your moving sets. Train the bagua movements by placing the bricks on the ground in the shape of the bagua circle.

The first thing that will become apparent will be the constant falling off the bricks with any leaning away from your centerline. In fact, in the beginning, you probably will not want to make the motions large. Over time, however, you will feel comfortable and be able to increase your movements. Just be patient and allow enough time for your body, breath, mind, qi, and spirit to be regulated.

Eventually, set the bricks on their sides and continue the same patterns. Finally, place the bricks in the upright position and repeat all the patterns. You see, the training is endless. After one brick, use two, then three. It is up to you how far you want to go. If you can train all the patterns on three bricks, your rooting is considered exceptionally good.

6.4.2 Taijiquan Patterns with Taiji Ball (Taiji Qiu Zai Taijiquan Jia De Ying Yong, 太極球在太極拳架的應用)

The taijiquan patterns exercise is simply practicing the taijiquan sequence while holding the ball. Of course, there are certain patterns in the sequence for which you

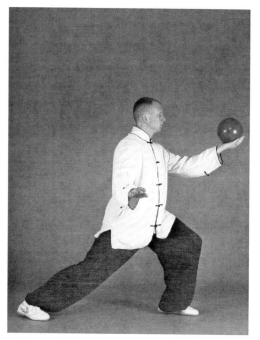

Figure 6-63. Grasp the sparrow's tail: left (zuo lan que wei).

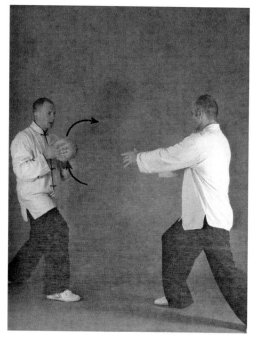

Figure 6-64

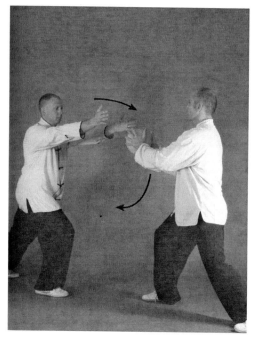

Figure 6-65

may need to separate the hands (i.e., grasp sparrows tail left). In such cases, place the ball in one of your hands (Figure 6-63).

Practicing these movements with your taiji ball will help you focus on twisting the waist as well as demonstrate a compact, rounded feeling for your postures.

6.4.3 Ball Tossing (Tou Qiu Lian Xi, 投球練習)

The final exercise is the two-person jin pattern, also known as ball tossing. This exercise will help develop your fa jin skills as well as assist you in intercepting, yielding, and neutralizing jins. To begin, face each other in si liu bu stance, approximately six feet apart. With the taiji ball initially in your hands, begin the yang vertical circling pattern while rocking. Your partner will start the vertical circling pattern in the yin direction without the ball. Once you have reached your maximum range of motion, you toss the ball. Toss the ball as it moves over the top of the circle and forward. With the proper timing, your partner will catch the ball without disrupting the flow of his pattern (Figures 6-64 and 6-65).

Your partner will continue with his pattern for a few repetitions, and then toss the ball back to you. While your partner is moving the ball, you should continue your pattern simulating a ball in between the hands. If you can do this successfully, back and forth, increase the distance between you and continue the exercise. Eventually you should add the yin-yang exchange while intercepting the ball. You may also include stepping.

Conclusion

(結論)

This book has revealed many of the training secrets that have been passed down to us from the ancient Chinese martial arts society. The theories and concepts explained in the first four chapters open the door to understanding how taiji ball qigong practice is able to condition your energetic (qi) body and physical body, and how this qi can be more effectively manifested into power through a focused mind. This is one of very few traditional qigong practices that combine internal gong (*nei gong*, 內功) and external gong (*wai gong*, 外功) on a very deep level.

If you are a martial artist, taiji ball qigong training can bring your energy to a profound level and develop your ability to move in one line, as described in the taiji classics. This energy, applied to the physical body correctly, can be as soft as water and also can be as hard as steel. Even if you are not a martial artist, there are many benefits to be derived from taiji ball qigong training. It can strengthen your guardian qi (*wei qi*, 衛氣) to boost your immune system and recondition your physical body, and taiji ball qigong training can direct abundant qi to nourish your bone marrow. This is the crucial key of longevity.

We hope that after you have studied the taiji ball basic training patterns introduced in this book, you will ponder and develop your own applications. Taiji ball qigong is an art that was created through deep feeling. As an art, it should be creative and alive and can be continuously developed, without limitation. If you have an opportunity, you should teach others. This will bring other people a healthier life and give you the opportunity to think about what you think you know. Learning through teaching is the best way of self-teaching.

We hope those who have learned other styles of taiji ball qigong will write down their ideas and publish what they have learned from their teachers and discovered in their training. *Knowledge should be shared or the art will be lost.*

Together,
Preserve the Past,
Value the Present,
Create the Future.

Translations and Glossary of Chinese Terms

(中文術語之翻譯與解釋)

ai (哀). Sorrow.

ai (愛). Love, kindness.

Ba Duan Jin (八段錦). Eight Pieces of Brocade. A wai dan qigong practice which is said to have been created by Marshal Yue Fei during the Southern Song Dynasty (A.D. 1127-1279).

Ba Kua Chang (Baguazhang) (八卦掌). Means "eight trigram palms." The name of one of the Chinese internal martial styles.

ba mai (八脈). Referred to as the eight extraordinary vessels. These eight vessels are considered to be qi reservoirs, which regulate the qi status in the primary qi channels.

ba shi (八勢). Means "eight standing postures." These eight basic fundamental stances are commonly used in Northern styles of Chinese martial arts.

bagua (八卦). Literally, "eight divinations." Also called the eight trigrams. In Chinese philosophy, the eight basic variations; shown in the *Yi Jing* as groups of single and broken lines.

Baguazhang (Ba Kua Zhang) (八卦掌). Means "eight trigram palms." The name of one of the Chinese internal martial styles.

Bai He (白鶴). Means "White Crane." One of the Chinese southern martial styles.

Bai, Yu-feng (白玉峰). A well-known Chinese martial artist during the Song Dynasty (Southern and Northern A.D. 960-1278). Later, he and his son joined the Shaolin Temple. His monk's name was Qiu Yue Chan Shi.

baihui (Gv-20, 百會). Literally, "hundred meetings." An important acupuncture cavity located on the top of the head. The baihui cavity belongs to the governing vessel.

Batuo (跋陀). An Indian Buddhist monk who came to China to preach Buddhism in A.D. 464.

bei kao (背靠). Using any part of the back to bump someone off balance is called bei kao.

Cai (採). Plucking.

Canton (Guangdong) (廣東). A province in southern China.

ce kao (側靠). To bump someone off balance from the side.

chan (ren) (禪) (忍). A Chinese school of Mahayana Buddhism, which asserts that enlightenment can be attained through meditation, self-contemplation and intuition, rather than through study of scripture. Chan is called ren in Japanese.

chan (纏). To wrap or to coil. A common Chinese martial arts technique.

Chen, Wilson (陳威伸). Dr. Yang, Jwing-Ming's friend.

Cheng, Gin-gsao (曾金灶). Dr. Yang, Jwing-Ming's White Crane master.

chi (qi) (氣). The energy pervading the universe, including the energy circulating in the human body.

chi kung (qigong) (氣功). The gongfu of qi, which means the study of qi.

chin na (qin na) (擒拿). Literally means "grab control." A component of Chinese martial arts, which emphasizes grabbing techniques, to control your opponent's joints, in conjunction with attacking certain acupuncture cavities.

chong mai (衝脈). Thrusting vessel. One of the eight extraordinary qi vessels

Confucius (孔子). A Chinese scholar, during the period of 551-479 B.C., whose philosophy has significantly influenced Chinese culture.

Da Mo (達摩). The Indian Buddhist monk who is credited with creating the *Yi Jin Jing* and *Xi Sui Jing* while at the Shaolin monastery. His last name was Sardili and he was also known as Bodhidarma. He was once the prince of a small tribe in southern India.

da zhou tian (大周天). Literally, "grand cycle heaven." Usually translated grand circulation. After a nei dan qigong practitioner completes small circulation, he will circulate his qi through the entire body or exchange the qi with nature.

da (打). To strike. Normally, to attack with the palms, fists or arms.

dan tian qi (丹田氣). Usually, the qi which is converted from original essence and is stored in the lower dan tian. This qi is considered "water qi" and is able to calm down the body. Also called xian tian qi (pre-heaven qi).

dan tian (丹田). "Elixir field." Located in the lower abdomen. It is considered the place which can store qi energy.

Dao De Jing (道德經). *Morality Classic*. Written by Lao Zi.

Dao Jia (道家). The Dao family. Daoism. Created by Lao Zi during the Zhou dynasty (1122-934 B.C.). In the Han dynasty (c. A.D. 58), it was mixed with Buddhism to become the Daoist religion (Dao Jiao).

Dao (道). The "way," by implication is the "natural way."

Deng Feng Xian Zhi (登封縣志). Deng Feng County Recording. A formal historical recording in Deng Feng County, Henan, where the Shaolin Temple is located.

deng shan bu (蹬山步). Means "mountain climbing stance." One of the eight basic fundamental stances.

di li shi (地理師). Di li means "geomancy" and shi means "teacher." Therefore, di li shi is a teacher or master who analyzes geographic locations according to the formulas in the *Yi Jing* (*Book of Changes*) and the energy distributions in the earth. Also called feng shui shi.

di (地). The earth. Earth, heaven (tian), and man (ren) are the "three natural powers" (san cai).

dian mai (dim mak) (點脈). Mai means "the blood vessel" (xue mai) or "the qi channel" (qi mai). Dian mai means "to press the blood vessel or qi channel."

dian qi (電氣). Dian means "electricity" and so dian qi means "electrical energy" (electricity). In China, a word is often placed before "qi" to identify the different kinds of energy.

dian xue massages (點穴按摩). One of Chinese massage techniques in which the acupuncture cavities are stimulated through pressing. Dian xue massage is also called acupressure and is the root of Japanese *shiatsu*.

dian xue (點穴). Dian means "to point and exert pressure" and xue means "the cavities." Dian xue refers to those qin na techniques, which specialize in attacking acupuncture cavities to immobilize or kill an opponent.

dian (點). To point or to press.

dim mak (dian mai) (點脈). Cantonese of "dian mai."

du mai (督脈). Usually translated "governing vessel." One of the eight extraordinary vessels.

Emei Da Peng Gong (峨嵋大鵬功). Da peng means "roc," a lengendary bird in ancient China. Emei Da Peng Gong is a qigong style developed under this name.

Emei (峨嵋). Name of a mountain in Sichuan Province, China.

fa jin (發勁). Emitting jin. Jin is a martial power in which muscular power is manifested to its maximum from mental concentration and qi circulation.

fan fu hu xi (反腹呼吸). Reverse abdominal breathing. Also commonly called "Daoist breathing."

fan tong hu xi (返童呼吸). Back to childhood breathing. A breathing training in nei dan qigong through which the practitioner tries to regain control of the muscles in the lower abdomen. Also called "abdominal breathing."

feng shui shi (風水師). Literally, "wind water teacher." Teacher or master of geomancy. Geomancy is the art or science of analyzing the natural energy relationships in a location, especially the interrelationships between "wind" and "water," hence the name. Also called di li shi.

feng (封). To seal or to cover.

fu hu bu (伏虎步). Means "tame the tiger stance." One of the eight basic fundamental stances.

fu shi hu xi (腹式呼吸). Literally, "abdominal way of breathing." As you breathe, you use the muscles in the lower abdominal area to control the diaphragm. It is also called "back to (the) childhood breathing."

Fu Xi (伏羲). A legendary Chinese ruler (c. 2852-2738 B.C.) who is credited with the introduction of farming, fishing, and animal husbandry. Fu Xi is also credited as the creator of taiji and bagua theory.

fu (夫). Fu has many meanings by itself. When it is placed together with gong, such as in "gongfu," it means any effort that requires patience and time to accomplish.

Fujian Province (福建). A province located in southeast China.

gong (kung) (功). Energy or hard work.

gong jian bu (弓箭步). Means "bow-arrow stance," one of the eight basic fundamental stances in Northern Chinese martial arts.

gongfu (kung fu) (功夫). Means "energy-time." Anything that will take time and energy to learn or to accomplish is called gongfu.

gu shen (固神). Valley spirit. The shen (spirit) that resides at the space, or valley, between the two hemispheres of the brain.

gu (固). To coalesce and to firm.

guan xin (觀心). Defined as observing the xin. Paying attention to the activities of the emotional mind.

Guang Cheng-zi (廣成子). An ancient Daoist qigong master.

gui qi (鬼氣). The qi residue of a dead person. It is believed by the Chinese Buddhists and Daoists that this qi residue is a so-called ghost.

guohuen (國魂). Country soul or spirit.

guoshu (國術). Abbreviation of "Zhongguo wushu," which means "Chinese martial techniques."

ha (哈). A qigong sound that is commonly used to lead an over-abundance of qi from inside the body to outside, and therefore reduces over-accumulated qi.

haidi (海底). Means "sea bottom." This is a name given by martial artists to the huiyin cavity (Co-1) in Chinese medicine. Perineum.

Han (漢). A dynasty in Chinese history (206 B.C.-A.D. 221).

Han, Ching-tang (韓慶堂). A well-known Chinese martial artist, especially in Taiwan in the last forty years. Master Han is also Dr. Yang, Jwing-Ming's Long Fist Grand Master.

he (和). Harmony or peace.

hen (哼). A yin qigong sound, which is the opposite of the 'ha' yang sound.

hen (恨). Hate.

Henan (河南省). The province in China where the Shaolin Temple is located.

hou tian fa (后天法 (後天法). Means "post-heaven techniques." An internal qigong style dating from A.D. 550.

Hsing Yi Chuan (Xingyiquan) (形意拳). A style of internal Chinese martial arts.

hua quan (化拳). Means "neutralizing style." Taijiquan is also called hua quan because it specializes in neutralizing the opponent's force into nothing.

Hua Tuo (華佗). A well-known doctor in the Chinese Three Kingdoms Period (A.D. 221-265).

hua (化). To neutralize.

huan (緩). Slow.

Huang Ting Ching (黃庭經). Means *Yellow Yard Classic*, the name of an ancient qigong book.

Hubei Province (湖北). A province in China.

huo qi (活氣). Vital qi. Also means the qi circulating in a living person.

huo (火). Fire. One of the five elements.

ji (擠). Means "to squeeze" or "to press."

jia dan tian (假丹田). False dan tian. Daoists believe that the lower dan tian located on the front side of the abdomen is not the real dan tian. The real dan tian corresponds to the physical center of gravity. The false dan tian is called qihai (qi ocean) in Chinese medicine.

jian kao (肩靠). Shoulder bump. Refers to the use of the shoulder to bump someone off balance.

jin (jing) (勁). Chinese martial power. A combination of "li" (muscular power) and "qi."

jin gong (勁功). Gongfu which specializes in the training of jin manifestation.

Jin Zhong Zhao (金鐘罩). Literally, "golden bell cover." A higher level of iron shirt training.

jin (金). Metal. One of the five elements.

Jin, Shao-feng (金紹峰). Dr. Yang, Jwing-Ming's White Crane grand master.

jing (jin) (勁). Chinese martial power. A combination of "li" (muscular power) and "qi."

jing (精). Essence. The most refined part of anything.

jing (靜). Calm.

jing-shen (精神). Literally, "essential spirit." The meaning is the spirit of vitality.

Jueyuan (覺遠). The monk name of a Shaolin priest during the Chinese Song dynasty (A.D. 960-1278).

Jun Qing (君倩). A Daoist and Chinese doctor during the Chinese Jin dynasty (A.D. 265-420). Jun Qing is credited as the creator of the Five Animal Sports Qigong set.

kan (坎). One of the eight trigrams.

Kao Tao (高濤). Master Yang, Jwing-Ming's first taijiquan master.

kao (靠). Means "bump." One of the taijiquan thirteen postures.

King Wen of Zhou (周文王). King Wen of Zhou. He was six feet tall, and it was he who interpreted the *Book of Changes* (*Yi Jing*).

kong qi (空氣). Air.

kung (gong) (功). Means "energy" or "hard work."

kung fu (gongfu) (功夫). Means "energy-time." Anything that will take time and energy to learn or to accomplish is called kung fu.

Lan Zhou (蘭州). Name of a county in ancient times. Exact location unknown to the author.

Lao Zi (老子). The creator of Daoism, also called Li Er.

laogong (P-8, 勞宮). Cavity name. On the pericardium channel in the center of the palm.

le (樂). Joy or happiness.

Li Er (李耳). Nickname of Lao Zi.

li (力). The power that is generated from muscular strength.

li (離). One of the eight trigrams.

Li, Mao-ching (李茂清). Dr. Yang, Jwing-Ming's Long Fist master.

Li, Qing-an (李清庵). An ancient Chinese qigong master.

Li, Shi-ming (李世民). The first Tang emperor.

lian qi (練氣). Lian means "to train, to strengthen, and to refine." A Daoist training process through which your qi grows stronger and more abundant.

Liang Wu (梁武). An emperor of the Chinese Liang dynasty.

Liang (梁). A dynasty in Chinese history (A.D. 502-557).

li-qi (力氣). When you use li (muscular power) you also need qi to support it. However, when this qi is led by a concentrated mind, the qi is able to manifest the muscular power to a higher level and is therefore called jin. Li-qi (or qi-li) is a general definition of jin and commonly implies manifested power.

liuhebafa (六合八法). Literally, "six combinations eight methods." One of the Chinese internal martial arts, its techniques are combined from taijiquan, xingyi, and baguazhang

luo (絡). The small qi channels that branch out from the primary qi channels and are connected to the skin and to the bone marrow.

ma bu (馬步). Horse stance. One of the basic stances in Chinese martial arts.

mai (脉). Means "vessel" or "qi channel."

Mencius (孟子). A well-known scholar (372-289 B.C.) who followed the philosophy of Confucius during the Chinese Zhou dynasty (909-255 B.C.).

mian quan (綿拳). Means soft style. Taijiquan is also called mian quan because it is soft and relaxed.

mian (綿). Soft.

mingmen (Gv-4, 命門). Cavity located on the back between L2 and L3 vertebrae. One of two cavities connected to the real dan tian.

mu zi xiang he (母子相合). Mutual harmony of mother and son. Shen training key used in regulating the spirit.

mu (木). Wood. One of the five elements.

na (拿). Means "to hold" or "to grab." Also an abbreviation for chin na or qin na.

Nanking Central Guoshu Institute (南京中央國術館). A national martial arts institute organized by the Chinese government in 1926.

nei dan (內丹). Literally, internal elixir. A form of qigong in which qi (the elixir) is built up in the body and spread out to the limbs.

nei gong (內功). Internal gongfu. This implies those practices that involve internal qi training.

nei jia (內家). Internal family. Those styles that emphasize internal qi training.

nei shi gongfu (內視功夫). Nei shi means "to look internally," so nei shi gongfu refers to the art of looking inside yourself to read the state of your health and the condition of your qi.

ni fu hu xi (逆腹呼吸). Reverse abdominal breathing. Also called fan fu hu xi or Daoist breathing. Commonly practiced in Chinese martial arts and Daoist qigong.

ni wan (泥丸). Daoist term meaning "mud pill." Namely, the brain, or upper dan tian.

ning (凝). To concentrate, condense, refine, focus, and strengthen.

nu (怒). Anger

pin (牝). Refers to female animals and means mothers. When combined with the word xuan(玄), meaning original, the word refers to the origin, or root of our lives.

ping (平). Peace and harmony.

Putian (浦田). Name of a county in China's Fujian Province.

qi (chi) (氣). Chinese term for universal energy. A current popular model is that the qi circulating in the human body is bioelectric in nature.

Qi Hua Lun (氣化論). *Qi Variation Thesis.* An ancient treatise that discusses the variations of qi in the universe.

qi huo (起火). To start the fire. In qigong practice, when you start to build up qi at the lower dan tian.

qi qing liu yu (七情六欲). Seven emotions and six desires. The seven emotions are happiness, anger, sorrow, joy, love, hate, and desire. The six desires are the six sensory pleasures associated with the eyes, nose, ears, tongue, body, and mind.

qi shi (氣勢). Shi means the way something looks or feels. Therefore, the feeling of qi as it expresses itself.

qigong (chi kung) (氣功). The gongfu of qi, which means "the study of qi."

qihai (Co-6, 氣海). Means "qi ocean." An acupuncture cavity belonging to the conception vessel.

qin (chin) (擒). Means "to catch" or "to seize."

qin na (chin na) (擒拿). Literally means "grab control." A component of Chinese martial arts that emphasizes grabbing techniques to control your opponent's joints, in conjunction with attacking certain acupuncture cavities.

Qing dynasty (清朝). A dynasty in Chinese history; The last Chinese dynasty (A.D. 1644-1912).

Qiu Yue Chan Shi (秋月禪師). A Shaolin monk during the Chinese Song dynasty (A.D. 960-1278). His layman name was Bai, Yu-feng.

re qi (熱氣). Re means "warmth or heat." Generally, re qi is used to represent heat. It is used sometimes to imply that a person or animal is still alive since the body is warm.

ren (chan) (忍). Means "to endure." A Chan Buddhist meditation passed down by Da Mo.

ren mai (任脈). Conception vessel. One of the eight extraordinary vessels.

ren qi (人氣). Human qi.

ren shi (人事). Literally, human relations. Human events, activities, and relationships.

ren (人). Man or mankind.

ren (仁). Humanity, kindness or benevolence.

ru jia (儒家). Literally, "Confucian family." Scholars following Confucian thoughts; Confucianists.

san bao (三寶). Three treasures: essence (jing), energy (qi), and spirit (shen). Also called "san yuan" (three origins).

san cai shi (三才勢). Three power posture. A standing meditation posture in taijiquan practice.

san cai (三才). Three powers: heaven, earth, and man.

san gong (散功). Literally, "energy dispersion." A state of premature degeneration of the muscles where the qi cannot effectively energize them. It can be caused by earlier overtraining.

san yuan (三元). Three origins. Also called "san bao" (three treasures). Human essence (jing), energy (qi), and spirit (shen).

Sardili (沙地利). The last name of Da Mo. Also known as Bodhidarma.

seng bing (僧兵). Monk soldiers. The monks who also trained martial arts to protect the property of the temple.

shang dan tian (上丹田). Upper dan tian. Located at the third eye, it is the residence of the shen (spirit).

Shao Yuan (邵元和尚). A Japanese Buddhist monk who went to Shaolin Temple in A.D. 1335.

Shaolin Temple (少林寺). A monastery located in Henan Province, China. The Shaolin Temple is well known because of its martial arts training.

shaolin (少林). "Young woods." Name of the Shaolin Temple.

shen qi xiang he (神氣相合). Mutual harmony of shen and qi. Training key of regulating the shen where one uses the spirit (shen 神) to direct the circulation and distribution of qi.

shen xi (神息). Spirit breathing. Spirit and breathing match each other.

shen (深). Deep.

shen (神). Spirit. According to Chinese qigong, the shen resides at the upper dan tian (the third eye).

shi er jing (十二經). The twelve primary qi channels in Chinese medicine.

shi er zhuang (十二庄). Twelve postures. The name of a qigong training style.

Shi Xiang Zu (師襄子). Name of Confucius' music teacher.

Shi, You-san (石友三). A military warlord during the Chinese civil war in the 1920s. He was known as the one who burned the Shaolin Temple in 1928.

shou shen (守神). Training that uses the regulated mind to direct, nurse, and keep the spirit in its residence.

shou (守). To keep and protect

shui (水). Water. One of the five elements

shun fu hu xi (順腹呼吸). Smooth abdominal breathing. Also called "normal abdominal breathing." Also called "Buddhist breathing."

si ji gong (四季功). Four seasons gong. A type of qigong practice which helps make the body's seasonal qi transition more smooth.

si liu bu (四六步). Four-six stance. One of the eight basic fundamental stances.

si qi (死氣). Dead qi. The qi remaining in a dead body. Sometimes called "ghost qi" (gui qi).

si xin hu xi (四心呼吸). A qigong nei dan practice in which a practitioner uses his mind with the coordination of the breathing to lead the qi to the centers of the palms and feet.

Song (宋). A dynasty in Chinese history (A.D. 960-1278).

Southern Song dynasty (南宋). After the Song was conquered by the Jin race from Mongolia, the Song people moved to the south and established another country, called Southern Song (A.D. 1127-1278).

suan ming shi (算命師). Literally, "calculate life teacher." A fortune teller who is able to calculate your future and destiny.

Sui dynasty (隋). A dynasty in China during the period A.D. 589-618.

sui qi (髓氣). "Marrow qi". The qi circulating in the bone marrow.

Sun, Lu-tang (孫祿堂). Well-known martial artist (1861-1932) in the early 1920s. He mastered many styles, such as baguazhang, xingyiquan, and taijiquan. He is also the creator of Sun Style Taijiquan.

Sun, Yat-sen (孫中山). Father of China.

Tai Chi Chuan (Taijiquan) (太極拳). A Chinese internal martial style that is based on the theory of taiji (grand ultimate).

Tai Xi (胎息). Embryo Breathing. One of the final goals in regulating the breath, Embryo Breathing enables you to generate a "baby shen" at the huang ting (yellow yard).

taiji qigong (太極氣功). A qigong training specially designed for taijiquan practice.

taiji (太極). Means "grand ultimate." It is this force that generates two poles, yin and yang.

Taijiquan (Tai Chi Chuan) (太極拳). A Chinese internal martial style that is based on the theory of taiji (grand ultimate).

Taipei (台北). The capital city of Taiwan located in the north.

Taiwan University (台灣大學). A well-known university located in northern Taiwan.

Taiwan (台灣). An island to the southeast of mainland China. Also known as "Formosa."

Taizuquan (太祖拳). A style of Chinese external martial arts.

Tamkang College Guoshu Club (淡江國術社). A Chinese martial arts club founded by Dr. Yang when he was studying in Tamkang College.

Tamkang (淡江). Name of a university in Taiwan.

Tang dynasty (唐). A dynasty in Chinese history during the period A.D. 713-907.

tang (趟). A martial sequence. Normally, a sequence is constructed from many techniques and becomes a routine practice form. Also commonly called "taolu."

taolu (套路). A martial sequence. Normally, a sequence is constructed from many techniques and becomes a routine practice form. Also commonly called "tang."

ti sui xi (体髓息). Skin marrow breathing.

ti xi (体息). Body breathing or skin breathing. In qigong, the exchanging of qi with the surrounding environment, through the skin.

Tian Mountain (天山). Literally, "sky mountain." The name of a mountain located in Xinjiang Province, China.

tian mu (天目). Heavenly eye. Called the third eye by Western society. The Chinese believe that prior to our evolution into humans, our race possessed an additional sense organ in our forehead. This third eye provided a means of spiritual communication between one another and with the natural world. As we evolved and developed means to protect ourselves from the environment, and as societies became more complex and human vices developed, this third eye gradually closed and disappeared.

tian qi (天氣). Heaven qi. It is now commonly used to mean the weather, since weather is governed by heaven qi.

tian ren he yi (天人合一). Literally, "heaven and man unified as one." A high level of qigong practice in which a qigong practitioner, through meditation, is able to communicate his qi with heaven's qi.

tian shi (天時). Heavenly timing. The repeated natural cycles generated by the heavens, such as seasons, months, days, and hours.

tian (天). Heaven or sky. In ancient China, people believed that heaven was the most powerful natural energy in this universe.

tianron (SI-17, 天容). An acupuncture cavity belonging to the small intestine primary qi channel.

tiantu (Co-22, 天突). Heaven's prominence. Acupuncture cavity located on conception vessel in the front of body. Controls vocal cords and generates "hen" and "ha" sounds for manifestation of qi.

tiao qi (調氣). To regulate the qi.

tiao shen (調神). To regulate the spirit.

tiao shen (調身). To regulate the body.

tiao xi (調息). To regulate the breathing.

tiao xin (調心). To regulate the emotional mind.

tu (土). Earth. One of the five elements.

tui bu (退步). Means "step backward." One of the taijiquan thirteen postures. Taijiquan is constructed from eight basic moving patterns (eight doors) and five strategic steppings (five steppings). Tui bu is one of the five steppings.

tui na (推拿). Means "to push and grab." A category of Chinese massages for healing and for injury treatment.

tuo tian shi (托天勢). Holding up the heaven posture. A common qigong posture that is used to stretch the torso and raise up the spirit of vitality

wa shou (瓦手). Tile hand. The hand form of taijiquan is also called tile hand because it resembles the shape of a Chinese roof tile.

wai dan chi kung (wai dan qigong) (外丹氣功). External elixir qigong. In wai dan qigong, a practitioner will generate qi to the limbs and then allow the qi to flow inward to nourish the internal organs.

wai dan (外丹). External elixir. External qigong exercises in which a practitioner will build up the qi in his limbs and then lead it into the center of the body for nourishment.

wai jia (外家). External family. Those martial schools that practice the external styles of Chinese martial arts.

wai jin (外勁). External power. The type of jin where the muscles predominate and only local qi is used to support the muscles.

Wang, Zong-yue (王宗岳). A well-known taijiquan master in the 1920s.

wei qi (衛氣). Protective qi or guardian qi. The qi at the surface of the body that generates a shield to protect the body from negative external influences, such as colds.

Wen Wang Cao (文王操). A piece of music composed by King Wen of Zhou.

wu bu (五步). Five steppings. Taijiquan is constructed from eight basic moving patterns and five steppings.

Wu Qin Shi (五禽戲). Five Animal Sports. A set of medical qigong practice created by Jun Qing during Chinese Jin dynasty (A.D. 265-420).

wu tiao (五調). Five regulations. This includes regulating the body, breathing, mind, qi, and spirit.

wu xin hu xi (五心呼吸). One of the qigong nei dan practices in which a practitioner uses his mind in coordination with breathing to lead the qi to the center of the palms, feet, and head.

wu xin (五心). Five centers. The face, the laogong cavities in both palms, and the yongquan cavities on the bottoms of both feet.

Wu Zhen Ren (伍真人). An ancient Daoist qigong master.

wu (武). Means "martial."

Wu, Jian-quan (吳鑒泉). A famous taijiquan master (1870-1942) in the 1930s. He is credited as the creator of Wu Style Taijiquan.

Wudang Mountain (武當山). A mountain located in Fubei Province in China.

wuji qigong (無極氣功). A style of taiji qigong practice.

wuji (無極). Means "no extremity."

wushu (武術). Literally, "martial techniques."

wuxing (五行). Five elements

wuyi (武藝). Literally, "martial arts."

xi kao (膝靠). Means "knee bump." To use the knee to bump someone off balance.

xi sui gong (洗髓功). Gongfu for marrow and brain washing qigong practice.

Xi Sui Jing (洗髓經). Literally, *Washing Marrow/Brain Classic*, usually translated *Marrow/Brain Washing Classic*. A qigong training that specializes in leading qi to the marrow to cleanse it or to the brain to nourish the spirit for enlightenment.

xi (喜). Joy, delight, and happiness.

xi (細). Slender.

xia dan tian (下丹田). Lower dan tian. Located in the lower abdomen, it is believed to be the residence of water qi (original qi).

xian jin (顯勁). The jins which are manifested externally and can be seen.

xian tian qi (先天氣). Pre-birth qi or pre-heaven qi. Also called dan tian qi. The qi that is converted from original essence and is stored in the lower tian. Considered to be "water qi," it is able to calm the body.

Xiao Jiu Tian (小九天). Small Nine Heaven. A qigong style created around A.D. 550.

xiao zhou tian (小周天). Literally, "small heavenly cycle." Also called "small circulation." In qigong, when you can use your mind to lead qi through the conception and governing vessels, you have completed "xiao zhou tian."

xiao (孝). Filial piety.

xin (信). Trust.

xin (心). Means "heart." Xin means "the mind generated from emotional disturbance."

xingyi (形意). An abbreviation of xingyiquan.

Xingyiquan (Hsing Yi Chuan) (形意拳). One of the best-known Chinese internal martial styles created by Marshal Yue Fei during the Chinese Song dynasty (A.D. 1103-1142).

Xinjiang Province (新疆). A Chinese province located in western China.

Xinzhu Xian (新竹縣). Birthplace of Dr. Yang, Jwing-Ming in Taiwan.

xiu qi (修氣). Cultivate the qi. Cultivate implies to protect, maintain, and refine. A Buddhist qigong training.

xu bu (虛步). Means "false stance." One of the eight basic fundamental stances. Also called xuan ji bu.

xu mi (須彌). Daoist term for the spiritual being in the fullness of human virtue.

xu wu (虛無). Nothingness.

xuan ji bu (玄機步). Tricky stance. One of the eight basic fundamental stances. Also called xu bu.

yan (言). Talking or speaking.

yang shou (陽手). Yang hand. Any time the palm is facing outward in taijiquan.

yang (陽). Too sufficient. One of the two poles. The other is yin.

Yang, Jwing-Ming (楊俊敏). Author of this book.

Yang, You-ji (養由基). A famous archer during the Chinese Spring and Autumn period (722-481 B.C.).

Yi Jin Jing (易筋經). Literally, *Changing Muscle/Tendon Classic*, usually called the *Muscle/Tendon Changing Classic*. Credited to Da Mo around A.D. 550, this book discusses wai dan qigong training for strengthening the physical body.

Yi Jing (易經). *Book of Changes*. A book of divination written during the Zhou dynasty (1122-255 B.C.).

yi shou dan tian (意守丹田). Keep your yi on your lower dan tian. Keeping your mind at the lower dan tian in order to build up qi.

yi yi yin qi (以意引氣). Use your yi (wisdom mind) to lead your qi. A qigong technique. Yi cannot be pushed, but it can be led. This is best done with the yi.

yi (意). Wisdom mind. The mind generated from wise judgment.

yi (義). Justice or righteousness.

yin shou (陰手). Yin hand. Any time the palm is facing inward in taijiquan. Also implied are the techniques that are hidden and not obvious to the opponent.

yin shui (陰水). Yin water. Qi stored in the real dan tian.

yin (陰). Deficient. One of the two poles. The other is yang.

ying bian (硬鞭). A hard whip, usually made from a hard wood.

ying gong (硬功). Hard gongfu. Any Chinese martial training that emphasizes physical strength and power.

yinjiao (Co-7, 陰交). Yin junction. The junction of two vessels, conception vessel and thrusting vessel. Yinjiao is on the conception vessel on the front of the body in the proximity of the dan tian. It is paired with the mingmen cavity (Gv-4, 命門).

yintang (m-hn-3, 印堂). Seal hall. Recognized by medical society as an acupuncture cavity located in the proximity of the third eye.

yongquan (K-1, 湧泉). Bubbling well. Name of an acupuncture cavity belonging to the kidney primary qi channel.

you (悠). Long, far, meditative, continuous, slow and soft.

yu men (玉門). Known by religious societies as the "jade gate". Location of spiritual residence.

yu (欲). Desire.

Yuan dynasty (元代). A Chinese dynasty during the period A.D. 1206-1368.

yuan jing (元精). Original essence. The fundamental, original substance inherited from your parents, it is converted into original qi.

yuan qi (元氣). Original qi. The qi created from the original essence inherited from your parents.

Yue Fei 岳飛). A Chinese hero in the Southern Song dynasty (A.D. 1127-1279). Said to have created Ba Duan Jin, Xingyiquan, and Yue's Ying Zhua.

yun (勻). Uniform or even.

Zhang Dao-ling (張道陵). A Daoist who combined scholarly Daoism with Buddhist philosophies and created religious Daoism (Dao Jiao) during the Chinese Eastern Han dynasty (A.D. 25-221).

Zhang, Xiang-san (張詳三). A well known Chinese martial artist in Taiwan.

zhen dan tian (真丹田). The real dan tian, which is located at the physical center of gravity.

zheng fu hu xi (正腹呼吸). Normal abdominal breathing. Also called shun fu hu xi, which means "smooth abdominal breathing."

zheng hu xi (正呼吸). Formal breathing. More commonly called Buddhist breathing.

zheng qi (正氣). Righteous qi. When a person is righteous, it is said that he has righteous qi, which evil qi cannot overcome.

zhi guan (止觀). Buddhist term meaning stop observation, which implies stopping the observation of the activities of the xin. One of the methods of cultivating the mind to reach ultimate goodness.

zhi (止). Stop.

zhong dan tian (中丹田). Middle dan tian. Located in the area of the solar plexus, it is the residence of fire qi.

zhong ding (中定). "Firm the center." One of the taijiquan thirteen postures.

Zhong Guo wushu (中國武術). Chinese wushu.

Zhong Guo (中國). Literally, "central country." This name was given by the neighboring countries of China. China was considered the cultural and spiritual center from the point of view of the Asian countries in ancient times.

zhong (忠). Loyalty.

zhou (周). Roundness or completeness.

zhou (肘). Means "elbow." To use the elbow to execute defensive or offensive techniques in taijiquan.

Zhuang Zhou (莊周). A contemporary of Mencius who advocated Daoism.

Zhuang Zi (莊子). Zhuang Zhou. A contemporary of Mencius who advocated Daoism. Zhuang Zi also means the works of Zhuang Zhou.

zuo dun (坐蹲). Means "squat stance." One of the eight fundamental stances in Northern Chinese martial arts training.

zuo pan bu (坐盤步). Literally, "sitting on crossed legs stance." One of the eight basic fundamental stances in Northern Chinese martial arts training.

zuowan (坐腕). Called "settling the wrist." When taijiquan uses the palm to strike, right before contact the wrist is settled to firm the posture and alignment of the palm.

Tai Chi Ball Qigong DVD 1 & 2

This appendix offers a simple navigation guide to using the companion DVDs and this book. Using this book and the two DVDs for learning is an excellent way to deepen your knowledge and improve your skills. The columns below: **Techniques (DVD Edition)** are the chapters names found on the DVDs. **This Book Section** identifies the location in this book for the DVD techniques. **Book Pages** refer to the pages in this book.

Tai Chi Ball Qigong 1 DVD contains courses 1 and 2.
Tai Chi Ball Qigong 2 DVD contains courses 3 and 4.

Techniques (DVD Edition)	This Book Section	Book Page(s)
About Taiji Balls	5.1–5.2	97–101
Understanding TJB Qigong	3.1	57
Internal Foundation	5.4	119-120
–Wuji Breathing		121
–Youngquan Breathing		122
–Laogong Breathing		123
–Four Gates Breathing		123
–TJ Grand Circulation Breathing		124
–TJ Ball Breathing		125
Part II		
Taiji Ball Qigong Circle Practice	5.2	
–Internal Skin/Bone Marrow		102
–External (with the ball)		103
–Unification of Internal & External		104
Disc One Course 1		
Vertical Circling–Forward (Yang)	5.6	128–129
–Stationary		130–133
–Rocking		134–135
–Walking (Straight Line Stepping—Book)		136–138
–Bagua Circle		139–140

Techniques (DVD Edition)	This Book Section	Book Page(s)
Vertical Circling–Backward (Yin)	5.6	
–Stationary		141–142
–Rocking		143–144
–Walking		145–146
–Bagua Circle		147
Horizontal Circle—Clockwise (Yang)	5.6	
–Stationary		154–155
–Rocking		155–156
–Walking		156–159
–Bagua Circle		160–161
Horizontal Circle—Counterclockwise (Yin)	5.6	
–Stationary		162
–Rocking		162–164
–Walking		164
–Bagua Circle		164
Disc One Course 2		
Vertical Rotation—Forward (Yang)	5.6	
–Stationary		172–174
–Rocking		174–175
–Walking		175–178
–Bagua Circle		179–180
Vertical Rotation—Backward (Yin)	5.6	
–Stationary		181–182
–Rocking		182–183
–Walking		184
–Bagua Circle		184
Horizontal Rotation—Clockwise (Yang)	5.6	
–Stationary		188–190
–Rocking		190–191
–Walking		192–193
–Bagua Circle		194
Horizontal Rotation—Counterclockwise (Yin)		
–Stationary	5.6	194
–Rocking		194–195
–Walking		196
–Bagua Circle		196
Disc Two Course 3		
Wrap Coiling	5.6	204–205
Vertical Wrap Coiling—Forward (Yang)	5.6	
–Stationary		206-207

Techniques (DVD Edition)	**This Book Section**	**Book Page(s)**
–Rocking		208
–Walking		208-210
–Bagua Circle		210-211
Vertical Wrap Coiling—Backward (Yin)	5.6	
–Stationary		211-212
–Rocking		212
–Walking		213
–Bagua Circle		213
Horizontal Wrap Coiling—Clockwise (Yang)	5.6	
–Stationary		217-218
–Rocking		219
–Walking		219
–Bagua Circle		219
Horizontal Wrap Coiling—Counterclockwise (Yin)	5.6	
–Stationary		220
–Rocking		220
–Walking		220
–Bagua Circle		221
Disc Two Course 4		
Self Practice		
–Yin Yang exchange 1 (vert./horiz.)	5.6	147–153, 164–172
2 (rotating)		185-188, 196–203
3 (wrap coiling)		213–217, 221–225
–Changing Directions (return the ball)	6.2	228–229
Attaching to the Ball 1 (pick it up)		231–233
2 (forward/back)		234–235
–Rotating		235–236
–Wrap-Coiling (Rolling)		236
–Adhere/Connecting		236
Flying Dragon Plays with the Ball	6.2	237
Along the Edge Practice	6.2	237
–Right Angle		237
–Disk		(not in book)
–Point		238
–Wall		239–243
Practice with a Partner	6.3	
–Straight		243–255
–Rotate		256–261
–Capture		264–265

Index

abdomen
    massaging 41
abdominal breathing 83
    exercises 120
    producing qi 41
abdominal muscles 29, 84, 116
abundant qi 63, 76
adhering jin 227, 239
adhering to the ball 228
aging 14, 22, 27, 28, 60
alertness 93
along the wall horizontal 239
arthritis 14
attaching jin 227
attaching to the ball 231
awakening 52
awareness 93
Ba Duan Jin 10
bagua stepping 139, 172
    horizontal circling 160
    horizontal rotation 194
    vertical-horizontal, yin-yang, circling-rotating mixed training 203
    vertical-horizontal, yin-yang, circling-rotating-wrap-coiling mixed training 225
    vertical-horizontal yin-yang exchange circling 172
    vertical-horizontal, yin-yang exchange rotating 200
    vertical-horizontal, yin-yang exchange wrap-coiling 223
    yang vertical rotation 179
    yang wrap-coiling 210, 219
    yin circling 147
    yin horizontal circling 164
    yin rotation 196
    yin vertical rotation 184
    yin wrap-coiling 213, 221
    yin-yang exchange 153, 188
    yin-yang exchange circling 168

yin-yang exchange horizon tal rotating 198
yin-yang exchange wrap-coiling 217
baihui 78, 87, 89
baihui breathing 88
balance stepping 138, 200, 210
ball tossing 267
Bao-Xi 66
ba shi 125
bio-battery 34, 43, 45, 79, 82
bioelectricity 2, 15
Bodhidarma 59, 84
body
    excess yang 14
    ligament, muscle, and tendon conditioning 76
    regulating 26, 104
    relaxed 27
body breathing 29, 34
body structure 62
bone 75
bone density 75, 104
bone marrow
    qi entry 75
bow and arrow stance 126
bows 114
brain
    control of body 21
    leading qi to 5, 12, 40
    limbic system 37
    lower dan tian 21
    xin and yi 37
Brain/Marrow Washing Qigong 75
brains
    two in humans 80
    upper and lower 22
breathing
    adjusting kan and li 17
    coordinating actions 63
    embryonic 32, 43

four gates 88, 123
harmonizing body and mind 38
harmonizing the mind 39
increasing qi 82
kan and li 15
kan-li method 27
laogong 123
martial grand circulation 124
methods 29
normal 29
normal abdominal 29
pre-heaven 41
purpose of regulating 27
regulating 27, 41, 104
regulating and 27
regulating exercises 119
reverse abdominal 30
shen and 50
skin 34
spiritual 88
taiji ball 125
techniques in taiji ball training 60
wuji 121
yongquan 122
brick training 266
Buddhahood 52, 85
    observations 52
    qi circulation 40
    religious qigong 11
bumping 264
calmness 52, 78
calm shen 17
capturing the ball from a partner 264
cavities
    four gates 88
    leading qi to 45
    pointing 12
cell replacement 27
central energy 89

channels
    qi channels 22
    qigong and 5
Cheng, Bi 59
Cheng, Ling-xi 59
chest
    thrusting and arcing the 118
chest breathing 29
Chinese medical qigong 14
circling
    horizontal 154
    partner practice 245
    yang 130
    yin 141
    yin-yang exchange 147
circling on a point 238
circling pattern 129
circling the waist 116
coiling 69
concealed qi 43
conditioning
    Taiji Ball Qigong 62
    taiji ball training 63
Confucius 10
connecting jin 239
conscious mind 52
cultivating qi 11, 42, 43
Da Mo 12, 17, 19, 59, 84, 85
dancing 6
dan tian
    keeping mind in 44
Dao
    achieving true 54
    human qi 4
    taiji and 67
Dao De Jing 10, 44, 46, 67
Daoism 10
Daoist breathing 30, 39
Dao-Yin 4
dead qi 2
deep feeling 94
desires 11, 53
dian mai 12
dian xue 12
ding shen 49

double-hands
    vertical yin-yang circling partner practice 245
dual cultivation 43
earth power 1
earth qi 1, 3
Eight Pieces of Brocade 10
eight reservoirs 5
eight stances 125
eight trigrams 66, 67, 139
    kan and li 13
    Yi Jing and 3
eight vessels 5, 9
    qi accumulation 22
electromagnetic energy 2
electromotive force (EMF) 22, 81
elixir
    external 7
    internal 8
    nei dan 8
    wai dan 7
elixir field 5
elixir qi 21
embracing singularity 77
Embryonic Breathing 27, 121
    self-awakening 52
embryonic state 54
emotional bondage 22, 51
emotional mind 14, 15, 37, 87
    regulating 36, 39, 42
    regulating benefits 38
emotional mud 51, 52
emptiness 52
endurance 59
    improving 63
energy 1, 71
    as qi 2, 4
    electromagnetic 2
    ha sound 30
    vital 34
energy center 21
energy dispersion 13
energy field 1
energy patterns 69
energy state 2

energy status 40
enlightenment 23
    cultivating spiritual 51
    observations 52
    qi circulation 40
    regulating shen 50
    religious qigong 11
essence 83
exercises
    breathing 119
    loosening 107
    spinal warm-up 114
    stretching 111
    taiji ball training 128
exhalation 15, 28, 30, 92
    fire activity 15
external elixir 7
external gong 97, 105
external styles 13, 85
fa jin 267
false lower dan tian 29
Faraday, Michael 54
feeling xv, 7, 25, 54, 61, 94, 97, 102, 103
    gong fu of inner vision 44
    of opponent 105
    roundness 58
    self-awareness 51
    training 62
feng shui 3, 43
fire 13, 14
fire mind 16
fire qi 14, 40, 48
Five Animal Sports 4, 9
Five Gates Breathing 34
Five Regulatings 25
flying dragon plays with the ball 237
following jin 227, 228
foods
    producing qi 40
forearms (on the)
    rotating the ball 236
forward-backward attaching 234
Four Gates Breathing 36, 88, 123

four phases 68

four-six stance 127

ghost qi 2

gong 3

gongfu 3

gongfu of inner vision 44

grand cyclic heaven circulation 45

Grand Cyclic Heaven Circulation 45

grand extremity 71

grand qi circulation 36, 61, 86

grand transportation gong 91

grand ultimate 71

gu 49

guan xin 51

guan zhi 51

guardian qi 28, 104

gu shen 49

hands

    holding taiji ball 128

Han, Gong-yue 59

Hao, Tang 60

hard gong 13

hard styles 6

harmonization 15, 62

    body and mind 38

    breathing and mind 39

    mind and body 27

    shen and qi 18, 44

    yi and qi 45

    yin and yang 21

ha sound 30, 87

health 18

    regulating shen 50

heart mind 15

heaven eye 47

heavenly cycle 46

heavenly timing 3

heaven power 1

heaven qi 1

hen sound 30, 87

herbs 82

    producing qi 40

holy embryo 43

horizontal circling 154

horizontal rotation 188

horizontal single-hands rotating
    the ball with a partner 259

horizontal single-hand wrap-coiling with a partner 262

horizontal wrap-coiling 217

hormones 19, 21, 41

horse stance 126

huiyin 78, 84, 87, 89

human emotional matrix 54

human energy 20

human power 1

human qi 1, 4

human qigong 6

human suffering 11

imaginary opponent 90

immune system 34, 85, 103

inhalation 15, 28, 30, 92

    water activity 15

inner feeling xv, 25

intention 37

internal elixir 8

internal gong 97, 104

internal gongfu 119

internal martial qigong 13

internal organs

    Taiji Ball Qigong 76

internal qi 12

internal styles 85

jin 90, 227

    storing and emitting 90

    two-person ball tossing 267

jin manifestation 89, 90, 91, 104

jin skills 227, 243

joints 14, 61, 62, 75, 93

kan 13

    mind and 26

kan-li

    water and fire 13

kong qi 2

Kong Zi 10

laogong 88

laogong breathing 35, 123

Lao Zi 10, 67

leading the qi 45

li 13

lian qi 11

Li, Dao-zi 59

lifestyle

    health and 18

    regulating 41

Li, Shi-zhen 5

listening jin 227

Liu, De-kuan 60

logical mind 23

longevity 20, 44, 61

    breathing 34

    Daoists and 20

    key points 20

    reaching 21

    regulating shen 50

    spiritual cultivation and 22

loosening exercises 107

lotus seed

    original shen 52

lower dan tian 9, 60, 64, 82

    brain 21

    elixir field 5

    storing qi 32

man power 1

marrow 85

Marrow/Brain Washing Classic 59, 85

Marrow/Brain Washing Qigong 82

marrow breathing 32

marrow qi 31, 104

Marshal Yue, Fei 10

Martial Grand Circulation Breathing 124

martial grand qi circulation 86, 87

martial qigong 12

martial styles 12

massage 82

massaging the abdomen 41

material bondage 53

medical qigong 9, 14
medical taiji ball qigong training 57
meditation
    internal 59
    natural energy 43
    scholar qigong 11
meditation 60
meditative mind 38
Mencius 10
Meng Zi 10
mental bondage 53
mental health
    mental healthyin side 18
mental relaxation 26
meridians 91
    regular 5
    strange 5
metabolism 60
mind
    dan tian 44
    emotional 14
    foundation of power 59
    guan zhi 51
    in qigong practice 7
    kan and li 15
    key to practice 97
    qi and regulating the 42
    qi and the 21
    qi circulation and the 40
    regulating 11, 104
    xin and yi described 37
mind training 86
mingmen 87, 91
momentum stepping 151, 156, 158, 192, 198, 203, 219
monkey mind 39
mountain climbing stance 126
mud pill 47
Mud Pill Palace 47, 54, 79
muscles 111, 114
    power and efficiency 12
muscle/tendon change 59, 85
Muscle/Tendon Changing 75

Muscle/Tendon Changing Classic 19, 59, 85
Muscle/Tendon Changing Qigong 82
muscle/tendon changing theory 85
muscular power 227
mutual harmony 50
mu zi xiang he 50
natural energy 43, 76
    nourishing qi 43
natural force 1
natural shen 47
nei dan 8
    internal martial arts 13
nei dan qigong practice 8
nei gong 97
    breathing exercises 119
ning 49
ni wan 47
ni wan gong 47
no-ball practice 102
no extremity 44, 71
normal breathing 29
normal qi 2
nothingness 44
observations 51
Ohm's Law 81
original shen 52
pagoda 47
partner practice 243
    capturing the ball 264
    circling the ball 245
    straight line listening and following 243
    yin-yang circling 245
    yin-yang horizontal circling training 252
passions 11, 53
patterns
    taiji ball training 128
    vertical and horizontal 105
physical body
    conditioning 103

Taiji Ball Qigong and 75
physical health
    yang side 18
physical relaxation 26
piezoelectric material 75
pin 47
pivotal force 71
pointing cavities 12
pointing vessels 12
post-heaven qi 40
post-heaven techniques 59
practice methods
    patterns 105
pre-heaven practice 52
producing qi 40
qi
    as bioelectricity 2
    bone marrow 75, 104
    bone marrow and 21
    breathing and 41
    building for endurance 64
    Chinese characters 2
    connection with yi 44
    cultivating 11, 42
    definition in China 2
    fire 40
    fire and water 14
    foods 40
    general concept 1
    harmonized with shen 17
    in sick person 5
    keeping mind in dan tian 44
    leading 7, 13, 45, 64
    methods of producing 40
    mind and 21
    mutual harmony with shen 50
    narrow definition 4
    natural cycles 3
    nourishing 41
    post-birth 27
    post-heaven 40
    preserving 42
    producing extra 82
    protecting the 41

regulating 105

storing 43, 45

Taiji Ball Qigong 60

training 11

transporting 44

qi ball 102

qi channels 5, 28

qi circulation 9, 45, 46, 77

abdominal breathing 32

arthritis 14

manifestation 84

using the mind 40

qi field 102

qi flow 5

breathing 15

qi gates 87

qigong

breathing methods 27

categories 9

channels 5

Daoist and Buddhist society 5

energy and time 3

general definition 4

martial 12

martial arts society 6

medical 9

origins in dancing 6

qi circulation 6

regulating processes 25

religious 11

scholar society 5

spinal warm-up 114

tu-na 4

qigong practice 7, 59

five regulatings 26

goals 44

health and 18

health benefits 60

spiritual cultivation 61

Taiji Ball Qigong 74

qigong training 28

shen 16

the general 15

qi manifestation 86

qi ocean 78

qi reservoirs 22

qi residence 78

qi rivers 22

qi storage 89

qi transport 46

qi vessels 21, 28

raised shen 17

real dan tian 70

real lower dan tian 21, 27, 32, 34, 40–45, 50, 54, 76–82, 88, 92, 121

regulating of no regulating 101

regulating qi 40

regulatings 25, 104

regulating shen 50

regulating the body 26

regulating the mind 11, 36, 38

relaxation 26, 86

religious belief 18

religious qigong 11

reverse abdominal breathing 83

exercises 121

righteous qi 2

rocking 162

horizontal rotation 190

horizontal single-hand rotating the ball with a partner 260

horizontal single-hand wrap-coiling with a partner 263

single-hand yin-yang horizontal circling training with a partner 254

vertical double-hands rotating with a partner 256

vertical-horizontal, circling-rotating mixed training with a partner 261

vertical-horizontal, yin-yang, circling-rotating mixed training 202

vertical-horizontal, yin-yang, circling-rotating-wrap-coiling mixed training 224

vertical-horizontal yin-yang

exchange circling 170

vertical-horizontal, yin-yang exchange rotating 199

vertical-horizontal, yin-yang exchange wrap-coiling 223

vertical-horizontal, yin-yang mixing circling with a partner 255

vertical single-hand rotating with a partner 258

vertical single-hand wrap-coiling with a partner 262

vertical yin-yang circling partner practice 250

vertical yin-yang circling with partner 246

yang circling 155

yang vertical rotation 174

yang wrap-coiling 208, 219

yin circling 143

yin rotation 194

yin vertical rotation 182

yin wrap-coiling 212, 220

yin-yang exchange 150, 186

yin-yang exchange circling 165

yin-yang exchange horizontal rotating 197

yin-yang exchange wrap-coiling 214, 222

yin-yang horizontal circling training with a partner 252

rocking pattern 134

rooting training 266

rotating pattern 172

rotating the ball 235

rotating the ballon the forearms 236

rotating the ball with a partner 258

roundness 58, 59

Sardili 84

sea bottom 89

self-awakening 52

self-awareness 51

self-recognition 51

seven passions 11, 53

Shaolin monks 59

    training 12

Shaolin Temple 59

shen 16, 78

    awakening 52

    breathing 17, 50

    condensing 49

    control kan and li 17

    harmonized with qi 17

    lotus seed 52

    mutual harmony with qi 50

    natural 47

    protecting 48

    raising the 48

    regulating 47

    stabilizing the 49

    trainings for regulating 47

shen cultivation 47

shen qi xiang he 17, 50

shen training 46

shen xi 17, 50

shen xi xiang yi 17

shou 48

shou shen training 48

sideways attaching 232

single-hand

    vertical yin-yang circling part-
        ner practice 248

sitting on crossed leg stance 126

six desires 11, 53

skin breathing 32, 34

small circulation 45

small cyclic heaven circulation 45

small nine heaven 59

soft martial skills 64

softness 13, 59, 93

soft styles 13

spine 93

    qi vessels 21

    waving the 117

spine muscles

    exercising 114

spiraling 69

spirit

    regulating 105

    residence 46

spirit of vitality 22, 38, 61

spiritual bondage 54

    freedom from 53

spiritual cultivation 12, 23, 61

    four steps 51

spiritual cultivation triangle 80

spiritual embryo 43

spiritual enlightenment 6, 7, 61

    cultivating 51

    practice 45

spiritual mountain 52

spiritual valley 46

stances 125

stationary

    horizontal double-hands rotat-
        ing the ball with a partner
        259

    horizontal rotation 189

    horizontal single-hand rotating
        the ball with a partner 260

    horizontal single-hand wrap-
        coiling with a partner 263

    single-hand yin-yang horizon-
        tal circling training with a
        partner 254

    vertical double-hands rotating
        with a partner 256

    vertical-horizontal, circling-
        rotating mixed training
        with a partner 261

    vertical-horizontal, yin-yang,
        circling-rotating mixed
        training 201

    vertical-horizontal, yin-yang,
        circling-rotating-wrap-coil-
        ing mixed training 224

    vertical-horizontal, yin-yang
        exchange rotating 199

    vertical-horizontal, yin-yang
        exchange wrap-coiling 222

    vertical-horizontal, yin-yang

mixing circling with a part-
    ner 255

vertical single-hand rotating
    with a partner 257

vertical single-hand wrap-coil-
    ing with a partner 262

vertical yin-yang circling part-
    ner practice 250

vertical yin-yang circling with
    partner 245

yang vertical rotation 173

yang wrap-coiling 206, 218

yin rotation 194

yin vertical rotation 181

yin wrap-coiling 211, 220

yin-yang exchange 185

yin-yang exchange circling
    164

yin-yang exchange horizontal
    rotating 196

yin-yang exchange wrap-coil-
    ing 214, 221

yin-yang horizontal circling
    training with a partner 252

stationary circling

    yang 148, 154

    yin 162

stepping

    balance method 178

    horizontal double-hands rotat-
        ing the ball with a partner
        259

    horizontal single-hand rotating
        the ball with a partner 260

    horizontal single-hand wrap-
        coiling with a partner 263

    straight line 136

    vertical double-hands rotating
        with a partner 257

    vertical-horizontal, circling-
        rotating mixed training
        with a partner 261

    vertical-horizontal, yin-yang
        mixing circling with a part-
        ner 255

vertical single-hand rotating
with a partner 258

vertical single-hand wrap-coiling with a partner 262

vertical yin-yang circling partner practice 251

vertical yin-yang circling with partner 247

yin-yang horizontal circling training with a partner 253, 254

storing qi 43

straight line listening and following 243

straight line stepping
horizontal circling 156
horizontal rotation 192
vertical-horizontal, yin-yang, circling-rotating-wrap-coiling mixed training 224
vertical-horizontal yin-yang exchange circling 171
vertical-horizontal, yin-yang exchange rotating 200
vertical-horizontal, yin-yang exchange wrap-coiling 223
yang vertical rotation 175
yang wrap-coiling 208, 219
yin 145
yin horizontal circling 164
yin rotation 196
yin vertical rotation 184
yin wrap-coiling 213, 220
yin-yang exchange 151, 187
yin-yang exchange circling 167
yin-yang exchange horizontal rotating 198
yin-yang exchange wrap-coiling 216, 222

strange meridians 5

strengthing 76

stretching exercises 107, 111

strokes 264

subconscious mind

yin 52

supernatural divine light 47

table (on the)
adhering to the ball 228
rotating the ball 235
wrap-coiling the ball 236

taiji 65
Dao and 67
theory 71
xin and yi 74
xuan pin 47
yin-yang symbol 76

taiji ball
adhering-connecting 236
adhering to 228
attaching to the 231
flying dragon plays with 237
forward-backward attaching 234
jins 228
material 98
rolling along the right edge 237
sideways attaching to the 232
sizes 100
solo maneuvering 228
taijiquan sequence and 266
tossing with partner 267
up and down the wall 239
walking along the edge practice 237

Taiji Ball Breathing 125

taiji ball qigong
history 58
training purposes 58

Taiji Ball Qigong
theory 65

taiji balls 58

taiji ball training
exercises 128
history 60
internal benefits 60
rules 101
strengthening 61

taiji palm 128

taijiquan sequence
holding the ball 266

taiji yin-yang symbol 148

The Book of Changes 3

Theory of Qi's Variation 3

third eye 50, 55, 88
natural shen 47

thirty-seven postures 59

thought 16, 22, 52, 54, 81

three dimensions
spiraling 68

three powers 1, 3

thrusting vessel 87

tian mu 47

tiantu 87

tiao 25

tile hand 128

torso
conditioning 62, 102

training methods
Taiji Ball Qigong 57

training rules 101

triple burner 112

true Dao 54

trunk muscles
exercising 114

two gates 91

two-person jin 267

two polarities 66, 76, 79, 87
human body 76

upper dan tian 21, 46, 47, 52, 76, 79

upper dan tian breathing 36

valley spirit 46, 47

vertical circling 129

vertical-horizontal, yin-yang, circling-rotating mixed training 200

vertical-horizontal, yin-yang, circling-rotating mixed training with a partner 260

vertical-horizontal, yin-yang, circling-rotating-wrap-coiling mixed training 224 vertical-horizontal, yin-yang, circling-rotating-wrap-coiling mixed training with a partner 264

vertical-horizontal, yin-yang exchange rotating 199

vertical-horizontal, yin-yang exchange wrap-coiling 222

vertical-horizontal, yin-yang mixing circling with a partner rotating 256

vertical-horizontal, yin-yang mixing circling with a partner 255

vertical rotation 173

vertical single-hand rotating with a partner 257

vertical wrap-coiling with a partner 261

vessels 5, 21
  pointing 12
  qi accumulation 22

vitality 22, 38, 40, 61

vital qi 2

wai dan 7

wai dan qigong practice 8

wai dan training 13

waist
  circling 116
  rotating 172

walking along the edge practice 237

Wang, Zong-yue 70

warm-up
  spinal 114

warm-up exercises 107

water 13, 14
  inhaling 15

water mind 16

water qi 14

White Crane Waves its Wings 118

wind water 3

wisdom mind 26, 39

without ultimate 71

wood balls 58

wrap-coiling 204
  ball on table 236
  vertical-horizontal with a partner 261

Wudang Mountain 60

wuji 44, 66, 71

wuji breathing 121

wuji point 148, 157

wuji state 73

Wu Tiao 25

xin 14, 15, 26, 37, 39
  Taiji Ball Qigong 74

Xi Sui Jing 59, 85

xiu qi 11

xuan 47

xuan pin 46, 47

xu mi 42

xu wu 44

Xu, Xuan-ping 59

yang
  conscious mind 52
  excess in body 14
  sprialing 69

yang 48

yang circling 130

yang fountain 76

yang shen 48, 78, 89

yang wrap-coiling 206, 218

yi 14, 15, 26, 37, 39
  connection with qi 44
  Taiji Ball Qigong 74

Yi Jing 3

Yi Jin Jing 59, 85

yin
  spiraling 69
  subconscious mind 52

yin circling 141

yinjiao 87, 91

Yin, Li-heng 59

yin rotation 194

yin shui 78

yin spirit 77

yintang 87

yin vertical rotation 181

yin-yang
  Taiji Ball Qigong 73

yin-yang circling
  vertical 245

yin-yang derivation 68

yin-yang exchange
  circling 147
  freestyle circling 169
  rotating the ball 185
  vertical-horizontal, yin-yang, circling-rotating mixed training 200

yin-yang exchange horizontal rotating 196

yin-yang exchange wrap-coiling 213, 221

yin-yang horizontal circling training with a partner 252

yin-yang polarities 69

yin-yang spiral derivation 69

yi shou dan tian 43

yongquan 88

yongquan breathing 122

yu men 47

Zhang, Dao-ling 10

zhi guan 51

Zhou Wen Wang 66

Zhuang Zhou 10

Zhuang Zi 34, 122

About the Author
Dr. Yang, Jwing-Ming (楊俊敏博士)

Dr. Yang, Jwing-Ming was born on August 11, 1946 in Xinzhu Xian, Taiwan, Republic of China (新竹縣,台灣,中華民國). He started his wushu (武術) and kung fu (gongfu, 功夫) training when he was fifteen years old in Shaolin White Crane (少林白鶴) under Master Cheng, Gin-gsao (曾金灶, 1911-1976). As a child, Master Cheng learned Taizuquan (太祖拳) from his grandfather. When he was fifteen years old, he started learning White Crane Style from Master Jin, Shao-feng (金紹峰) and followed him for 23 years until Master Jin's death.

After thirteen years of study, from 1961 to 1974, under Master Cheng, Dr. Yang became an expert in the White Crane Style of Chinese martial arts, including the bare hand and various weapons such as saber, staff, spear, trident, two short rods, and many others. Under Master Cheng, he also studied White Crane Qigong (氣功), qin na (or chin na, 擒拿), he (推拿), dian xue (點穴按摩) massage, and herbal treatment.

At the age of sixteen, Dr. Yang began the study of Yang Style Taijiquan (楊氏太極拳) under Master Gao, Tao (高濤). He later continued his study of taijiquan under several other masters and senior practitioners, such as Master Li, Mao-ching (李茂清) and Mr. Wilson Chen (陳威伸) in Taipei (台北). Master Li learned taijiquan from the well-known Master Han, Ching-tang (韓慶堂), and Mr. Chen learned from Master Zhang, Xiang-san (張祥三). Under these masters, Dr. Yang mastered the taiji bare-hand sequence, the two-man fighting sequence, pushing hands, taiji sword, taiji saber, and taiji qigong.

When Dr. Yang was eighteen years old, he entered Tamkang College (淡江學院) in Taipei Xian to study physics. During this time, he began studying traditional Shaolin Long Fist (少林長拳) under Master Li, Mao-ching in the Tamkang College Guoshu Club (淡江國術社) from 1964 to 1968 and eventually became an assistant instructor to Master Li. From Master Li, he learned northern-style wushu, including bare-hand and kicking techniques, and numerous weapons. In 1971, he completed his Master of Science degree in physics at National Taiwan University (台灣大學) before serving in the Chinese Air Force from 1971 to 1972. He taught physics at the Junior Academy of the Chinese Air Force (空軍幼校) while also teaching wushu. Honorably discharged in 1972, he returned to Tamkang College to teach physics and resume his study under Master Li, Mao-ching.

Dr. Yang moved to the United States in 1974 to study mechanical engineering at Purdue University. At the request of a few colleagues, he began to teach gongfu, founding the Purdue University Chinese Gongfu Research Club in 1975. He also taught college-credit-courses in taijiquan. In May 1978, he was awarded a Ph.D. in mechanical engineering from Purdue University.

In 1980, Dr. Yang moved to Houston to work for Texas Instruments and also founded Yang's Shaolin Kung Fu Academy, now under the direction of his disciple Jeffery Bolt. In 1982, he moved to Boston and founded Yang's Martial Arts Academy. In 1984, he gave up his engineering career to devote his time to research, writing, and teaching of Chinese martial arts. In 1986, he moved YMAA to the Jamaica Plain area of Boston and established this location as Yang's Martial Arts Association (YMAA) headquarters. YMAA became a division of Yang's Oriental Arts Association, Inc. (YOAA, Inc.) in 1989.

Dr. Yang has been involved in Chinese wushu since 1961, studying Shaolin White Crane, Shaolin (*Bai He*) Long Fist, and Taijiquan (*Chanqquan*) under several different masters. He has taught for more than 40 years: 7 years in Taiwan, 5 years at Purdue University, 2 years in Houston, 26 years in Boston, and 5 years at his YMAA California Retreat Center. He has taught seminars all around the world, sharing his knowledge of Chinese martial arts and qigong: in Argentina, Austria, Barbados, Botswana, Belgium, Bermuda, Canada, China, Chile, England, Egypt, France, Germany, Holland, Hungary, Iran, Ireland, Italy, Latvia, Mexico, Poland, Portugal, Saudi Arabia, Spain, South Africa, Switzerland, and Venezuela.

YMAA has grown into an international organization that includes 60 schools spread across 19 countries: Argentina, Belgium, Canada, Chile, France, Holland, Hungary, Iran, Ireland, Italy, Poland, Portugal, Qatar, Spain, South Africa, Sweden, Switzerland, the United Kingdom, and the United States. YMAA publications, books, and videos have been translated into French, Italian, Spanish, Polish, Czech, Bulgarian, Russian, Hungarian, and Farsi.

In 2005, Dr. Yang established the YMAA California Retreat Center (楊氏武藝協會特訓中心), a dedicated training ground for a small committed group of selected students. Located in the mountainous regions of northern California, the center was formed to host a 10-year training program, directed and taught by Dr. Yang himself, beginning in September 2008. It is Dr. Yang's wish that through this effort, he will be able to preserve traditional Chinese martial arts to the same standards and quality of ancient times. He remains the chief supervisor of YMAA International and in January 2008, his youngest son Nicholas has succeeded him as president of YMAA.

Dr. Yang has authored other books and videos on martial arts and qigong:
1. *Shaolin Chin Na,* Unique Publications, Inc., 1980
2. *Shaolin Long Fist Kung Fu,* Unique Publications, Inc., 1981
3. *Yang Style Tai Chi Chuan,* Unique Publications, Inc., 1981
4. *Introduction to Ancient Chinese Weapons,* Unique Publications, Inc., 1985
5. *A Martial Arists Guide to Ancient Chinese Weapons,* revised edition, YMAA Publication Center, 1999
6. *Chi Kung for Health and Martial Arts,* YMAA Publication Center, 1985
7. *Qigong—Health and Martial Arts,* revised edition, YMAA Publication Center, 1998
8. *Northern Shaolin Sword,* YMAA Publication Center, 1985
9. *Advanced Yang Style Tai Chi Chuan Vol. 1—Tai Chi Theory and Martial Power,* YMAA Publication Center, 1986
10. *Tai Chi Theory and Martial Power,* revised edition, YMAA Publication Center, 1996
11. *Advanced Yang Style Tai Chi Chuan Vol. 2—Tai Chi Chuan Martial Applications,* YMAA Publication Center, 1986
12. *Tai Chi Chuan Martial Applications,* revised edition, YMAA Publication Center, 1996

13. *Analysis of Shaolin Chin Na*, YMAA Publication Center, 1987, 2004
14. *The Eight Pieces of Brocade—Ba Duan Jin*, YMAA Publication Center, 1988
15. *Eight Simple Qigong Exercises for Health*, revised edition, YMAA Publication Center, 1997
16. *The Root of Chinese Qigong—The Secrets of Qigong Training*, YMAA Publication Center, 1989, 1997
17. *Muscle/Tendon Changing and Marrow/Brain Washing Chi Kung—The Secret of Youth*, YMAA Publication Center, 1989
18. *Qigong the Secret of Youth, Da Mo's Muscle Tendon Changing and Marrow Brain Washing Qigong*, revised edition, YMAA Publication Center, 2000
19. *Hsing Yi Chuan—Theory and Applications*, YMAA Publication Center, 1990
20. *Xingyiquan—Theory and Applications*, revised edition, YMAA Publication Center, 2003
21. *The Essence of Tai Chi Chi Kung—Health and Martial Arts*, YMAA Publication Center, 1990
22. *The Essence of Taiji Qigong—Health and Martial Arts*, revised edition, YMAA Publication Center, 1998
23. *Qigong for Arthritis*, YMAA Publication Center, 1991
24. *Arthritis Relief*, revised edition, YMAA Publication Center, 2005
25. *Chinese Qigong Massage—General Massage*, YMAA Publication Center, 1992
26. *Qigong Massage—Fundamental Techniques for Health and Relaxation*, revised edition, YMAA Publication Center, 2005
27. *How to Defend Yourself*, YMAA Publication Center, 1992
28. *Baguazhang—Emei Baguazhang*, YMAA Publication Center, 1994
29. *Baguazhang—Theory and Applications*, revised edition, YMAA Publication Center, 2008
30. *Comprehensive Applications of Shaolin Chin Na—The Practical Defense of Chinese Seizing Arts*, YMAA Publication Center, 1995
31. *Taiji Chin Na—The Seizing Art of Taijiquan*, YMAA Publication Center, 1995
32. *The Essence of Shaolin White Crane*, YMAA Publication Center, 1996
33. *Back Pain—Chinese Qigong for Healing and Prevention*, YMAA Publication Center, 1997
34. *Back Pain Relief—Chinese Qigong for Healing and Prevention*, revised edition, YMAA Publication Center, 2004
35. *Taijiquan Classical Yang Style—The Complete Form and Qigong*, YMAA Publication Center, 1999
35. *Tai Chi Chuan—Classical Yang Style,* revised edition, YMAA Publication Center, 2010
36. *Taijiquan Theory of Dr. Yang, Jwing-Ming—The Root of Taijiquan*, YMAA Publication Center, 2003
37. *Qigong Meditation—Embryonic Breathing*, YMAA Publication Center, 2003
38. *Qigong Meditation—Small Circulation,* YMAA Publication Center, 2006
39. *Tai Chi Ball Qigong—Health and Martial Arts,* YMAA Publication Center, 2010
   DVD Videos by Dr. Yang, Jwing-Ming
1. *Chin Na In Depth Courses 1–4*, YMAA Publication Center, 2003
2. *Chin Na In Depth Courses 5–8*, YMAA Publication Center, 2003
3. *Chin Na In Depth Courses 9–12*, YMAA Publication Center, 2003
4. *Eight Simple Qigong Exercises for Health—The Eight Pieces of Brocade*, YMAA Publication Center, 2003

5. *Shaolin White Crane Gong Fu Basic Training Courses 1 & 2*, YMAA Publication Center, 2003

6. *Shaolin White Crane Hard and Soft Qigong*, YMAA Publication Center, 2003

7. *Tai Chi Chuan Classical Yang Style (long form Taijiquan)*, YMAA Publication Center, 2003

8. *Analysis of Shaolin Chin Na*, YMAA Publication Center, 2004

9. *Shaolin Kung Fu Fundamental Training*, YMAA Publication Center, 2004

10. *Baguazhang (8 Trigrams Palm Kung Fu)*, YMAA Publication Center, 2005

11. *Essence of Taiji Qigong*, YMAA Publication Center, 2005

12. *Qigong Massage*, YMAA Publication Center, 2005

13. *Shaolin Long Fist Kung Fu Basic Sequences*, YMAA Publication Center, 2005

14. *Taiji Pushing Hands Courses 1 & 2*, YMAA Publication Center, 2005

15. *Taiji Sword, Classical Yang Style*, YMAA Publication Center, 2005

16. *Taiji Ball Qigong Courses 1 & 2*, YMAA Publication Center, 2006

17. *Taiji Fighting Set—88 Posture, 2-Person Matching Set*, YMAA Publication Center, 2006

18. *Taiji Pushing Hands Courses 3 & 4*, YMAA Publication Center, 2006

19. *Understanding Qigong DVD 1—What is Qigong? Understanding the Human Qi Circulatory System*, YMAA Publication Center, 2006

20. *Understanding Qigong DVD 2—Keypoints of Qigong & Qigong Breathing*, YMAA Publication Center, 2006

21. *Shaolin Saber Basic Sequences*, YMAA Publication Center, 2007

22. *Shaolin Staff Basic Sequences*, YMAA Publication Center, 2007

23. *Simple Qigong Exercises for Arthritis Relief*, YMAA Publication Center, 2007

24. *Simple Qigong Exercises for Back Pain Relief*, YMAA Publication Center, 2007

25. *Taiji & Shaolin Staff Fundamental Training*, YMAA Publication Center, 2007

26. *Taiji Ball Qigong Courses 3 & 4*, YMAA Publication Center, 2007

27. *Understanding Qigong DVD 3—Embryonic Breathing*, YMAA Publication Center, 2007

28. *Understanding Qigong DVD 4—Four Seasons Qigong*, YMAA Publication Center, 2007

29. *Understanding Qigong DVD 5—Small Circulation*, YMAA Publication Center, 2007

30. *Understanding Qigong DVD 6—Martial Arts Qigong Breathing*, YMAA Publication Center, 2007

31. *Five Animal Sports Qigong*, YMAA Publication Center, 2008

32. *Saber Fundamental Training*, YMAA Publication Center, 2008

33. *Shaolin White Crane Gong Fu Basic Training Courses 3 & 4*, YMAA Publication Center, 2008

34. *Taiji 37 Postures Martial Applications*, YMAA Publication Center, 2008

35. *Taiji Saber, Classical Yang Style*, YMAA Publication Center, 2008

36. *Taiji Wrestling— Advanced Takedown Techniques*, YMAA Publication Center, 2008

37. *Taiji Yin/Yang Sticking Hands*, YMAA Publication Center, 2008

38. *Xingyiquan (Hsing I Chuan)*, YMAA Publication Center, 2008

39. *Northern Shaolin Sword*, YMAA Publication Center, 2009

40. *Sword Fundamental Training*, YMAA Publication Center, 2009

41. *Taiji Chin Na in Depth*, YMAA Publication Center, 2009

42. *YMAA 25-Year Anniversary*, YMAA Publication Center, 2009

43. *Shuai Jiao–Kung Fu Wrestling*, YMAA Publication Center, 2010

About the Author
David W. Grantham

David Grantham was born on September 22, 1965, in Dorchester, Massachusetts and raised in Weymouth, Massachusetts from the age of three. At the age of eighteen, he attended Bridgewater State College to pursue his dream and currently is employed by Continental Airlines as a pilot based in New Jersey.

Mr. Grantham began his martial art training at the age of twenty-four, studying Liuhebafaquan under the tutelage of instructor David Zucker. Mr. Zucker studied under the late Master John Chung Li. He also trained in a fighting form taught only to advanced students. After training for one year with Mr. Zucker, Mr. Grantham was encouraged to further his knowledge of Chinese martial arts and was recommended to attend Yang's Martial Arts Association headquarters in Boston. He joined YMAA and started training under the Shaolin curriculum. Over the years of training at the school and attending seminars abroad, Mr. Grantham expanded his studies to include taiji-quan and qigong. On January 28, 2000, he was awarded assistant instructor of chin na and on January 30, 2007, he was awarded the rank of chin na instructor. In 2008, Mr. Grantham was awarded a coach instructor position by Nicholas Yang.

David Grantham has been training in martial arts for twenty-one years. He continues to train the YMAA curriculum and currently teaches at the Hunterdon Health and Wellness Center in Clinton, New Jersey. David Grantham resides in Hunterdon County, New Jersey with his wife, Jenifer, and two children, Jillian and Alexander.

ᴀɪJɪ Bᴀʟʟ Qɪɢᴏɴɢ DVD 1

:epen Your Taiji Training with Taiji Ball Qigong

formed by Dr. Yang, Jwing-Ming and Senior Students

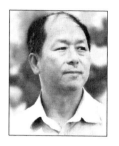

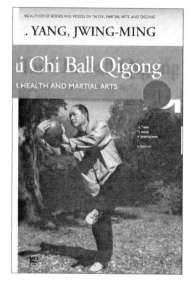

Ball training is common practice in both :rnal and internal martial arts in China. It strengthen the torso, condition the mus-, and increase physical power by using the mind ead the Qi. In Taijiquan (Tai Chi Chuan), Taiji Qigong training was once a major training tool nhance Pushing Hands ability. However, due to ;ecrecy, fewer and fewer people have learned it. ay the art of Taiji Ball training is almost nown.

Course 1, Dr. Yang, Jwing-Ming teaches funda-ıtal Taiji Ball breathing techniques, and 16 basic erns of stationary and moving Taiji Ball Circling, both Vertical and Horizontal.

Breathing patterns demonstrated:

- Wuji breathing
- Yongquan breathing
- Laogong breathing
- Four Gates breathing
- Taiji Grand Circulation breathing

ırse 2 focuses on 16 basic patterns of stationary and moving Taiji Rotating, both Vertical and Horizontal.

Yang offers detailed instruction as students demonstrate in the sroom, accompanied by an easy-to-follow demonstration of each ern shown in a lush outdoor setting, with beautiful classical nese music.

ular Qigong practice accelerates the health benefits of Taiji. You'll ⁚y reduced stress, a stronger immune system, and a deeper aware-; of breath and body coordination. This authoritative guide can be l with any style of Taijiquan, and it is a great way for anyone to rgize the body, raise the spirit, and deepen your understanding of ong and Taiji.

cial Features: Over 100 Scene Selections • Narration: English, French [ulti-Language Menus and Subtitles: English, French, Spanish, tuguese, Polish • Bonus DVD-Outtakes Segment • Interactive YMAA duct catalog with Previews of Other YMAA Videos

minutes • DVD9-NTSC • all regions • Code: D0517 • N-13: 1-59439-051-7 • UPC: 822003002023

 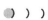

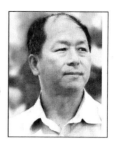

TAIJI BALL QIGONG DVD 2

Deepen Your Taiji Training with Taiji Ball Qigo

performed by Dr. Yang, Jwing-Ming and Senior Students

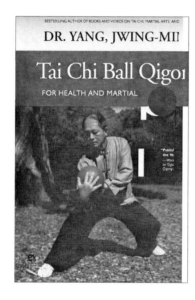

T aiji Ball training can strengthen the torso, c dition the muscles, and teach the practitio to use the mind to lead the Qi. In Taijiqu Taiji Ball training was once a major training too enhance Pushing Hands ability, but it is ra taught in modern times. Dr. Yang, Jwing-M teaches more advanced Taiji Ball techniques, bu ing upon the foundation taught in Tai Chi Qigong DVD 1.

In **Course 3**, Dr Yang teaches 16 patterns of Taiji Wrap-Coiling, including vertical and horizontal.

Course 4 focuses on solo and partner applicatio which improve coiling and neutralizing taiji sk and develop "listening jing", or sensitivity. Dr. Y offers detailed instruction as you follow along v the demonstration, including:

- Self-practice Exercises
- Flying Dragon Plays with the Ball
- Taiji Ball Along the Edge
- Two-person Matching Drills.

Regular Qigong practice accelerates the health benefits of Taiji. Yo enjoy reduced stress, a stronger immune system, and a deeper aw ness of breath and body coordination. This authoritative guide ca used with any style of Taijiquan, and it is a great way for anyon energize the body, raise the spirit, and deepen your understanding Qigong and Taiji.

Special Features: Over 100 Scene Selections • Narration: Engl French • Multi-Language Menus and Subtitles: English, Frer Spanish, Portuguese • Interactive YMAA Product catalog w Previews of YMAA Videos

191 minutes • DVD9-NTSC • all regions • Code: D0777 •
ISBN-13: 1-59439-077-7 • UPC: 822003002023

BOOKS FROM YMAA

6 HEALING MOVEMENTS	B906
101 REFLECTIONS ON TAI CHI CHUAN	B868
108 INSIGHTS INTO TAI CHI CHUAN	B582
A WOMAN'S QIGONG GUIDE	B833
ADVANCING IN TAE KWON DO	B072X
ANCIENT CHINESE WEAPONS	B671
ANALYSIS OF SHAOLIN CHIN NA 2ND ED	B0002
ART OF HOJO UNDO	B1361
ARTHRITIS RELIEF 3RD ED.	B0339
BACK PAIN RELIEF 2ND ED.	B0258
BAGUAZHANG 2ND ED.	B1132
CARDIO KICKBOXING ELITE	B922
CHIN NA IN GROUND FIGHTING	B663
CHINESE FAST WRESTLING	B493
CHINESE FITNESS	B37X
CHINESE TUI NA MASSAGE	B043
COMPLETE CARDIOKICKBOXING	B809
COMPREHENSIVE APPLICATIONS OF SHAOLIN CHIN NA	B36X
CROCODILE AND THE CRANE	B0876
CUTTING SEASON (CLTH)—A XENON PEARL MARTIAL ARTS THRILLER	B0821
CUTTING SEASON (PBK)—A XENON PEARL MARTIAL ARTS THRILLER	B1309
DR. WU'S HEAD MASSAGE	B0576
EIGHT SIMPLE QIGONG EXERCISES FOR HEALTH, 2ND ED.	B523
ESSENCE OF SHAOLIN WHITE CRANE	B353
ESSENCE OF TAIJI QIGONG, 2ND ED.	B639
EXPLORING TAI CHI	B424
FACING VIOLENCE	B2139
FIGHTING ARTS	B213
INSIDE TAI CHI	B108
KAGE—THE SHADOW	B2108
KATA AND THE TRANSMISSION OF KNOWLEDGE	B0266
LITTLE BLACK BOOK OF VIOLENCE	B1293
LIUHEBAFA FIVE CHARACTER SECRETS	B728
MARTIAL ARTS ATHLETE	B655
MARTIAL ARTS INSTRUCTION	B024X
MARTIAL WAY AND ITS VIRTUES	B698
MEDITATIONS ON VIOLENCE	B1187
MIND/BODY FITNESS	B876
MUGAI RYU	B183
NATURAL HEALING WITH QIGONG	B0010
NORTHERN SHAOLIN SWORD, 2ND ED.	B85X
OKINAWA'S COMPLETE KARATE SYSTEM—ISSHIN RYU	B914
POWER BODY	B760
PRINCIPLES OF TRADITIONAL CHINESE MEDICINE	B99X
QIGONG FOR HEALTH & MARTIAL ARTS 2ND ED.	B574
QIGONG FOR LIVING	B116
QIGONG FOR TREATING COMMON AILMENTS	B701
QIGONG MASSAGE	B0487
QIGONG MEDITATION—EMBRYONIC BREATHING	B736
QIGONG MEDITATION—SMALL CIRCULATION	B0673
QIGONG, THE SECRET OF YOUTH—DA MO'S CLASSICS	B841
QUIET TEACHER (PBK)—A XENON PEARL MARTIAL ARTS THRILLER	B1262
ROOT OF CHINESE QIGONG, 2ND ED.	B507
SHIHAN TE—THE BUNKAI OF KATA	B884
SIMPLE CHINESE MEDICINE	B1248
SUDDEN DAWN (PBK)—THE EPIC JOURNEY OF BODHIDHARMA	B1989
SUNRISE TAI CHI	B0838
SUNSET TAI CHI	B2122
SURVIVING ARMED ASSAULTS	B0711
TAEKWONDO—ANCIENT WISDOM FOR THE MODERN WARRIOR	B930
TAEKWONDO—A PATH TO EXCELLENCE	B1286
TAE KWON DO—THE KOREAN MARTIAL ART	B0869
TAEKWONDO—SPIRIT AND PRACTICE	B221
TAO OF BIOENERGETICS	B289
TAI CHI BALL QIGONG—FOR HEALTH AND MARTIAL ARTS	B1996
TAI CHI BOOK	B647
TAI CHI CHUAN—24 & 48 POSTURES	B337
TAI CHI CHUAN CLASSICAL YANG STYLE (REVISED EDITION)	B2009
TAI CHI CHUAN MARTIAL APPLICATIONS, 2ND ED.	B442
TAI CHI CONNECTIONS	B0320
TAI CHI DYNAMICS	B1163
TAI CHI SECRETS OF THE ANCIENT MASTERS	B71X
TAI CHI SECRETS OF THE WU & LI STYLES	B981
TAI CHI SECRETS OF THE WU STYLE	B175
TAI CHI SECRETS OF THE YANG STYLE	B094
TAI CHI THEORY & MARTIAL POWER, 2ND ED.	B434

more products available from . . .

YMAA Publication Center, Inc. 楊氏東方文化出版中心

1-800-669-8892 • info@ymaa.com • www.ymaa.com

YMAA
PUBLICATION CENTER

BOOKS FROM YMAA (continued)

TAI CHI WALKING	B23X
TAIJI CHIN NA	B378
TAIJI SWORD—CLASSICAL YANG STYLE	B744
TAIJIQUAN THEORY OF DR. YANG, JWING-MING	B432
TENGU—THE MOUNTAIN GOBLIN	B1231
THE WAY OF KATA	B0584
THE WAY OF KENDO AND KENJITSU	B0029
THE WAY OF SANCHIN KATA	B0845
THE WAY TO BLACK BELT	B0852
TRADITIONAL CHINESE HEALTH SECRETS	B892
TRADITIONAL TAEKWONDO	B0665
WESTERN HERBS FOR MARTIAL ARTISTS	B1972
WILD GOOSE QIGONG	B787
WISDOM'S WAY	B361
XINGYIQUAN, 2ND ED.	B416

DVDS FROM YMAA

ADVANCED PRACTICAL CHIN NA IN-DEPTH	D1224
ANALYSIS OF SHAOLIN CHIN NA	D0231
BAGUAZHANG 1, 2, & 3—EMEI BAGUAZHANG	D0649
CHEN STYLE TAIJIQUAN	D0819
CHIN NA IN-DEPTH COURSES 1—4	D602
CHIN NA IN-DEPTH COURSES 5—8	D610
CHIN NA IN-DEPTH COURSES 9—12	D629
EIGHT SIMPLE QIGONG EXERCISES FOR HEALTH	D0037
ESSENCE OF TAIJI QIGONG	D0215
FIVE ANIMAL SPORTS	D1106
KUNG FU BODY CONDITIONING	D2085
KUNG FU FOR KIDS	D1880
NORTHERN SHAOLIN SWORD —SAN CAI JIAN, KUN WU JIAN, QI MEN JIAN	D1194
QIGONG MASSAGE	D0592
QIGONG FOR LONGEVITY	D2092
SABER FUNDAMENTAL TRAINING	D1088
SANCHIN KATA—TRADITIONAL TRAINING FOR KARATE POWER	D1897
SHAOLIN KUNG FU FUNDAMENTAL TRAINING—COURSES 1 & 2	D0436
SHAOLIN LONG FIST KUNG FU—BASIC SEQUENCES	D661
SHAOLIN LONG FIST KUNG FU—INTERMEDIATE SEQUENCES	D1071
SHAOLIN LONG FIST KUNG FU—ADVANCED SEQUENCES	D2061
SHAOLIN SABER—BASIC SEQUENCES	D0616
SHAOLIN STAFF—BASIC SEQUENCES	D0920
SHAOLIN WHITE CRANE GONG FU BASIC TRAINING—COURSES 1 & 2	D599
SHAOLIN WHITE CRANE GONG FU BASIC TRAINING—COURSES 3 & 4	D0784
SHUAI JIAO—KUNG FU WRESTLING	D1149
SIMPLE QIGONG EXERCISES FOR ARTHRITIS RELIEF	D0890
SIMPLE QIGONG EXERCISES FOR BACK PAIN RELIEF	D0883
SIMPLIFIED TAI CHI CHUAN—24 & 48 POSTURES	D0630
SUNRISE TAI CHI	D0274
SUNSET TAI CHI	D0760
SWORD—FUNDAMENTAL TRAINING	D1095
TAI CHI CONNECTIONS	D0444
TAI CHI ENERGY PATTERNS	D0525
TAI CHI FIGHTING SET	D0509
TAIJI BALL QIGONG—COURSES 1 & 2	D0517
TAIJI BALL QIGONG—COURSES 3 & 4	D0777
TAIJI CHIN NA—COURSES 1, 2, 3, & 4	D0463
TAIJI MARTIAL APPLICATIONS—37 POSTURES	D1057
TAIJI PUSHING HANDS—COURSES 1 & 2	D0495
TAIJI PUSHING HANDS—COURSES 3 & 4	D0681
TAIJI WRESTLING	D1064
TAIJI SABER	D1026
TAIJI & SHAOLIN STAFF—FUNDAMENTAL TRAINING	D0906
TAIJI YIN YANG STICKING HANDS	D1040
TAI CHI CHUAN CLASSICAL YANG STYLE	D645
TAIJI SWORD—CLASSICAL YANG STYLE	D0452
UNDERSTANDING QIGONG 1—WHAT IS QI? • HUMAN QI CIRCULATORY SYSTEM	D069X
UNDERSTANDING QIGONG 2—KEY POINTS • QIGONG BREATHING	D0418
UNDERSTANDING QIGONG 3—EMBRYONIC BREATHING	D0555
UNDERSTANDING QIGONG 4—FOUR SEASONS QIGONG	D0562
UNDERSTANDING QIGONG 5—SMALL CIRCULATION	D0753
UNDERSTANDING QIGONG 6—MARTIAL QIGONG BREATHING	D0913
WHITE CRANE HARD & SOFT QIGONG	D637
WUDANG SWORD	D1903
WUDANG KUNG FU—FUNDAMENTAL TRAINING	D1316
WUDANG TAIJIQUAN	D1217
XINGYIQUAN	D1200
YMAA 25 YEAR ANNIVERSARY DVD	D0708

more products available from . . .

YMAA Publication Center, Inc. 楊氏東方文化出版中心

1-800-669-8892 • info@ymaa.com • www.ymaa.com